Palliative Care Within Mental Health

Palliative Care Within Mental Health: Ethical Practice explores the comprehensive concerns and dilemmas that occur surrounding people experiencing mental health problems and disorders. Working beyond narrow, stereotypical definitions of palliative care as restricted to terminal cancer patients, this balanced and thought-provoking volume examines the many interrelated issues that face the individual, families, and caregivers, setting the groundwork for improved, ethical relationships and interventions. Chapters by experts and experienced practitioners detail the challenges, concerns, and best practices for ethical care and responses in a variety of individual and treatment contexts. This is an essential and thoughtful new resource for all those involved in the fast-developing field of palliative mental health.

David B. Cooper has specialized in mental health and substance use for over 36 years. He is currently an associate editor for the *Journal of Substance Use*, and has served as editor-in-chief of *Mental Health and Substance Use.*

Jo Cooper spent 16 years as a palliative care specialist, initially working in a hospice inpatient unit, and then for 12 years as a Macmillan Clinical Nurse Specialist in palliative care.

D11932555

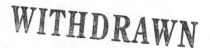

WITHDRAWN

WITHDRAWN

Palliative Care Within Mental Health

Ethical Practice

Edited by

DAVID B. COOPER AND JO COOPER

TOURO COLLEGE LIBRARY
Kings Hwy

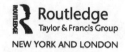
Routledge
Taylor & Francis Group

NEW YORK AND LONDON

4616 KH

First published 2019
by Routledge
711 Third Avenue, New York, NY 10017

and by Routledge
2 Park Square, Milton Park, Abingdon, Oxon, OX14 4RN

Routledge is an imprint of the Taylor & Francis Group, an informa business

© 2019 Taylor & Francis

The right of David B. Cooper and Jo Cooper to be identified as
the authors of the editorial material, and of the authors for their
individual chapters, has been asserted in accordance with sections
77 and 78 of the Copyright, Designs and Patents Act 1988.

All rights reserved. No part of this book may be reprinted or
reproduced or utilised in any form or by any electronic, mechanical,
or other means, now known or hereafter invented, including photocopying
and recording, or in any information storage or retrieval system,
without permission in writing from the publishers.

Trademark notice: Product or corporate names may be trademarks
or registered trademarks, and are used only for identification
and explanation without intent to infringe.

Library of Congress Cataloging-in-Publication Data
Names: Cooper, David B. (Mental health nurse), editor. |
Cooper, Jo, 1949– editor.
Title: Palliative care within mental health. Ethical practice/edited by
David B. Cooper and Jo Cooper.
Other titles: Ethical practice
Description: New York, NY: Routledge, 2018. | Includes bibliographical
references and index.
Identifiers: LCCN 2018015639 (print) | LCCN 2018016296 (ebook) |
ISBN9780429465666 (eBook) | ISBN 9781138609815 (hbk) |
ISBN 9781138609822 (pbk.) | ISBN 9780429465666 (ebk)
Subjects: | MESH: Mental Health Services | Palliative Care—ethics |
Palliative Care—methods
Classification: LCC R725.5 (ebook) | LCC R725.5 (print) | NLM WM 30.1 |
DDC174.2/96029—dc23
LC record available at https://lccn.loc.gov/2018015639

ISBN: 978-1-138-60981-5 (hbk)
ISBN: 978-1-138-60982-2 (pbk)
ISBN: 978-0-429-46566-6 (ebk)

Typeset in Minion Pro
by Florence Production Ltd, Stoodleigh, Devon, UK

2/22/19

Dedication

This book is dedicated to Professor Larry Purnell. Larry is and has been a very dear friend and confidant over many years and has greatly enriched our lives by offering his constant friendship. Always willing to help and support both professionally and personally Larry has contributed to several of our books and has been a board member of journals we have edited. Thank you.

Also, in the final book we edit, we would sincerely like to thank all the people who we have worked alongside over the years, some colleagues, some of whom became close friends. Their guidance, support, help, and advice has not gone unnoticed over the years . . . and we wholeheartedly thank them all.

Contents

About the Editors

David B. Cooper
Sigma Theta Tau International: Honor Society of Nursing
Outstanding Contribution to Nursing
Associate Editor – nursing and dual diagnosis: *Journal of Substance Use*

David has specialized in mental health and substance use for over 36 years. He has worked as a practitioner, manager, researcher, author, lecturer, and consultant. He has served as editor, or editor-in-chief, of several journals, most recently as editor-in-chief of *Mental Health and Substance Use*. David is currently an Associate Editor: nursing and dual diagnosis for the *Journal of Substance Use*. He has published widely and is 'credited with enhancing the understanding and development of community detoxification for people experiencing alcohol withdrawal' (Nursing Council on Alcohol; Sigma Theta Tau International citations). Seminal work includes *Alcohol Home Detoxification and Assessment* and *Alcohol Use*, both published by Radcliffe Publishing, Oxford. David co-edited with Jo Cooper a three-book series titled *Palliative Care within Mental Health*.

Jo Cooper
Macmillan Clinical Nurse Specialist in Palliative Care (retired)

Jo spent 16 years in Specialist Palliative Care, initially working in a hospice inpatient unit, then 12 years as a Macmillan Clinical Nurse Specialist in Palliative Care. She gained a Diploma in Oncology at Addenbrooke's Hospital, Cambridge, and a BSc (Hons) in Palliative Nursing at The Royal Marsden Hospital, London, and an Award in Specialist Practice. Jo edited *Stepping into Palliative Care* (2000) and the 2nd edition, *Stepping into Palliative Care 1: relationships and responses* (2006) and *Stepping into Palliative Care 2: care and practice* (2006), both published by Radcliffe Publishing, Oxford. Jo has been involved in teaching for many years and her specialist subjects include management of complex pain and symptoms, terminal agitation, communication at the end-of-life, therapeutic relationships, and breaking bad news. Jo co-edited with David B. Cooper a three-book series titled *Palliative Care within Mental Health*.

List of Contributors

Professor Cynthia M.A. Geppert
Chief of Consultation Psychiatry & Ethics, New Mexico Veterans Affairs Health Care System and Director, Graduate Certificate Program in Health Care Ethics, Department of Veterans Affairs National Centre for Ethics in Health Care, U.S.A.

Cynthia Geppert is Chief of Consultation Psychiatry and Ethics at the New Mexico Veterans Affairs Health Care System and acting health care ethicist at the Department of Veterans Affairs National Center for Ethics in Health Care. She is also Professor in the Departments of Psychiatry and Internal Medicine and Director of Ethics Education at the University of New Mexico School of Medicine as well as Adjunct Professor of Bioethics at Alden March Bioethics Institute Albany Medical College. Professor Geppert is board certified in general psychiatry, psychosomatic medicine, hospice and palliative medicine, and addiction medicine and holds credentials in pain management. She holds master's degrees in religious ethics and health and hospital law masters and doctoral degrees in bioethics. Professor Geppert's research interests are in religious and clinical ethics, addiction ethics, ethics education and consultation and she has written over 200 articles, chapters and other texts in these areas.

Professor Nel Noddings
Lee Jacks Professor of Child Education Emerita, Stanford University, U.S.A.

Nel Noddings is Lee Jacks Professor of Education, Emerita, at Stanford University. She is a past president of the National Academy of Education, the Philosophy of Education Society, and the John Dewey Society. In addition to 22 books, she is the author of more than 300 articles and chapters on topics ranging from the ethics of care to mathematical problem solving. Her latest book (co-authored with daughter Laurie Brooks) is Teaching Controversial Issues.

Professor Tony Warne
Professor of Mental Health and Associate Pro-Vice Chancellor, University of Salford, England

Tony Warne is a Professor in Mental Health Care and Associate Pro Vice Chancellor at the University of Salford. He has worked in N.H.S. mental health care services since

1975, both as a practitioner and service manager. After leaving the N.H.S. in 1995 he joined Manchester Metropolitan University, gaining his Ph.D. in 2000. In 2006, Tony was appointed Professor at the University of Salford. The focus of Tony's research interest is on inter-personal, intra-personal, and extra-personal relation-ships, using a psychodynamic and managerialist analytical discourse. He has published extensively in these areas and is co-editor of and author in the books Using Patient Experience in Nurse Education and Creative Approaches to Health and Social Care Education. Tony was the former Nurse Representative on the Council of Deans (Health) Executive Committee, which represent the 85 U.K. universities providing health care education. He is currently a Non-Executive Director for the Wrightington, Wigan and Leigh N.H.S. Trust, with a special interest in improving the quality and safety of patient care.

Dr. Sue McAndrew
Reader in Mental Health, University of Salford, England

Sue McAndrew is a Reader in Mental Health [M.H.] at the University of Salford, U.K. and an active researcher. Sue has worked in mental health nursing since 1972. In 1992 she became a lecturer at the University of Leeds, where she worked for 17 years, during which time she continued to work one day per week in primary M.H. care. After attaining her Ph.D. in 2008, in 2009 Sue took up post as Research Fellow [M.H.] at University of Salford, and was promoted to her current position in 2014. Sue has published extensively and co-edited three books; Sexual Health: Foundations for Practice; Using Patient Experience in Nurse Education; and Creative Approaches in Health and Social Care Education and Practice: Knowing me, understanding you. Her research interests include young carers and service users; childhood sexual abuse and its impact on mental health; self harm and suicide; therapeutic engagement and preparation for the emotionality inherent in mental health nursing practice. Sue is associate editor for the International Journal of Mental Health Nursing and currently is Chair of the Post Graduate Research, Innovation and Enterprise Ethics Panel.

Professor Michael Hazelton
Professor of Mental Health Nursing, University of Newcastle, Australia

Mike Hazelton is Professor of Mental Health Nursing at the University of Newcastle, Australia. He has published widely on mental health nursing and mental health, is a past editor of the International Journal of Mental Health Nursing and a current member of the Editorial Advisory Board of the Australian and New Zealand Journal of Psychiatry. Mike has supervised 18 Ph.D. students to successful completion, received various awards for research, and in 2003 was made a Life Member of the Australian College of Mental Health Nurses, the highest award conferred by that professional organization. Mike has a longstanding interest in improving treatment and support for people with lived experience of mental illness. He was a member of the expert committee that guided the development of the 2013 National Health and Medical Research Council (N.H.M.R.C.) Clinical Practice Guideline for the Management of Borderline Personality Disorder.

Dr. Roxanne Amerson
Associate Professor, Clemson University, U.S.A.

Roxanne Amerson is an associate professor at Clemson University, where she teaches community-based care, nursing education, and global health. The Transcultural Nursing Society recognizes her as a Transcultural Nursing Scholar. Her research interests focus on cultural competence among nursing students and health education via promotoras (community health workers) among indigenous populations in Guatemala and Peru. The National Institutes of Health funded her previous work in Guatemala. Her current project involves anaemia screenings and anaemia prevention among Quechua infants and children in Peru.

Dr. Lyn Merryfeather
Instructor, University of Victoria and Hospice Volunteer, Cowichan Valley Hospice, Canada

I have been interested in gender issues since childhood when I discovered that being identified as female meant I was restricted to certain circumscribed activities and excluded from others. I eventually put away all the joyful trappings of my tomboy youth and succumbed to those restrictions. As an adult, I performed my gender as a person of the female sex and did all the expected feminine things until I awoke from my long alcohol-fueled sleep and discovered my lesbianism and feminism and became immersed in the world of alternate sexuality. On an academic level, I studied my experience, as well as that of other women as partners of transsexual men, in a dissertation titled, Stories of Women Who Support Trans Men: An autoethnographic voyage (2014). I went on to revise this work into something that would appeal to both the general public as well as scholars and named it, You've Changed: An evocative autoethnography (2016). My life as a woman, lesbian, nurse, trans supporter, and autoethnographer, all minority positions in Western culture, has inspired an activist mentality where the ethical treatment of all people is a cherished goal.

Scott Macpherson
Lecturer in Mental Health, Robert Gordon University, Scotland

Scott Macpherson is a lecturer in mental health and Ph.D. student at Robert Gordon University in Aberdeen. Scott has an academic background in psychology and cognitive behavioral psychotherapy. Scott qualified as a mental health nurse from Dundee University in 1999 and worked primarily in the field of substance use prior to moving into teaching in 2013. During that time Scott worked in both private and statutory organizations. Scott has presented work on stigma at conferences at both a national and international level. Scott's teaching and research interests include film and mental health, substance use, spirituality, and cognitive behavioral therapy. Alongside Dan Warrender, he is a co-founder of R.G.U.'s Mental Health Movie Monthly, which aims to promote empathy and understanding of mental health issues by providing free showings of relevant films to staff, students, and the general public, and hosting facilitated discussion.

Dan Warrender
Lecturer in Mental Health, Robert Gordon University, Scotland

Further to an M.A. in philosophy and a working background in learning difficulties, Dan qualified as a mental health nurse from Robert Gordon University in September 2011 and chose to work in acute mental health. Gaining a place on the Early Clinical Career Fellowship (E.C.C.F.) 2012, he completed an M.Sc. in nursing, undertaking primary research and disseminating this nationally and internationally before joining R.G.U. as a lecturer in 2014 and commencing Ph.D. study in 2016.

As well as his teaching and research interests, Dan is a registered mentalization based therapist with the British Psychoanalytic Council and continues to practice this within the N.H.S., as well as providing clinical supervision for mental health staff. He has also been involved with strategic groups regarding the care of people with personality disorders at local and national level.

Alongside Scott Macpherson, he is a co-founder of R.G.U.'s Mental Health Movie Monthly.

Dr. John Richard Ashcroft
Locum Consultant Psychiatrist in Adult A.D.H.D. and Neurodevelopment, Mersey Care N.H.S. Trust, England

John is a Consultant Psychiatrist with special interests in mental health rehabilitation and brain injury medicine. He graduated from Imperial College London in 2000 after earning a B.Sc. in neurosciences with basic medical sciences in 1997. John obtained membership of the Royal College of Psychiatrists in 2005. He was awarded a Ph.D. in clinical neuropsychiatry from the University of Birmingham in 2008 and a Ph.D. in mental health law from Northumbria University in 2017. John has authored a number of book chapters published by Radcliffe and Routledge. John is approved by the Secretary of State as having special experience in the diagnosis and treatment of mental disorder under Section 12(2) of the Mental Health Act 1983 (as amended 2007) and is an Approved Clinician. John is on the General Medical Council Specialist Register and is the responsible clinician and clinical lead for Ash House Rehabilitation Unit in Warrington, Cheshire.

Laura Henry
Occupational Therapist, Ash House Rehabilitation Hospital, England

Laura is a qualified and experienced occupational therapist working at Ash House Rehabilitation Unit in Warrington, Cheshire, a locked unit for men with complex mental health needs. Prior to joining Ash House Laura worked as an O.T. across both secure inpatient and specialist community services, these experiences developing her knowledge and practice skill sets. Laura is very clear that in addition to clinical therapeutic engagement individuals need to develop a range of occupational capabilities whilst in a rehabilitation service to ensure a successful and sustainable transition to less restrictive services.

Subia Parveen Rasheed
Former Assistant Professor, Shifa College of Nursing, Shifa Tameer e Milat University, Pakistan

Subia Rasheed is a Former Assistant Professor at Shifa College of Nursing, Shifa Tameer e Milat University, Islamabad, Pakistan. Her main area of teaching included mental health-psychiatric nursing, critical care nursing and evidence based nursing practice. She has recently completed International Teacher Education Program from JAMK University of Applied Science, Finland. Presently she is an independent researcher. She has published in national and international peer reviewed journals. Her research interests include, self-awareness and self-knowing, nurse client relationship, teaching learning pedagogies, simulation, and crisis resource management.

Ahtisham Younas
Developmental Support Worker, The CareGivers, Canada and Former Junior Lecturer, Shifa College of Nursing, Pakistan

Ahtisham Younas has been a Junior Lecturer at Shifa College of Nursing in Islamabad, Pakistan where he taught the courses on theoretical models of nursing and mental health nursing. Currently, he is pursuing a doctoral degree in Nursing at Memorial University of Newfoundland, Canada. He has published both in national and international peer reviewed journals and presented papers at conferences. His research interests include, relational inquiry-based practice; self-knowing and self-consciousness; reflective practice, knowledge translation, building relational capacities of nurses, men in nursing, and teaching learning pedagogies.

Nicole Newman
Ph.D. student in Clinical Psychology, Palo Alto University, U.S.A.

Nicole Newman graduated from the University of Southern California in 2015 with a B.A. in psychology. She continued her education at University of Pennsylvania where she earned her M.Sc. in Counseling and Mental Health Services. In 2016, she began the Ph.D. in Clinical Psychology program at Palo Alto University and is completing the Neuropsychology Area of Emphasis in preparation for becoming a clinical neuro-psychologist. She currently assists the Palo Alto VA's Defense Veterans Brain Injury Center with research on traumatic brain injury and psychological disorders using neurobehavioral inventories and cognitive assessments. She is working toward furthering her understanding of the biomechanisms and neuropsychological effects of trauma, especially transgenerational and systematic trauma.

Professor Lisa M. Brown
Professor/Director of Trauma Program, Palo Alto University, U.S.A.

Dr. Lisa Brown is a tenured Professor, Director of the Trauma Program, and Director of the Risk and Resilience Research Lab at Palo Alto University. Her clinical and research focus is on aging, trauma and resilience, global mental health, and vulnerable populations. As a researcher, she is actively involved in developing and evaluating mental health programs used nationally and internationally, crafting recommendations aimed at enhancing health and quality of life of individuals and communities, facilitating participation of key stakeholders, and improving access to resources and services. Her research experience and her collaborative relationships with first responder groups and long-term care organizations led to the development of the 2nd edition of the Psychological First Aid Field Guide for Nursing Home Residents. Dr. Brown is a Fellow of the American Psychological Association Division 20, and the Gerontological Society of America. She was the recipient of two Fulbright Specialist awards with the University of the West Indies, Mona, Jamaica (2014) and with Massey University, Palmerston North, New Zealand (2015).

Dr. Geraldine S. Pearson
Associate Professor of Medicine, University of Connecticut, U.S.A.

Dr. Pearson has been an advanced practice registered nurse in child and adolescent psychiatry for over 40 years. Her B.S.N. and M.S.N. are from the University of Cincinnati, College of Nursing and Health and her Ph.D. was received from the University of Connecticut School of Nursing. She is also the editor of the Journal of the American Psychiatric Nurses Association. She is currently an associate professor in the U.C.O.N.N. School of Medicine and the co-chairperson of the Committee on Publication Ethics. Her clinical practice is in an outpatient community mental health clinic with children and adolescents.

Dr. Siân Bensa
Clinical Psychologist, Cheshire and Wirral Partnership N.H.S. Foundation Trust, England

Dr. Siân Bensa is an experienced clinical psychologist working in inpatient acute and rehabilitation mental health settings in the North West of England. Her particular interests are around trauma, psychosis, and psychological formulation. She holds bachelor and master degrees in psychology and health psychology respectively, and obtained a doctorate in clinical psychology from Royal Holloway, University of London. She is also a trained systemic practitioner.

W.J. Wayne Skinner
Assistant Professor of Psychiatry and Adjunct Senior Lecturer in the Faculty of Social Work, University of Toronto, Canada

Wayne Skinner is an assistant professor in the Department of Psychiatry and as adjunct senior lecturer in the Faculty of Social Work at the University of Toronto, with adjunct faculty appointments in social work at York and Trent universities. He is a member of the Motivational Interviewing Network of Trainers. Wayne played a lead role in the development of treatment services for people with co-occurring mental health and substance use problems at the Center for Addiction and Mental Health in Toronto for over 20 years. He is active as an educator, trainer, and consultant, supporting professionals nationally and internationally in their work with people and families affected by addiction and mental health concerns.

Marilyn White-Campbell
Geriatric Addictions Specialist, St. Josephs Health Care Guelph Behavioral Response Team and Provincial Lead for Geriatric Addiction, Behavioral Supports
Ontario Substance Use Collaborative, Canada

Marilyn White-Campbell is the provincial lead and co-chair of the Older Adult Substance Use Collaborative with Behavioral Supports Ontario and a principal investigator for the Canadian Coalition for Seniors Mental Health Geriatric Addictions Best Practice Guidelines. She is currently on secondment to the Community Responsive Behavioral Team and Specialized Geriatric Services and Geriatric Addiction Specialist for the COPA program in Toronto, one of Canada's first addictions treatment programs for older adults. She is recognized as a Canadian pioneer in the treatment of substance use issues in older adults.

Carl A. Kent
Community Outreach Worker in Toronto, Canada

Carl Kent has been a clinical leader in a number of innovative programs for people with addiction and mental health programs for many years, supervising students and staff in multidisciplinary settings. At the Addiction Research Foundation, he co-developed and was clinical supervisor in the first brief outpatient treatment program for people with substance use problems in Ontario. As a community consultant at the Center for Addiction and Mental Health, he co-lead projects to build better primary and secondary care services and supports of people and families affected by mental health and substance use problems. Most recently he has been a community-based clinician and then a board member at C.O.P.A., a unique outreach treatment program for older adults in Toronto.

Dr. Patrick Ryan
Director of Clinical Psychology, University of Limerick, Ireland

Patrick Ryan is Head of Psychology at the University of Limerick, Ireland, where is also the Director of Clinical Psychology. A practising clinician, researcher, author, and academic, his main area of interest lies in understanding psychological distress through a lifespan trauma lens.

Julie Lynch
Research Psychologist, Royal College of Physicians, Ireland

Julie Lynch is a research psychologist with the Royal College of Physicians of Ireland. She completed her undergraduate training in Trinity College Dublin. She completed her Masters in Psychological Science at University College Dublin. Julie's primary research interest is the psychological benefits of choral singing across the lifespan.

Dr. Lottie Morris
Clinical Psychologist, Hospice Isle of Man, Isle of Man, U.K.

Dr. Lottie Morris is a clinical psychologist who has worked in oncology and palliative care for several years, within third sector organizations. Dr. Morris works with people across the lifespan, from children through to older people. She is committed to a compassionate and collaborative approach to supporting individuals and their families, drawing from empirically grounded psychological therapies. She completed her doctorate in clinical psychology at the University of Bath and has published research on a range of topics relating to both mental and physical health. Having worked predominantly with children and families prior to training as a clinical psychologist, Dr. Morris values a holistic, family-based approach. In addition, she has a keen interest in staff well-being and the impact this has on patient care. She has been instrumental in setting up Schwartz Rounds in her local area to improve staff well-being and compassionate care, alongside research relating to this topic.

Jacqueline Talmet
Advanced Nurse Clinical Services Coordinator and Regional Manager, D.A.S.S.A. Northern Service, Australia

Jacky Talmet is a registered nurse with a mental health nursing background with over 35 years' experience working in drug and alcohol nursing and mental health. Jacky has a special interest in ethical practice and how it relates to people with alcohol and other drug and mental health comorbidity. Over many years, Jacky has worked with colleagues to improve the standards of assessment and care provision to people with AOD problems and to address discrimination and stigmatization to ensure people's rights are upheld for equitable access to health services and to receive supportive and appropriate care. For some years Jacky has identified palliative care as a valid component of the continuum of service provision to people with severe A.O.D. dependence and has been involved in supporting this form of care.

Professor Charlotte Francis Champion de Crespigny
Retired Adjunct Professor of Nursing, University of Adelaide, Australia

Professor Charlotte de Crespigny is a registered nurse and has a Ph.D. She has been a clinician, educator and researcher for 30 years. Charlotte is a strong advocate for young and older people who experience dependence wherever they seek help, and health care. She has also worked with the Aboriginal community for over 20 years. She has written many research and other articles, and educational and practice guidelines. Charlotte has conducted nationally and local funded research into service access for people aged 12 years and over with comorbidity, including refugees and Aboriginal people; young women drinking in pubs; older women and medications; and Aboriginal people's experiences with over-the-counter analgesics.

Annessa Rebair
Senior Lecturer in Mental Health, Northumbria University, England

Annessa Rebair is a Senior Lecturer and Executive and Leadership Coach at the University of Northumbria, Newcastle upon Tyne. Annessa has an interest in the subject of suicide and her doctoral research is concerned with co-constructing conversations about suicide in nursing contexts. Annessa is also a Trustee for the national charity PAPYRUS (prevention of young suicide) and represents the Royal College of Nursing on national suicide prevention groups.

Dr. Geralyn Hynes
Associate Professor in Palliative Care, Trinity College Dublin, Ireland

Geralyn Hynes has interests in palliative care, action, and evaluation research. She has published methodological papers and has a particular interest in the specialist/non-specialist palliative care interface, and implementation of palliative care policy in everyday practice. Her research has spanned people with different conditions (including C.O.P.D., paediatric oncology, intellectual disability, and dementia) and service development in different care settings. She has undertaken a number of action research initiatives using a variety of innovative methods that focus on the idea of participation being both epistemological and political. This means that how we engage with the notion of participation will determine the kind of knowledge that is produced and the privileging of certain kinds of knowledge over others. With her interest in palliative care as a public health concern, she has collaborated with Dr. Suresh Kumar, Institute of Palliative Medicine, Kerala both in Dublin and Kerala, all of which focuses on the idea of compassionate care. In her doctoral work she brought together nurses from respiratory and palliative care teams to explore non-specialist palliative care. A key finding from this work was the importance of meetings with a focus on sharing experiences of caring and compassion.

Professor Agnes Higgins
Professor of Mental Health, Trinity College Dublin, Ireland

Agnes is a registered mental health nurse and general nurse who has worked in both mental health and hospice/palliative care. Her research interest is in the area of mental health recovery, service user and family engagement, and peer support. She has undertaken a number of studies using participatory methodologies that focus on building a body of work that enables service users and family members to feel empowered, and provides a template for service user and family involvement as co-producers of knowledge and partners in service development and reform. She has also completed research in the area of peer support, illuminating the role of expertise by experience in people's personal recovery journeys. In addition to challenging the discourse around people who experience severe mental health problems from one of professional pessimism and chronicity to one of hope and recovery, her work is challenging traditionally-held views that people who experience enduring mental health problems are 'poor collaborators and poor research informants.' Agnes is Professor of Mental Health at the School of Nursing and Midwifery, Trendy College Dublin Ireland.

Professor Sarah Galvani
Professor of Adult Social Care, Manchester Metropolitan University, England

Sarah's research and teaching focuses on alcohol and other drug use in association with a range of social and health care issues, e.g. domestic violence, older people, sight loss, and substance use in specific minority ethnic communities. Sarah is currently leading and on a large exploratory study focusing on end-of-life and palliative care for people with alcohol and other drug problems. Her heart lies in qualitative research methods, but she works well with quantitative specialists for her mixed methods research.

In addition to her academic role, Sarah is a registered social worker with a practice background in adult services, particularly working with people experiencing mental distress, homeless people, and people with alcohol and other drug problems. She has led research and policy work in the U.K. on substance use in social work education and practice including her recent document 'Alcohol and other drug use: the roles and capabilities of social workers.' She is widely published, including practice guidance, online learning, peer reviewed journals, professional magazines and books. Sarah is a trustee of a number of national charities including Alcohol Research U.K., A.V.A. (Against Violence and Abuse), and Cumbria Alcohol and Drug Advisory Service. She chairs the British Association of Social Work's Special Interest Group in Alcohol and Other Drugs. She also sits on the editorial board of the journal Drugs: Education, Prevention and Practice.

Dr. Gemma Anne Yarwood
Strategic Partnership Lead, Manchester Metropolitan and Pennine Care Foundation Trust and Senior Lecturer in Social Care and Social Work, Manchester Metropolitan University, England

Gemma Anne Yarwood, Ph.D., senior lecturer in social care and social work at Manchester Met University. She is strategic partnership lead for Manchester Met University and Pennine Care N.H.S. Foundation Trust (P.C.F.T.). Her work focuses on research, workforce development, and curriculum innovation to improve service delivery for practitioners, services users, and their families.

Professor Sue Read
(Acting) Head of School and Professor of Learning Disability Nursing, School of Nursing and Midwifery, Keele University, England

Dr. Sue Read is Professor of Learning Disability Nursing and (Acting) Head of School, School of Nursing and Midwifery, Keele University, Staffordshire. Sue's professional area of interest for many years has been loss, death, end-of-life care and bereavement for marginalized populations, but particularly people with an intellectual disability, from a psycho therapeutic, counselling, and support perspective. Sue is interested in applied research, particularly qualitative approaches, which make a demonstrable impact on practice.

Dr. Sotirios Santatzoglou
Teaching Fellow in the School of Law, Keele University, England

Dr. Sotirios Santatzoglou is a Teaching Fellow in the Law School, Keele University, U.K. Sotirios has a strong interest in loss, palliative, and end-of-life care and bereavement, particularly from the legal perspective and its application into practice initiatives. He is currently undertaking research into bereavement support among young people across the criminal justice system.

Dr. Anthony Wrigley
Senior Lecturer in Ethics and Faculty Director of Taught Postgraduate Studies, Centre for Professional Ethics (PEAK), Keele University, England

Dr. Anthony Wrigley is senior lecturer in ethics, Centre for Professional Ethics, School of Law, Keele University, U.K. His work focuses on ethical dilemmas and philosophical problems at the margins of life, with a particular interest in issues surrounding vulnerability, authority, and consenting for others, personhood, and end-of-life care.

REFERENCE

Merryfeather, L (2014) Women who support trans men: An autoethnographic voyage. Ph.D. thesis. University of Victoria BC Canada.

Merryfeather, L (2016) You've changed: An evocative authoethnography. Victoria BC Canada: Friesen Press.

Preface
About *Palliative Care Within Mental Health*

This book is not just about caring for the dying within mental health, but about applying the quality care and practice of the palliative care approach within mental health practice. The book focuses on intervention, treatment, care and practice, and the similarities in practice between palliative care and mental health.

The common ground is an excellent foundation in care and practice for integrating palliative care, now recognized as best-practice end-of-life care, into mental health care, practice, and service delivery. In short, the shared practice values and vision between these two disciplines provide a starting point for integrated intervention, treatment, care, and practice using best practices from both palliative care and mental health.

The book came into being when we (the editors) were talking and the discussion led on to the need for more information/direction when applying humanness and the issues of adopting a palliative care approach within mental health practice. Whilst we acknowledge that mental health has a lot to offer palliative care, we both felt that palliative care could offer this approach within mental health practice, in that it is a neglected area. There was little, or no literature related to palliative care within mental health practice, and that which does exist relates to care of the dying in terms of cancer.

What struck us was that several chapters covered within the series Mental Health-Substance Use, edited by this editor (Published by CRC) could equally apply to palliative care within mental health care and practice. In the time it took us to drink our coffee we had developed a contents list! As the title *Palliative Care within Mental Health: Ethical Practice* suggests, the whole approach would be on the human aspects of care and practice.

Is there a place for palliative care within mental health? At the mention of palliative care, there is a general assumption that:
➤ the person has a cancer diagnosis; and
➤ the person is dying.

However, this is not the true meaning of palliation. A simple understanding might be that if one has ill health that is serious and enduring (even with periods of respite) then that person needs careful and continuous symptom management, together with skilled emotional support, so that she or he can achieve the best quality of life, with managed symptom control, as effectively as possible – that is – palliative care. Attention to detail is a prime principle, for the individual and family members.

We have combined our different skills (Jo – palliative care; David – mental health) to edit this book and a highly qualified team were invited to contribute. We hope we have edited a thought provoking and informative text on *Palliative Care Within Mental Health: Ethical Practice.*

Acknowledgments

We are grateful to all the contributors for having the faith in us to produce a valued text and we thank them for their hard work, support, and encouragement. We hope that faith proves correct. Thank you to those who have commented along the way, and whose patience has been outstanding.

Many people have helped us along our career paths and life – too many to name individually. Most do not even know what impact they have had on us. Most were individuals who touched our professional lives and who contributed most to our knowledge and understanding, leading us to appreciate the importance of compassion in care, and our effort to move towards this in practice and life.

Our sincere thanks to our friends and colleagues along our career paths: those who have touched our life in a positive way – and a minority, in a negative way (for we can learn from the negative to ensure we do better for others).

A final heartfelt statement: any errors, omissions, inaccuracies, or deficiencies within these pages are our sole responsibility.

Terminology

Whenever possible, the following terminology has been applied. However, in certain instances, when referencing a study and or specific work, when an author has made a specific request, or for the purpose of additional clarity, it has been necessary to deviate from this applied 'norm.'

PROBLEM(S), CONCERNS, AND DILEMMAS OR DISORDERS

The terms *problem(s)*, *concerns, and dilemmas* and *disorders* can be used interchangeably, as stated by the author's preference. However, where possible, the term 'problem(s)' or 'concerns and dilemmas' has been adopted as the preferred choice.

INDIVIDUAL, PERSON, PEOPLE

There seems to be a need to label the individual – as a form of recognition. Sometimes the label becomes more than the person. We refer to patients, clients, service users, customers, consumers, and so on. Yet, we feel affronted when we are addressed as anything other than what we are – individuals. We need to be mindful that every person we see during our professional day is an individual – unique. Symptoms are in many ways similar (e.g. delusions, hallucinations), some need interventions and treatments are similar (e.g. specific drugs, psychotherapy techniques), but people are not. Alan may experience an illness labelled schizophrenia, and so may John, Beth, and Mary, and you or me. However, each will have his or her own unique experiences – and life. None will be the same. To keep this constantly in the mind of the reader, throughout the book we shall refer to the *individual, person,* or *people* – just like us, but different to us by their uniqueness.

PROFESSIONAL

In the eyes of the individual, we are all professionals, whether students, nurses, doctors, social workers, researchers, clinicians, educationalists, managers, service developers, religious ministers – and so on. However, the level of expertise may vary from one professional to another. We are also individuals. There is a need to distinguish between the person experiencing a mental health problem and the person interacting professionally (at whatever level) with that individual. To acknowledge and to differentiate between those who experience – in this context – and those who intervene, we have adopted the term *professional.* It is indicative that we have had, or are receiving, education and training related specifically to help us meet the needs of the individual. We may or may not have experienced palliative care and or mental health problems, but we have some knowledge that may help the individual – an expertise to be shared. We have a specific knowledge that, hopefully, we wish to use to offer effective intervention and treatment to another human being. It is the need to make a clear differential, and for that purpose only, that forces the use of 'professional' over 'individual' to describe our role – our input into another person's life.

CHAPTER 1

Why a Palliative Care Approach Within Mental Health?

Jo Cooper and David B. Cooper

Perhaps our human purpose is no more or less than that of providing warmth, companionship and acceptance of our fellow women and men, rather than trying to fix them.

(Barker & Buchanan-Barker 2008)

INTRODUCTION

Palliative care and mental health (and other health- and social-care fields) are driven, not only by knowledge, skills, and attitudes, but by compassion. We could say that all health and social care is driven by these elements, which are intrinsic in the skills needed to help in alleviating grief, hopelessness, and distress. All three of these elements feature widely in meeting both palliative care and mental health needs. There are many parallels to be drawn in our comparisons between palliative care and mental health. The two pathways traverse and intersect, whereby creating a need for active and heartfelt listening, and for us to act on what we hear. As health care professionals we have a mandate to provide ethically based care, regardless of diagnosis.

This book aims to improve, above all else, the relationships, responses, compassion, care, and practice necessary to be an effective professional in offering interventions and treatment for those experiencing mental health problems and the ethical dilemmas that we face on a daily basis. Ethics has a crucial importance in decision making. The emphasis throughout is on the individual *and* the family, compassion, and the appreciation of the stigma such problems bring to the individual and family. We look at ethical care, practice, intervention, and palliative treatment within mental health services. Helping to provide:

➤ person-centered practice
➤ relationship based connectedness
➤ care and practice
➤ cultural dilemmas
➤ ethical dilemmas
➤ a belief in compassion, respect, and dignity in care and practice
➤ respect for autonomy and choice
➤ quality of life issues

> the family as the unit of care
> the need for democratic and intra- and inter-disciplinary team work.

For the individual and family experiencing serious and enduring mental health, life presents many problems. The needs are complex and all encompassing. For the professional, educator, researcher, manager, and service providers/developers this presents multifaceted ethical challenges. To successfully, and innovatively, deliver interventions, treatment, care and practice responses, and comprehensive services, professionals need to continually explore, and update knowledge and skills. *Palliative Care within Mental Health: Ethical Practice* offers discussion and dissemination around the subject of palliative care within mental health. The book does not separate or address 'mental health' or 'palliative care' as individual subjects. Concerns raised relate not only to the individual and family, but to the future direction of care, practice, interventions, and treatment. Whilst presenting a balanced view of what is best practice today, we aim to challenge concepts and stimulate debate, exploring all aspects of the development of palliative care and practice within mental health and develop proper responses incorporating ethically-based research-led best practice. This book examines a dynamic approach to the ethics underpinning both palliative care and mental health.

WHAT IS PALLIATIVE CARE?

'Palliation' derives from the Latin word palliate or 'cloak' meaning to offer comfort, support, and to surround that person with a modified form of love, as well as the knowledge, skills, and attitudes needed to provide care, which encompasses family members. Care giving is not a 'one off' exercise in palliative expertise; it is continuous and will always remain as a person-centered approach.

> **KEY POINT 1.1**

> You matter because you are you. You matter to the last moment of your life, and we will do all we can to help you not only to die peacefully, but also to live until you die.
>
> (Saunders 1976)

Palliative care is widely accepted as best practice end-of-life care and is concerned with promoting and supporting the best possible quality of life. Connecting with the person is the central focus in both palliative care and mental health disciplines. The World Health Organization (WHO) defines palliative care as:

> An approach that improves the quality of life of patients and their families facing the problems associated with life threatening illness, through the *prevention and relief of suffering* by means of early identification and impeccable assessment and treatment of pain and other problems, physical, psychosocial and spiritual . . .
> Affirms life and regards dying as a normal process that:
> > provides relief from pain and other symptoms
> > intends neither to hasten nor postpone death
> > integrates psychological and spiritual aspects of care

- ➤ offers a support system to help patients to live as actively as possible until death
- ➤ offers a support system to help the family cope during the patient's [persons] illness and in their own bereavement
- ➤ uses a team approach to address the needs of patients and families, including bereavement counselling if indicated
- ➤ enhances the quality of life, and may also positively influence the course of illness
- ➤ is applicable early in the course of the illness, in conjunction with other therapies that are intended to prolong life, such as chemotherapy or radiotherapy, and includes those investigations needed to better understand and manage distressing clinical complications.

(WHO 1990)

KEY POINT 1.2

Every person has the right to receive high quality palliative care whatever the ill-health problems, regardless of the course and nature of that ill health.

KEY POINT 1.3

The principles and philosophy of palliative care can be applied to any condition, irrespective of the clinical setting (*See* Palliative Care within Mental health: principles and philosophy).

The goal of palliative care is to meet individual needs and to provide the best quality-of-life for the person and their family. This approach includes physical, psychological, emotional, social, and spiritual health, extending into bereavement, grief, and loss, which can occur before, during and after death.

WHY A PALLIATIVE CARE 'APPROACH' IN MENTAL HEALTH

As in mental health, palliative care relies on intra- and inter-disciplinary team working, an integral part of the philosophy of both disciplines, providing a responsive and sustained approach to person-centered care and practice. This engages the need to support a therapeutic relationship with each person we work alongside. This is not something we go and 'do' to a person, but it is very much a way of 'being'; a way of life. It is something we should strive for in our everyday lives when we relate to our medical and health- and social-care colleagues, the person we are engaged with, and their family. Our work should be about **being human with people** and not just being the 'nurse', 'doctor', or 'social worker'. People allow us into their lives, each having a story to tell and from that stems a connectedness, encouraging care always to be tailored to that persons' individual needs. In conditions where life is limited (palliative care) or quality life is compromised (mental health), it can be tempting for us [the professional] to feel that we know what is best for that person. This stems from our innate need to be the helper. As tempting as it may be to make our opinion known, we need to stand back, allowing the person to make choices of their own. Simple things like, choosing what he or she wants to wear that day, or what he or she would like to eat is as important as helping the individual to decide something which has potential impact on, and is important to their state of health. Our responsibility is **to motivate, to inspire, to be alongside**. To be there should things go wrong and to smooth the way forward. In today's health- and social-care world and culture, we proclaim loudly that 'it is the patients [persons] choice'. However, it takes huge courage for a person who is feeling vulnerable to make a choice which may conflict with those who are in the 'powerful' position of caring.

Using a palliative care approach reaches out to the specific needs of the person (rather than the service) experiencing mental health problems, and their families. The palliative care approach includes the management of complex and intractable symptoms, both physical, psychological, and emotional, and responds also to social, spiritual, and, if needed, bereavement needs of the individual (e.g. loss of employment, family, hope).

> ### KEY POINT 1.4
>
> The goal of a palliative care approach is to provide supportive care during all stages of a mental health problem and the latter stages of ill-health – and enables a life that is as comfortable and as meaningful as possible to that person and the family.

It is not just apposite to end-of-life care; palliative, relieving without cure. Where compassion often overrides science. It is about using the principles and philosophy of palliative care within the mental health care environment.

We have, within our power, spirit, and opportunity, to encourage change. To create an environment that is beneficial and restorative for, not only the individual and their families, but for our colleagues working in health and social care services, that generates many everyday ethical problems.

> ### KEY POINT 1.5
>
> There is no financial cost involved in changing workplace attitudes. From being unhelpful to helpful; from perverse to cheerful.

Being polite is not difficult, despite what may be arising in our own life. We are all 'somebody's patient'. We can all be on the receiving end of 'care'. No person will recover quickly if they feel a burden for just being there. It is more than disheartening; it is not ethical conduct, and does not promote a relationship that is therapeutic.

It is a natural part of human life that we experience suffering. Emotional, psychological, physical, and spiritual. Physical suffering inevitably creates emotional and psychological suffering. How we cope, depends on many variables, including 'who' we are and our own coping abilities learned from nature and nurture. It is only by recognizing and learning from our own difficult life experiences that we try to do our very best to help others to regain some palliation of their distress, pain, and grief. The moment that pain and sadness is shared with another, 'something happens'; being able to speak freely can be liberating. The helper has to carefully and diligently listen.

KEY POINT 1.6

One of the most meaningful and powerful gifts we can give is to listen. Its value is often not recognized.

People do not always want or need advice. But, simply someone who will listen, to hear their pain, and to show understanding and compassion.

> The most basic and powerful way to connect to another person is to listen . . . just listen. The most important thing we ever give each other is our attention. . . . When people are talking, there's no need to do anything but receive them. Just take them in. Listen to what they're saying. Care about it.
>
> (Rachel Naomi Remen 2006)

COMMUNICATION

Effective communication is a prime function and fundamental within mental health and palliative care. The essence of effective communication is our ability to listen carefully to what we are being told, if the person is to feel fully heard and understood. It is not only about our interpretation of the information in order to manage complex needs and symptoms. It is about ensuring that we convey, with empathy, the validity of the person and their story.

Communication is imperative with and between the families, so that they are in no doubt about what we are doing. If we are to give the person free choices, then they must be properly informed about what those choices are, and the consequences of the choices they make. The individual is facing strong feelings and emotions as a direct consequence of her or his ill-health, such as anger, sadness, fear, anxiety, and faces existential concerns, which demand exploration and sensitive approaches, to reduce and allay the many and varied emotions experienced. Improved awareness of palliative care is a first step toward reducing disparities in utilization of important and useful services for persons experiencing life-changing, life-limiting, mental ill-health. Lack of awareness may limit access to needed palliative care (Matsuyama et al. 2011).

HUMANITY IN CARING

> Humanity is the place where you will find someone who will enter into your suffering and never leave you there alone.
>
> (Roy 2004)

The human condition encompasses the experiences of being human. Human nature refers to certain characteristics that humans have in common: As 'Human Beings', we have certain characteristics, such as empathy, compassion, aggression, and fear.

Being human is about the acceptance of every human being for just being another human being, regardless of colour, religion, race, or gender (*See* Chapter 6 and 7 and Palliative Care within Mental Health: Principles and Philosophy, Chapter 3 and 9). When caring for people who are ill, we are constantly challenged to provide support and care in a human and compassionate way. The person-centered philosophy of mental health and palliative care is based on humanness and compassion. The focus is not just on the ill-health or the complex symptoms it produces, but is actively involved in finding out the needs of the whole person. In order to carry out this level of person-centered care, we must attend to the three indivisible facets of the human condition – the mind, body, and spirit of human kind (Hooper 2000).

THE ESSENCE OF CARING

REFLECTIVE PRACTICE EXERCISE 1.1

Time: 20 minutes
In your place of work, how do you, or how could you, use a palliative care approach to improve and maintain the quality of life for:
- the individual?
- their family?

What changes would you need to make?

Florence Nightingale (1946) firmly believed that the essence of nursing rested on the nurse's capacity to provide humane, sensitive care to the sick, which she believed would allow healing. The therapeutic relationship in mental health has its origins in the work of Peplau (1965) who introduced her Theory of Interpersonal Relations, which focused on the human connection between the professional and individual. In today's health and social care environment, the human relationship is in danger of being overlooked in deference to computerized technology and financial restraints. We acknowledge the beneficial advantages of technology, but this does not provide information relevant to the person as a 'human being'.

WARMTH, COMPANIONSHIP, AND ACCEPTANCE

Caring for someone should be a human activity, performed as humanly as possible, one person to another, an equal footing. We meet people at a time of emotional need. However, do we have the resources to meet that need? Do we, in fact, see that there is an emotional need to be met? The tricky situations that we meet may tempt us to run away from the emotional pain – it is often easier to deal with physical pain.

KEY POINT 1.7

In '*doing*', rather than '*being*' we can easily fail to reach the '*meaning*' of the situation, a meaning which will offer opportunity for us to discover how we can best help the person, in a compassionate way.

We need to have a genuine desire to help, to acknowledge the pain of another, make a human response.

SUFFERING

> Suffering is subjective, encompassing factors that diminish quality of life, a perception of distress, and an expression of a life not worth living.
>
> (Cherny, Coyle & Foley 1994)

Suffering can be physical, emotional, spiritual, psychological, or all of these. Relief of suffering is an important goal for all professionals and a mutual commitment exists to reduce and relieve suffering. However, no type of care can ever alleviate *all* suffering, and some issues will always defy explanation. It is not only the person themselves who suffers, feeling isolated and desperate, but also the family and often the professional. It takes time, human effort and attention to detail to help the person who is suffering. It can be fear provoking for the professional. We can feel tempted to 'run away'. Sometimes, 'just sitting' with the distress can be enough for the individual to know that someone cares. Suffering is all embracing; it affects us all. **It is part of life.**

A GENUINE DESIRE TO HELP

For us to try to help the person, we need to be fully present, to focus on the experience of that person – to listen fully to their story, for they will have one to tell, rather than be focused on ourselves, in order to protect us from the suffering of another. Watching someone suffer causes distress within ourselves and seeing this suffering does not leave us untouched. As helpers we make human responses, showing compassion, empathy and understanding, and the offering of hope. We need the desire and competence to act, to acknowledge and share in the other's suffering and to make worthwhile and purposeful responses to the person's pain.

The family are important. Watching someone you love in physical, psychological, and/or emotional pain and suffering, causes distress that goes far beyond words.

SELF-KNOWING

As adults, we have the capacity to *feel* and to *think*, as well as the capacity to think about feelings. Being able to imagine the feelings of others is the cognitive basis for empathy (Lendrum & Syme 2004). It is helpful to be self-aware and '*knowing*' oneself is the fundamental axiom in both mental health and palliative care. Ideally, we attempt to 'know' ourselves, our environment, truly observing, imagining the possibilities, deducing from what we observe and are continually learning (Gardiner 2016).

KEY POINT 1.8

Self-awareness enriches our own understanding of *who* we are.

Possessing self-awareness shows that we have a philosophical belief about life, death, and the human condition (Eckroth-Bucher 2001). It is important to examine our own beliefs in order to influence the way we interpret and make use of the person's story about him- her-self. When we have been touched, as human beings, by the pain of others, we may try to find strategies to distance ourselves from that pain, for us to survive, and move on to offer support to others within our care.

COMPASSION

Compassion becomes the dominant premise in provision and conservation of care and practice and the art of caring lies in the relationship with the person, the family and is inclusive of our colleagues within the intra- inter-disciplinary team. When offering a helping relationship, based on empathic understanding, it is important, as far as we can, to still be connected to that person. As we go through our own life, we learn to use our own experiences to help those we care for (Lendrum & Syme 2004). We all recognize and feel something about the benefits of compassion. In one way, we are all the same, we all want to avoid suffering. What then, is *compassion* (*See* Chapter 3 and Palliative Care within Mental Health: Principles and Philosophy, Chapter 6)? It is not simply a sense of sympathy or caring for the person suffering. Rinpoche explains it as a sustained and practical determination to do whatever is possible and necessary to help alleviate the suffering of another (Rinpoche 2008). Neither is it a sense of pity. Pity has its roots in fear, a sense of smugness, or arrogance, we need to move from pity to compassion. However, both sympathy and pity may be useful for a brief period; both may bring some comfort to the sufferer during episodes of extreme suffering. At best, it is still an expression of sadness for the person who is suffering. It can also help to confirm the person's suffering, as it can be so easy for a person's suffering to be minimized, for example, by being told to have a *positive attitude*!

KEY POINT 1.9

Compassion gives some sign of acceptance of the person's dilemma, it is strength giving and affords comfort. This is not to say that feeling compassionate is easy. It is often challenging and difficult, and causes suffering for ourselves, as we share in the suffering of another.

Those we care for are our teachers. If we stay open, with a sense of allowingness, we can learn to develop our compassion for others. Each person we meet who is ill, or who is dying, will teach us. *All we must do is . . . listen and reflect.*

PALLIATIVE CARE AND SUBSTANCE USE

The problems met by prolonged and excessive use of alcohol and other drugs (substance use) have an important consideration in the often long-term mental and physical health issues that accompany such use. Therefore, we need to be open to the types of problems we meet and our role in offering a palliative care approach to these individuals and family. The reader is asked to be open minded throughout this book to the problems that arise because of substance use and or of existing mental health problems amongst the people we care for.

HOW TO

Before we can begin with any intervention and treatment programme we have to acknowledge that people are unique individuals, each with his or her own thoughts, feelings, needs, losses, loves . . . We need to own the philosophy that one size does *not* fit all. Whilst there may be some similarities in the approaches used and the symptoms experienced, each person will need different interventions once these needs and expectations have been acknowledged. For example, pain for one person may be similar to that of another's' but the experience of pain is completely individual. Careful management and attention to detail is the key to improving the individual's experience and pain management. The person who complains of pain is not a weak person, a moaning person, but a unique individual with his or her own needs and expectations.

"Pain is what the patient says it is" (McCaffery 1998).

To begin the process of care and practice we must first appreciate *how* we can maintain and influence compassion, respect and dignity for that individual. This may involve many problems along our path and present us with numerous ethical dilemmas, often a minefield for the individual, family and professional. People need supporting through their care but more importantly *after* that care, what happens next is our responsibility as a professional on whom people depend. Additionally, we need to be culturally competent to appreciate the individual needs of the person and family, so that we can incorporate those needs and expectations into our care and practice. This involves not just knowing but acting upon that knowledge always.

ASSESSMENT

The professional cannot meet the needs of the individual or family without a thorough assessment. A quick five minutes is not enough! Having said that, assessment must be spread over time, as needs change, and not a one-off exercise to be '*done*' before the professional moves on. Sitting with the person or family filling out forms is not meaningful assessment. Such is perceived as impersonal and detached from that person's real life and needs (*See* Chapters 9 and 10).

SUICIDE

The person experiencing suicidal intent needs compassionate care and open assessment and intervention to understand the individual's needs. However, just as important are the needs of the family who are often confused and distressed as to why the person feels the need to end his or her life. For the family, it is not easy to understand why the person that you love has turned away from you and has been unable to seek your help.

LONG-TERM ILL-HEALTH

Long-term mental health problems bring a plethora of needs and expectations for the individual and family. Life will need to be revaluated to incorporate the impact of the ill-health. Explanations should be offered as to what interventions are available, and they will see that someone '*cares*' about them. Just as important is to ensure there is a network of support available to the person and family. If the person feels valued, then aiding him or her to accept something that has interfered with their life expectancy and future is integral to his or her daily living. A future can be achieved and a stable path developed with safety nets in place when needed, however, these should not be merely reactive but proactive.

DEMENTIA

Dementia is traumatic to the individual and family. The loss of someone we love is experienced when the person is still alive, which brings the emotions of guilt and anger. The person in the initial stages of dementia may have some insight, which may be frightening and they can feel lost. Moreover, there may be embarrassment and a feeling of foolishness for the person experiencing dementia. To work alongside and encourage an active mind is essential as is 'cupping/holding' the family in their grief (See Chapter 15 and Palliative Care within Mental Health: Care and Practice, Chapter 11).

CONCLUSION

The palliative care approach becomes important in mental health when we cannot offer a cure but can offer symptom management (See Chapter 9). It applies to both mental health and substance use problems. Mental health and substance use professionals may already offer such an approach; however, we all have a lot to learn from each other.

This series of books are a *beginning* and will need much building upon to influence changes in ethical care, practice, behaviour, and attitude of professionals. However, it can be done and costs nothing other than compassionate care and practice. Working *with* the individual and family, giving time to understand and appreciate their collective problems, the act to support, guide, and improve each person's quality of life. The person and their family should always remain the point on which our attention and activity is centred.

REFERENCES

Barker, P. and Buchanan-Barker, P. (2008) 'Mental health in an age of celebrity: the courage to care', *Journal of Medical Ethics*, 34, 110–14.

Cherny, N. I,. Coyle, C. and Foley, K. M. (1994) 'Suffering in the advanced cancer patient: a definition and taxonomy', *Journal of Palliative Care*, 10, 57–70.

Eckroth-Bucher, M. (2001) 'Philosophical basis and practice of self-awareness in psychiatric nursing', *Journal of Psychosocial Nursing*, 39, 32–9.

Gardiner, F. W. (2016) 'The art of self-knowledge and deduction in clinical practice', *Annals of Medicine and Surgery*, Available at: www.ncbi.nlm.nih.gov/pmc/articles/PMC4961678/ (Accessed 20 June 2017)

Hopper, A. (2000) 'Meeting the spiritual needs of patients through holistic practice', *European Journal of Palliative Care*, 7, 60–3.

Lendrum, S. and Syme, G. (2004) *Gift of Tears: A Practical Approach to Loss and Bereavement in Counselling and Psychotherapy*. 2nd edition. East Sussex: Routledge.

Matsuyama, R. K., Balliet, W., Ingram, K., Lyckholm, L. J. and Smith, T. S. (2011) 'Will patients want hospice or palliative care if they do not know what it is'? *Journal of Hospice and Palliative Nursing*, 13, 41–6.

McCaffery, M. (1968) *Nursing Practice Theories Related to Cognition, Bodily Pain, and Man-Environment Interactions*. Los Angeles: University of California at Los Angeles Student Store, p. 95.

Nightingale, F. (1946) *Notes of Nursing: What It Is and What It Is Not*. Philadelphia: J. P. Lippincott.

Peplau, H. E. (1965) 'The heart of nursing: interpersonal relations', *Canadian Nurse*, 61, 273–5.

Remen, R. N. (2006) *Kitchen Table Wisdom: Stories That Heal*. New York City, New York: Riverhead Books, p. 143.

Roy, D. J. (2004) 'Humanity: idea, image, reality', *Journal of Palliative Care*, 20, 131–2.

Rinpoche, S. (2008) *The Tibetan Book of Living and Dying: A Spiritual Classic from One of the Foremost Interpreters of Tibetan Buddhism to the West*. Classic ed. London: Rider.

Saunders, C. (1976) 'Care of the dying – the problem of euthanasia', *Nursing Times*, 1, 1003–5.

World Health Organisation (1990) *Definition of Palliative Care*, Geneva: World Health Organisation. Available at: www.who.int/cancer/palliative/definition/en/ (accessed 6 June 2017)

To Learn More

Broom D. M. (2003) *The Evolution of Morality and Religion.* Cambridge: Cambridge University Press.

Cooper, D. B. and Cooper, J. eds (2012) *Palliative Care within Mental Health: Principles and Philosophy.* New York/Oxon: Radcliffe Medical Press.

Cooper, D. B. and Cooper, J. eds (2014) *Palliative Care within Mental Health: Care and Practice.* New York/Oxford: Radcliffe Medical Press.

Jeffrey, D. (2006) *Patient-centred Ethics and Communication at the End of Life.* Oxon: Radcliffe Publishing Ltd.

Lendrum, S. and Syme, G. (2004) *Gift of Tears: A Practical Approach to Loss and Bereavement in Counselling and Psychotherapy.* 2nd edition. East Sussex: Routledge.

Rinpoche, S. (2008) *The Tibetan Book of Living and Dying: A Spiritual Classic from One of the Foremost Interpreters of Tibetan Buddhism to the West.* Classic ed. London: Rider.

CHAPTER 2

What Is Ethics?

Cynthia M.A. Geppert

INTRODUCTION

Ethics is among the most venerable branches of philosophy and religion. Yet ethics, unlike metaphysics or epistemology, is not the exclusive domain of philosophers and theologians, rather it is something every thinking person must seriously consider. The most fundamental answer to the question what is ethics is another question the ancient Greeks pondered first and still perhaps most profoundly, "what does it mean to live a good life?" For the purposes of this volume, "what does it mean to die a good death?" If the chapter is to provide the practical guidance to professionals working at the crossroads of mental health and palliative care as it aims to do, it must keep these two questions at the forefront. The ethical principles and virtues, theories that constitute the academic discipline of ethics the chapter discusses, will be reinterpreted when professionals are confronted with the real-time complex challenges of providing care that is both compassionate and competent for people experiencing mental health conditions also facing life-limiting ill-health.

REFLECTIVE PRACTICE EXERCISE 2.1

Time: 15 minutes
Spend a few moments reflecting on how you, personally and professionally, would answer these two questions about what makes a good life and a good death? Are there differences in your personal and professional responses? At the end of the chapter repeat this exercise and see if your views have changed.

BRIEF REVIEW OF ACADEMIC ETHICS FOR THE MENTAL HEALTH AND PALLIATIVE PROFESSIONAL

We often think and speak of ethics and morality as interchangeable. Philosophers often make a distinction between the two. Morality is the stuff of being human and of the humanities that express our condition. It is the ineluctable choices we must make every day between good and bad, right and wrong. It is personal and existential. It involves both beliefs and actions. Because we are all people before and after we are professionals, each of us brings our morality with us to health-care training and practice. One of the important lessons this chapter will try to convey is the necessity of developing an ethical awareness of our own moral principles, so that we can account for biases in judgment practice in a manner that is coherent with our deepest values and yet respects what may be the very different values of those we care for and with.

Ethics is then not the same as morality. Ethics is the scholarly study of our common morality as individuals and cultures using the analytic methods, technical vocabulary, and modes of reasoning of philosophy. Ethics is interested in establishing ethical theories to justify our moral intuitions, formulating ethical principles to direct our thinking and virtues to motivate our actions. In the concise definition of independent ethics scholar, Lewis Vaughn, "Thus ethics—also known as **moral philosophy**—is a reasoned way of delving into the meaning and import of moral concepts and issues and of evaluating the merits of moral judgments and standards" (Vaughn 2017, p. 4)

KEY POINT 2.1

Morality and ethics are different concepts: ethics being the study of our moral judgments and beliefs.

Descriptive, or, in bioethics, evidence-based or **empirical ethics** uses social scientific tools rather than logical thought to examine the actual attitudes and actions, opinions and choices of persons and communities (Gardner and Williams 2015). For example, surveys will be conducted with physicians and nurses at different times to determine how views of the moral acceptability of physician-assisted suicide have changed. This is as close as ethics gets to the facts of what kind of lives we actually lead and deaths we experience (Dickinson et al. 2002).

Three Major Branches of Ethics

Moral philosophers further divide ethics into three major branches (Vaughn 2017).

1. **Metaethics** is the examination of the nature and warrant of the most fundamental moral assumptions. This division asks what we mean by words like good, right, and true. How do we define suffering? How would we recognize a 'good' person? From whence do our ethical concepts derive especially outside a religious framework and how do we reasonably defend them. Although as professionals this is the least relevant division of ethics to us, it provides the ultimate intellectual grounding for the kind of applied ethics we all practice.

2. **Normative ethics** seeks to identify and justify moral maxims and principles, the standards of conduct to which we as individuals and professionals adhere and that are expressed in codes of ethics, in medical and nursing practice laws, in hospital regulations. Normative ethics seeks to establish and reasonably justify the ethical theories that are the basis of our practice philosophy, the models of decision making we follow, as we attempt to resolve ethical dilemmas, the approaches we take to weigh the various ethical principles and balance the respective virtues when these are in conflict or cannot all be equally satisfied.

3. **Applied ethics** is the third branch and the one most important for our study of palliative and mental health care. Applied ethics is about working through everyday real world problems using the skills and knowledge of normative ethics and

increasingly of empirical ethics. More professional subspecies are medical ethics, nursing ethics, and integral to this chapter are the grassroots clinical areas of palliative and mental health ethics. While medical ethics is at least as old as the Hippocratic Oath, bioethics is relatively new. As Daniel Callahan one of the founders of the field has written, "The word *bioethics*, of recent vintage, has come to denote not just a particular field of human inquiry—the intersection of ethics and the life sciences, but also an academic discipline, a political force in medicine, biology, and environmental studies; and a cultural perspective of some consequence" (Callahan 2004, p. 278).

Bioethics then is a species of this applied ethics genus having to do with the ethical concerns and issues that arise in the broad field of science and medicine and encompasses an ever-expanding range of concerns from genetics to resource allocation. For example, should an individual with end-stage dementia receive dialysis? (Ying, Levitt and Jassal 2014). Should a person with melancholic depression who has attempted suicide be allowed to refuse cardio-pulmonary resuscitation? (Campo-Engelstein, Jankowski and Mullen 2016).

KEY POINT 2.2

There are three main branches of ethics: metaethics, normative ethics, and applied ethics, of which bioethics is an example.

What Ethics is Not Yet is: Law, Religion, and Culture

Ethics, especially bioethics, is frequently and understandably confused and confounded with many other types of related domains such as the law, compliance, risk management government ethics, and most commonly clinical issues. In part this is due to the multi-linear genealogy of bioethics with its origins in philosophy, theology, law, sociology, anthropology, and other disciplines (Jonsen 1998). As the Venn diagram below shows (Figure 2.1), these and other areas are related to bioethics concerns but it is a crucial first step when being presented with a putative ethics concern to identify where the issue best fits, so it may be properly addressed (National Center for Ethics in Health Care 2015).

Particularly in the areas of mental health (Appelbaum and Gutheil 1992) and certain aspects of palliative care ethics for persons experiencing serious mental ill-health, legal aspects of an issue are often relevant factors. From the perspective of professionalism though, it is crucial to distinguish the two domains and recognize that the **must** of the law sets the floor for our decisions while it is the **should** of ethics that constitutes the moral ceiling for our aspirations. Put another way, the law circumscribes the ethically justifiable options in a specific situation. For example, physician-assisted suicide or euthanasia can only be an ethical possibility in those countries or states where the practice is legal. Even where it is lawful there will obviously be other medical, ethical, and often religious considerations.

Spirituality and religion are also more frequently and intrinsically aspects of the ethics of palliative and mental health care than other areas of medicine. A person who is an orthodox Jew may well have beliefs that influence decisions about withdrawing or

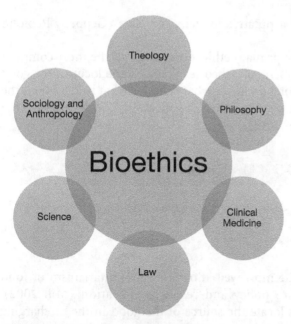

Figure 2.1 Contributions to Bioethics

withholding life-sustaining treatment that are different than those of a liberal Protestant or a spiritual but non-religious person (Baeke, Wils and Broeckaert 2011). Culture is also more closely involved in palliative care and mental health ethics decisions (*See* Chapter 6). Food and water are in some more traditional cultures strongly associated with nurturing, family, and caring than in others. Even when placing a feeding tube is medically contraindicated and what professionals consider a form of medical intervention, if a family or cultural group believes this is satisfying a basic human need, and obligation, this must be accounted for in ethical decision-making (Barrocas et al. 2010).

ETHICAL THEORY

The deliberations of moral philosophers and theologians over the centuries have given us several salient ethical theories that can inform the practical philosophy of mental health and palliative care. Each theory has strengths and limitations, but also offers a source of wisdom that may be more attuned to the beliefs and values of a professional or group or more applicable in a specific clinical situation or ethical dilemma (Kuhse and Singer 2012). Each ethical theory can be thought of as a different kind of map charting similar ethical terrain, yet giving a slightly different outlook on the territory. When a professional or the individual under their care is struggling with a difficult health care decision, feels morally lost or unable to see any way out of the situation, looking at the problem from the vantage point of several theoretical maps can often disclose a heretofore missed or unappreciated direction (Slote 2014).

For example, when an individual experiencing chronic schizophrenia is diagnosed with chronic obstructive pulmonary disease, his chief pleasure in life is smoking and drinking sodas on his walks. Successful treatment of the ill-health will require the person to stop smoking, wear oxygen at all times, and limit his activity. A virtue or care ethics approach might well find the cost of misery for this individual that treatment entails to be not worth the price of a putative longer time alive (Geppert, Rabjohn and Vlaskovits 2011).

There are several ways to group the primary ethical theories, but the most common one is to differentiate between consequentialist theories that find the locus of the good in the outcome of the action or decision and hence what is best is what brings about the optimal happiness or health for most people. Other classifications divide theories into duty-based and rights-based (Hinman 2013).

KEY POINT 2.3

Ethical theories may be grouped in several different ways based on different aspects of ethical action, character, and decision-making.

Consequentialist theories of which the most well known is the utilitarianism of John Stewart Mill is central to health-care policy and resource allocation (Mill 2002). Deontological or duty-based theories locate the source of the good in the discharging of the appropriate obligation. Theories of duty are as close as non-religious philosophy comes to universal obligations, in particular, near absolute respect for life and truth and individual dignity. The eighteenth-century philosopher Immanuel Kant is recognized as the founder of those ethical schools that emphasize the intention of moral agent (Kant 1998). Divine command theory also belongs in this category and holds that what is right and good is what God wills and ordains.

These two schools of thought concentrate on the duty of the moral agent while the oldest of the ethical theories, the virtue ethics of Aristotle is more interested in the character and habits of the moral agent (Aristotle 1976). We recognize and embody the good when we cultivate a virtuous character that displays moral excellence as seen in saints and heroes.

Care ethics is a newer theory that sees the personal and especially relational qualities of the individual as the wellspring of morality. In contrast to acute or intensive care the goals of palliative medicine and much of mental health treatment resonate with these theories for which the good life and death are consonant with human flourishing. Initially, the Harvard psychologist Carol Gilligan presented these theories as being more attuned to the values of women and as offering a much-needed counterbalance to the more rules-based theories of male philosophers (Gilligan 1993).

Philosophers disagree on whether principlism should be counted as a true ethical theory or as the next level of reasoning after ethical theory (Vaughn 2017). Because of its frequent use in clinical ethics as a theory, it is included here. Professors Beauchamp and Childress are the intellectual progenitors of this theory, which argues ethical dilemmas can be resolved through the balancing, weighing, and specification of cardinal ethical principles (Beauchamp & Childress 2013). The core four are:
1. autonomy
2. non-maleficence
3. beneficence
4. justice

Other experts would see these four principles and other more minor ones such as fidelity and veracity as the expression of a common language all theories can speak.

Casuistry is a case-based ethical theory derived from sixteenth-century Catholic moral theology that underwent resurgence in the 1980s thanks to Albert Johnsen, another of the pioneers of bioethics. It is familiar to, and favoured by many legally and medically trained professionals, as its case-based approach is the way they were educated. In contrast to the deductive logic of theories like principlism, casuistry is inductive in its approach. Decision-making regarding any case should begin with examining precedent cases and determining their respective bearing on the situation at hand. The principle of double-effect often utilized in palliative care to ethically justify the use of pain medication or palliative sedation, even when it may hasten death, derives from this school (Boyle, 2004). Table 2.1 applies the major theories to the Case Study 2.1 below and offers additional explication.

Ethical values, principles, and virtues

All ethical theories share a common language of values, principles, and virtues. At the most basic values are things we as individuals and societies decide are important to foster, worthwhile to defend, and meaningful to the good life and death. Some foundational values are listed below (Table 2.2).

SELF-ASSESSMENT EXERCISE 2.1

Time: 10 minutes
Using free-associations write down the five values that are most important to you. When you are finished glance at the inventory below and see if there is any overlap and whether you alter your choices based on this list.
- Peace
- Justice
- Family
- Faith
- Love
- Caring
- Safety
- Giving
- Comfort
- Dignity

Principles, viewed apart from theory, are what Beauchamp and Childress call 'action guides' and Kant called moral maxims. These are norms, standards, rules that inform ethical reasoning and that stipulate the kinds of decisions and actions that should be permitted, prohibited, or allowed in a specific situation. Non-maleficence is perhaps the oldest and most fundamental principle and most of us believe that we should try and minimize suffering in caring for each individual. Table 2.2 illustrates the function of virtues salient to mental health and palliative care in commonly encountered clinical scenarios.

Table 2.1 Ethical theories

Theory	Explication	Application to Case
Consequentialism	The good of the many outweighs the good of the one. The health care resources employed in Jack's care would have more utility in other settings/needs.	If Jean will not choose a palliative approach, then an administrative or legal order to compel the foregoing of life-sustaining treatment should be sought.
Deontology	The value of life is not dependent on the individual's ability to think or do, but simply to be. The wishes of a self-determining moral agent should be respected.	Jean's wishes for Jack should be honored. Professionals should respect Jack's life intrinsically.
Virtue Ethics	The virtuous professional will in any situation behave as would an exemplar of moral excellence. The professionals should respect, but need not endorse, Jean's belief that Jack is cognizant.	Palliative care and ethics should assist the health care professionals to act with fidelity and compassion and continue to seek a mutually acceptable solution. The professionals should continue empathically to communicate the medical recommendations for withdrawal of care.
Care Ethics	Relationships and emotions rather than rules and reasoning predominate in ethical decisions. Taking a legal or regulatory approach when values and interactions are what is primary will only further polarize the situation.	Palliative care consultants will help the professionals to focus on Jean's relationship to her son and its meaning for her and how foregoing aggressive care might affect the family unit. A family meeting will be held to provide support for Jean.
Principlism	While autonomy is **prima facie** it is not absolute. Moral reasoning using principles should determine ethical decision-making.	Jean's autonomy is not absolute and is based on a misunderstanding or refusal to accept the reality of the clinical situation. In the interest of justice, and to avoid non-maleficence the professionals may need to obtain the authorization to withdraw care and proceed with hospice.
Casuistry	Precedent cases determine the content of ethical principles. The particularity of each case should be compared to prior decisions for similarities and substantive differences and their applicability to the case at hand.	The ethics consultants should examine prior similar cases and how these have been handled. If life-sustaining treatment was foregone in those circumstances, then it may be justified to do so in Jack's case.

Case Study 2.1 – Jack

Jack is a 45-year-old man who has been in, what neurologists have identified as a continuous (persistent) vegetative state, for 20 years. Jack was a paramedic tending to an injured victim of a motor vehicle accident when a van speeding down the highway hit him. His mother Jean, who was trained as a psychologist, believes her son interacts with her in a meaningful way. Health-care professionals involved in Jack's care for years do not believe that he communicates or moves in any purposeful manner. Yet they all acknowledge that his mother has taken exquisite care of Jack, far superior to what he would receive in an institution. Like anyone in his condition, Jack has periodic health problems for which he must be hospitalized; usually an infection or the need to replace the intravenous lines and tubes that hydrate, feed, and medicate him. Each time Jack is hospitalized the health-care professionals request palliative consultation because they believe Jean should request a do-not-resuscitate order and discontinue life-sustaining treatment. The nursing professionals especially experience moral distress in caring for Jack believing he is "suffering" and "already dead." Some professionals have even gone so far as to say that Jean is "selfish" and "delusional." Yet Jean maintains her position that her son is "in there" and should thus continue to receive all life-sustaining treatments. The professionals currently responsible for Jack request an ethics consultation to identify a lawful means of ordering the withdrawal of life-sustaining treatment and provision of hospice.

Virtues are qualities of character like compassion, honesty, and trustworthiness that are essential to the professional-person relationship. We admire and try to emulate persons who habitually act virtuously. Table 2.3 illustrates the function of virtues salient to mental health and palliative care in commonly encountered clinical scenarios.

REFLECTIVE PRACTICE EXERCISE 2.2

Time: 30 minutes

Principles are concepts that help us think about what is good and reason about what is right. Virtues help us choose what is good and act on what we know is right. Principles without virtues may enable a person to know what is good but lack the character to act upon it. Conversely, a person of virtue may have the best of intentions yet make a misguided judgment not acting upon considered principles.

- Can you reflect on a situation or case in your mental health or palliative practice where decisions were made, or actions taken without the benefit of both principles and virtues being involved?
- How did this situation turn out?
- What would you do different in a future similar case?

Table 2.2 Ethical principles in mental health and palliative care

Principle	Definition	Mini-Case Application
Autonomy	Self-determination in health care decisions, literally 'self-rule'.	An individual with adjustment disorder and end-stage renal disease chooses to dialyze for briefer periods than medically recommended as it is less anxiety provoking for him.
Beneficence	'To do good'. The professional acting to promote the good of the people above all other priorities.	With his consent, a homeless individual with opioid use disorder and osteomyelitis receives his intravenous antibiotics as well as pain management on a rehabilitation unit of the hospital where he is less likely to relapse.
Non-maleficence	'To do no harm'. The goal of health care is to prevent, alleviate, and eliminate pain and suffering and to minimize the adverse effects of necessary treatment.	The surrogate of, and palliative care professional caring for, an elderly man experiencing advanced Alzheimer's dementia who is no longer eating choose hand-feeding over a feeding tube.
Justice	Treating like persons similarly, and persons differently only if the difference is substantive.	A person experiencing schizophrenia who has decision-making capacity receives cardiac bypass surgery for his three blocked-vessels.
Fidelity	'Faithfulness in the professional–individual relationship expressed in promise keeping, non-abandonment, and honoring trust.	An outpatient palliative care professional continues to visit a person experiencing ALS and weekly when he is transferred from home to an inpatient hospice.

ETHICAL ABSOLUTISM AND RELATIVISM

A contemporary controversy in ethics that has relevance for medical ethics is whether these values, principles, and virtues are universal or relative. If they are absolute, then they would be fundamental principles, like non-maleficence would vary with the culture and era. While if these core values are relative then they would change with time and demonstrate geographic and cultural diversity. Both absolutism and relativism are ethically fraught with difficulties, for example, practical health-care decision making. A purist form of universalism implies an objectivity that is likely not achievable in the applied sciences of both medicine and medical ethics. An extreme relativism would embrace individual subjectivity to a point where attaining an ethical consensus regarding shared moral sensibility would be nearly impossible (Macklin 1999).

Table 2.3 Key virtues in mental health and palliative care

Virtue	Definition	Mini–Case Application
Compassion/ Empathy	'Feeling with another's suffering' Active regard for the well-being of another person or animal and the corresponding response of kindness and mercy.	A mental health professional intervenes to arrange hospice care for a veteran individual with post-traumatic stress disorder and end-stage heart failure who wants to return home to be with his beloved dog.
Courage	Standing up for one's values and the defense of the vulnerable even at risk to one's livelihood or life.	A team of mental health and palliative care professionals work to provide care for individuals in a prison psychiatric unit who are nearing the end-of-life despite receiving death threats from conservatives.
Discernment	The exercise of moral intuition, ethical insight and professional judgment in decision-making.	The professional providing therapy for a person experiencing severe abuse and trauma realizes that she cannot advocate for herself when told the surgeons insist she needs a mastectomy for breast cancer and she would prefer a less aggressive approach.
Integrity	Soundness and coherence of intention and action that is expressed in fairness and consistency.	A palliative care professional declines a request from a person with a history of multiple suicide attempts and borderline personality disorder to discontinue life-sustaining treatment for sepsis until a mental health professional can evaluate them.
Respect	The virtue of respecting the dignity, individuality, and conscience of every person regardless of economics, ethnicity, religion, sexual orientation or any other external factor.	A transgender person with a heroin addiction is provided with new medications for hepatitis C.

KEY POINT 2.4

There is a spectrum of opinion among ethicists whether ethical values and principles are universal or relative each position presenting practical problems.

Even a cursory knowledge of the history of medicine demonstrates that even core principles like autonomy and beneficence are not immutable. Paternalism was, until the last 50 years, the dominant mode of professional-person relationship and variants of it still reign in the less developed world. While in the developed world there has been a steady progression of individual self-determination in medical decision making. Even in post-modern Anglo-American countries there are exceptions to this rule. A beneficence-based approach is far more appropriate for an elderly man experiencing dementia who needs a cardiac bypass, than for a young adult experiencing bipolar disorder and Type I diabetes whose preferences for care should be respected. Yet the latter individual may lose their ability to exercise their autonomy in a manic episode so severe they stop all their medications for both conditions and endanger their life. Here, soft paternalism is ethically justified and a failure to intervene might well violate the cardinal duty to do-no-harm (Ackerman 1982). Where the same soft paternalism in the first case may argue for the medical management of angina given that the person's neuropsychiatric condition renders him unable to understand and participate in what is painful and for this individual a frightening and painful intervention.

REFLECTIVE PRACTICE EXERCISE 2.3

Time: 20 minutes

Think about your own practice as a palliative or mental health-care professional particularly in a team or group. Do you generally handle disagreements about ethical issues as relativistic, 'ethics is whatever someone thinks is right for them', or as more universal, 'there are some values that just cannot be compromised ever'. What are some strengths and perhaps areas for growth you can identify in your personal approach?

Case Study 2.2.1 – Mrs. Yee

Mrs. Yee is an 88-year-old woman who two years ago moved to the United States from China to live with her son Sam (who is himself a physician), his wife and children. Mrs. Yee has had difficulty learning much English and has grown increasingly depressed trying to adapt to such a different culture. Two weeks ago, she began eating very little and began to lose weight and complain that her stomach hurts. Sam Yee, her son, takes her to a colleague, Dr. Davies who specializes in gastroenterology. Dr. Davies undertakes a thorough diagnostic work up that unfortunately reveals gastric cancer. Sam instructs his colleague not to disclose the diagnosis to his mother who will become despondent and quickly die. Sam asks Dr. Davies to just tell his mother that she had indigestion from eating American food and to stick to a more traditional diet. Dr. Davies bristles at the thought of not telling Mrs. Yee the truth and reminds Sam of their obligation as physicians to obtain informed consent for treatment. Sam says he does not want his mother to have any treatment but simply to live out her days comfortably. Dr. Davies threatens to report Sam to the ethics committee at their hospital for asking him to lie to Mrs Yee and withholding treatment without consent.

Analyzing and Resolving Ethical Dilemmas

When there is a clear clash between right and wrong there is no dilemma. If a person with decision-making capacity refuses surgery, we cannot tie them down and operate on them because as professionals we feel this is in their best interest. To do so would not only violate ethical codes but laws, and we would be committing battery.

The ethics committee asked to intervene would likely use one of many methods to work through the ethical question posed. One of the most frequently used models organizes information in a combination of the domains below (Jonsen, Seigler & Winslad 2010).

➤ Clinical information
➤ Individual preferences
➤ Third Party preferences
➤ Quality of life
➤ Contextual features
➤ Ethical knowledge

Ethical knowledge and skill are required to analyze and resolve these dilemmas and in no two areas of health care are there quite as many or as difficult conflicts of values. Ethicists first identify the ethically justifiable options. Those that are illegal or immoral like euthanasia in the United States and United Kingdom are not within this set, nor are medical interventions that do not meet a broadly understood standard of care. When an individual experiencing a schizotypal personality disorder and a life-threatening infection insists that the professional treat him with herbal medications rather than antibiotics, which he believes are dangerous because they are 'man-made,' this is also not an acceptable alternative (Schwartz 1992).

The ethically justifiable options are then weighed, specified, balanced in arguments and counter-arguments through a process of moral deliberation informed by expert opinion, precedent cases empirical ethics literature, codes of ethics, professional guidelines, and seminal articles (National Center for Ethics in Health Care 2015).

KEY POINT 2.5

The resolution of ethical dilemmas involves considering the arguments and counter-arguments in support of those options determined to be ethically justifiable.

Tensions and Ties Between Mental Health and Palliative Care Ethics

An intrinsic tension, at times almost a contradiction, manifests in the ethical dilemmas described in this text and experienced in practice at the intersection of mental health and palliative care. This tension is between the different ways in which specific core ethical theories, principles, and values are prized and prioritized compared to others in the two clinical circles of concern. The attitudes of health care professionals toward the principle of autonomy display the sharpest contrast and are thus used as an exemplar. A conscientious mental health professional will likely act to prevent a person with severe bipolar depression from committing suicide. To discharge their obligation to save life, they may well utilize the machinery of the law to forcibly hospitalize and even treat the

Case Study 2.2.2 – Mrs. Yee – Analysis

The members of the ethics committee, usually called ethics consultants, are called to resolve the conflict between Dr. Sam and Dr. Davies. Sam, as Mrs. Yee's son, knows her values and wishes and strongly believes she would not want to know she has a life-limiting illness. As a physician, he feels her depression will worsen with bad news. Dr. Davies feels individuals have autonomy and that since Mrs. Yee, even speaking through a hospital interpreter, clearly has decision-making capacity, she has a right to be told of her diagnosis and prognosis, and to be given the opportunity to ask questions and make treatment decisions. Dr. Davies feels that Dr. Sam is not respecting his mother when he unilaterally decides she should not be treated. The ethics consultants point out to both doctors that each of them is trying to avoid a different kind of harm. For Dr. Sam it is preventing psychological distress and for Dr. Davies the personal harm of not being allowed to exercise self-determination. They are also each expressing a different cultural worldview despite both valuing and honouring the fundamentals of medical ethics: avoiding harm and doing good, telling the truth and respecting persons. But they are weighing and balancing these values in conflicting ways.

The ethics consultant recommends a middle-way through the dilemma. The consultant persuades both doctors to agree that the available treatment options have little chance of cure and a strong likelihood of making Mrs. Yee very sick and more depressed. Both concede that neither has considered that palliative care is a form of treatment that could ease both her emotional and physical suffering.

The ethics consultant suggests the kindest strategy that respects all the values at play would be for the consultant, along with an interpreter, to meet with Mrs. Yee and let her know that Dr. Davies has important medical information to communicate and that some serious medical decisions will need to be made. They will then ask her would she prefer to speak to Dr. Davies herself about her care or defer to her son. Dr. Davies agrees this will fulfil his duty to obtain informed consent or refusal and Dr. Sam that this will enable his mother to express her actual wishes without directly subjecting her to the shock of learning she has only a few months to live (Tse, Chong and Fok 2003).

individual. Persons whom mental health and society have deemed incapable of acting according to their most authentic preferences and values, are constrained from carrying out their wishes. The duty of non-maleficence overrides the autonomous choice of the individual albeit with the assumption that they cannot exercise self-determination due to ill-health and that the justification of treatment is to restore that capacity.

The perspective of the caring palliative care professional to an individual at the end-of-life with capacity who decides to forego life-sustaining treatment, perhaps dialysis or mechanical ventilation is one of empathic support. In some jurisdictions, this palliative care professional may even assist the person with terminal ill-health to die. And if delirium or dementia has rendered the person incapable of making their own decisions to decline life-prolonging interventions, their wishes expressed in an advanced directive or through an authorized surrogate will be respected and facilitated. The autonomy of the individual outweighs almost all other ethical considerations.

Yet professionals in mental health and palliative care and the individuals who entrust their lives and well-being to them have more that unites than divides them as this brief listing of the common ethical ground suggests.

➤ Families intimately share in the care and distress of individuals at the end-of-life and with serious mental ill-health

➤ Spirituality is a source of strength and resilience for persons experiencing life-limiting conditions of body or mind

➤ Both serious mental ill-health and death and dying are historically and culturally stigmatized

➤ To deliver holistic person-centred care, palliative and mental health professionals must work in intra- inter-disciplinary teams (Cooper & Cooper 2014).

CONCLUSION

The importance of this chapter and even more this volume and the others in the series (Cooper & Cooper 2012), are its brave attempt to suggest that the lines between these two professional specialties are seldom distinct and bright and are often blurred and overlapping. Even more, the persons who are suffering, mentally, physically, and spiritually will often conceive harm and good in ways that challenge clinical standards, legal statutes, religious beliefs, and even our own personal moral stances.

REFERENCES

Ackerman, T. F. (1982) 'Why doctors should intervene'. *Hastings Central Report*, 12, pp. 14–17.

Appelbaum, P. and Gutheil, T. (1992) *Clinical Handbook of Psychiatry and the Law*, Baltimore: Williams & Wilkins.

Aristotle (1976) *The Ethics of Aristotle: The Nicomachean Ethics*. New York, NY: Penguin Books.

Baeke, G., Wils, J. P. and Broeckaert, B. (2011) 'Orthodox Jewish perspectives on withholding and withdrawing life-sustaining treatment.' *Nursing Ethics*, 18, pp. 835–46.

Barrocas, A., Geppert, C., Durfee, S. M., Maillet, J.O., Monturo, C., Mueller, C., Stratton, K. and Valentine, C. (2010) 'A.S.P.E.N. ethics position paper.' *Nutrician in Clinical Practice*, 25, pp. 672–9.

Beauchamp, T. L. and Childress, J. F. (2013) *Principles of Biomedical Ethics*, New York: Oxford University Press.

Boyle, J. (2004) 'Medical ethics and double effect: the case of terminal sedation.' *Theoretical Medicine and Bioethics*, 25, pp. 51–60.

Callahan, D. (2004) 'Bioethics,' in: Post, S. G. (ed.) *Encyclopedia of Bioethics*. 3rd edition. New York: Thompson-Gale.

Campo-Engelstein, L., Jankowski, J. and Mullen, M. (2016) 'Should health care providers uphold the dnr of a terminally ill patient who attempts suicide'? *HEC Forum*, 28, pp. 169–74.

Cooper, D. B. and Cooper, J. (eds) (2014) *Palliative Care Within Mental Health: Care and Practice*, London: Radcliffe Publishing.

Cooper, D. B. and Cooper, J. (eds) (2012) *Palliative Care Within Mental Health: Principles and Philosophy*, London: Radcliffe Publishing.

Dickinson, G. E., Lancaster, C. J., Clark, D., Ahmedzai, S. H. and Noble, W. (2002) 'U.K. physicians' attitudes toward active voluntary euthanasia and physician-assisted suicide.' *Death Studies*, 26, pp. 479–90.

Gardner, J. and Williams, C. (2015) 'Responsible research and innovation: A manifesto for empirical ethics?' *Clinical Ethics*, 10, pp. 5–12.

Geppert, C. M., Rabjohn, P. and Vlaskovits, J. (2011) 'To treat or not to treat: psychosis, palliative care, and ethics at the end-of-life: a case analysis.' *Psychosomatics*, 52, pp. 178–84.

Gilligan, C. (1993) *In a Different Voice*, Cambridge, MA: Harvard University Press.

Hinman, L. M. (2013) *Ethics: A Pluralistic Approach to Moral Theory*, Boston, MA: Wadsworth.

Jonsen, A. R. (1998) *The Birth of Bioethics*, New York, NY: Oxford University Press.

Jonsen, A. R., Seigler, M. and Winslade, W. J. (2010) *Clinical Ethics: A Practical Approach to Ethical Decisions in Clinical Medicine*, New York: McGraw-Hill, Inc.

Kant, I. (1998) 'Groundwork of the metaphysics of morals', in Gregory, M. (ed.) *Cambridge Texts in the History of Philosophy.* Cambridge: Cambridge University Press.

Kuhs, E. H. and Singer, P. (eds) (2012) *A Companion to Bioethics*, Oxford: Blackwell.

Macklin, R. (1999) *Against Relativism: Cultural Diversity and the Search for Ethical Universals in Medicine*, New York: Oxford University Press.

Mill, J. S. (2002) *The Basic Writings of John Stuart Mill: On Liberty, the Subjection of Women and Utilitarianism (Modern Library Classics).*New York, NY: Modern Library Classics.

National Center for Ethics in Health Care. (2015) *Ethics Consultation Responding to Ethics Questions in Health Care.* 2nd edition. Washington, DC: U.S. Department of Veterans Affairs.

Schwartz, R. L. (1992) 'Autonomy, futility, and the limits of medicine'. *Cambridge Quarterly pf Healthc Ethics*, 1, pp. 159–64.

Slote, M. A. (2014) 'History of ethics', in Jennings, B. (editor.) *Bioethics.* 4th edition. Farmington, MI: Gale, Cengage.

Tse, C. Y., Chong, A. and Fok, S. Y. (2003) 'Breaking bad news: a Chinese perspective'. *Palliative Medicine*, 17, pp. 339–43.

Vaughn, L. (2017) *Bioethics: Principles, Issues, and Cases*, New York: Oxford University Press.

Ying, I., Levitt, Z. and Jassal, S. V. (2014) 'Should an elderly patient with stage V CKD and dementia be started on dialysis'? *Clinical Journal of the American Society of Nephrology*, 9, pp. 971–7.

To Learn More

Pence, G. E. *The Elements of Bioethics.* New York: McGraw-Hill, 2007.

Weston, A. 'A practical companion to ethics'. New York: Oxford University Press, 1997.

Singer, P. A. and Viens, A. M. (2008) (eds). *The Cambridge Textbook of Bioethics.* Cambridge: Cambridge University Press, 2008.

CHAPTER 3

The Ethics of Care

Nel Noddings

INTRODUCTION

Care theory offers an ethic that strongly supports palliative care (Candib 1995; Gordon, Benner, & Noddings, 1996). It is a relational ethic, one that describes the roles of both the one caring (carer) and the one receiving care (cared-for) in encounters that may be single brief meetings or regular occasions in long-lasting relationships. We will begin with an overview of the basics of care theory and its application to palliative care and then discuss how it might relieve the current antagonistic divisions in our society, how it might provide a form of palliative care in the intellectual/social realm.

THE BASICS OF CARE ETHICS

Care ethics has been developing steadily over the past thirty-five years (Mayseless 2016). "First, the central focus of the ethics of care is on the compelling moral salience of attending to and meeting the needs of the particular others for whom we take responsibility" (Held 2006, p. 10). Here we are primarily interested in its use in nursing, mental health, and education. As a *relational* ethic, it holds special promise for application in these fields (Bishop & Scudder 1996).

Care ethics starts with natural caring, describing the relation between a carer and a cared-for. Both contribute to the caring relation. Indeed, if the cared-for does not recognize the efforts of the carer *as* caring either explicitly in words or implicitly in, say, a sigh of relief, there is no caring relation. Observers might credit the would-be carer's efforts and take note of the virtues displayed: "She worked so hard, she was honest . . ." But care ethics is different from virtue ethics. Virtues are strongly valued, but they are not the foundation or building blocks of care theory.

Sensitive parents and friends recognize that their own virtue by itself does not establish caring relations and try to adjust their efforts to meet the expressed needs of those for whom they care. There are some excellent—if enormously sad—examples in literature of parents who act only on the needs they assume for their children and exercise the virtues they suppose will meet those needs. In *The Way of All Flesh* (Butler 1944), the Pontifex family illustrates this way of 'caring' dramatically. The children are told exactly what they should do, what they should want, how they should feel. Butler passes along (with obvious disgust) the Pontifex-type advice to parents:

27

Tell them how singularly indulgent you are; insist on the incalculable benefit you conferred upon them, firstly in bringing them into the world at all, but more particularly in bringing them into it as your own children rather than anyone else's.

(1944, pp. 30–31)

One could hardly find a more painful contrast to genuine, natural caring. It is not hard for a reader to predict the deep unhappiness experienced by the Pontifex son, Ernest.

Care theory agrees with David Hume (1983/1751) that morality as an active virtue is rooted in feeling, not reason. Natural caring—the sensitive response to another's expressed needs—is fundamental, and remembrance of natural, caring responses provides the foundation for ethical caring.

This memory of our own best moments of caring and being cared for sweeps over us as a feeling—as an 'I must'—in response to the plight of the other and our conflicting desire to serve our own interests.

(Noddings 2013, pp. 79–80)

Care theory is clearly relational. It recognizes both the role of the cared-for and that of the one-caring. It may be contrasted with virtue ethics, an approach that prescribes the virtues that individuals should cultivate and exercise. Care theory does not ignore virtues, but it rests on the foundation of natural caring, and natural caring describes a relation, the interaction of carers and cared-fors. In this, care ethics follows Martin Buber who wrote: "In the beginning is the relation" (Buber 1970).

Ethical caring, like natural caring, requires attention to the expressed needs of the cared-for. It does not proceed directly from the assumed needs identified by the one-caring.

Concentration on the expressed needs of the cared-for does not imply neglect or denial of assumed needs. In nursing, for example, carers certainly do not ignore the patient needs identified by physicians and diagnostic testing. But they do more than simply follow directions. Indeed, the close attention of carers to the expressed needs of patients may add considerably to the initial diagnostic recommendations. Expressed needs—whether in words, sighs, grimaces, or bodily moves—induce a desire to respond in the one-caring.

In much of today's social and medical literature, the cognitive or affective response to someone's internal state or feelings is referred to as *empathy*. The word *empathy* came to us in the late nineteenth century through the art world where it referred to the understanding achieved by projecting oneself into a work of art. Notice that the original meaning was primarily cognitive. Over time, the emphasis has shifted to the affective, and many writers today define empathy in terms of a response that matches the feelings of another (Hoffman 2000). However, we have to be careful with this. How do we know when our feelings match those of another? The original, projective definition of empathy might well confuse our understanding of another's feelings with those we might feel in his or her situation, and indeed this confusion misguides us in many situations where others need help. Indeed, many of us almost prefer the older word, 'sympathy', to emphasize 'feeling with'.

Projective empathy, however, is not ethically useless. As parents and teachers, we often use it to get wrong-doers to rethink their acts: "How would you feel if someone did that to you"? is a question many of us have asked when a child has done something nasty to another. Consideration of that question can arouse compassion, sympathy, empathy, and the motivation to care—to respond to the pain, suffering, and expressed needs of others (Mayseless 2016). Therefore, care theory does not ignore the question of how I might feel in another's situation, but it advises us to concentrate on how the other *does* feel. Simone Weil conveyed the idea beautifully: 'The love of our neighbor in all its fullness simply means being able to say to him: "What are you going through?" It is a recognition that the sufferer exists . . . For this reason it is . . . indispensable to know how to look at him in a certain way. This way of looking is first of all attentive. The soul empties itself of all its own contents in order to receive into itself the being it is looking at, just as he is, in all his truth' (Weil 1977, p. 51).

This receptive attention is central in care theory. In caring, we put aside—at least temporarily—our preconceived notions, the possible objectives with which we might have entered the encounter, the temptation to change the cared-for's story into our own. We enter an affective–receptive mode: 'qualitatively different from the analytic-objective mode in which we impose structure on the world. It is a precreative mode characterized by outer quietude and inner voices and images, by absorption and sensory concentration. The one so engrossed is listening, looking, feeling' (Noddings 2013, p. 34).

This is a precreative mode in both intellectual work and interpersonal relations. We are peculiarly vulnerable in this mode, open to the beauty, pain, hope, or need of another. What emerges takes us back into the analytic–objective mode with an enlightened consciousness.

This affective–receptive mode is vital in the intellectual as well as the ethical domain. So often today, students listen to a lecture or read a chapter with the specific purpose of learning what must be learned to do well on a test of some sort. They have a definite objective at the outset. They remain unaware that the 'best' minds rarely approach a field of study this way. Rather, a vital intellectual experience requires an open-minded immersion in an affective–receptive mode that *receives*, one that does not impose an objective at the outset. So much intellectual wonder is lost in our schools because we do not encourage the affective–receptive approach to learning.

In human relations, too, we often simply refuse to enter the affective–receptive mode, and the outcome of our well-intentioned efforts to help is disappointing. George Orwell described how 'do-gooders' so often fail to connect with those they would help to rise to a higher standard. Instead, without working cooperatively with the people they want to help—without engaging in open dialogue—they preach at them and try to improve them: 'by means of hygiene, fruit-juice, birth-control, poetry, etc'. (1958, p. 162).

Michael Walzer (2015) notes failure of a similar sort in the efforts of liberators to free the oppressed; the liberators merely assume that the oppressed want what the privileged already have. And Paulo Freire (1970) warned us against the exclusive use of the 'banking method' in teaching—a pedagogical approach that largely ignores what the students are feeling and hoping for. In nursing, too, failure to enter the affective–receptive mode may result in unhappy, discontented patients who—in technical terms—are receiving the 'best care' (Candib 1995). In all of these cases, there is a failure to attend to *expressed* needs, usually because we are directed by technically established *assumed* needs.

We should not conclude, however, that carers must always satisfy expressed needs. Sometimes that is impossible, beyond our capabilities. And there are times when responding actively to an expressed need would violate the professional rules to which we are committed. At times like these, we would do better to talk things through and perhaps persuade the cared-for to reject or put aside the original expressed need. In such situations, we work to preserve the caring relation and continue to talk, listen, and feel for (if not with) the cared-for. One can see that critical thinking must be exercised in the evaluation of expressed needs, and we will explore that topic in the next section. All of us occasionally express needs that we later assess as unrealistic or even harmful. Certainly, this happens often with children and quite frequently with students of all ages. At these times, carers must remain in relation, make suggestions, listen, perhaps joke a bit, encourage the cared-for to consider other possibilities. The basic requirement in caring is to remain in relation.

Care theory emphasizes needs, not rights. In terms suggested by John Rawls, it is a non-ideal theory. According to Rawls, an ideal theory such as his *Theory of Justice* (1971) supplies a foundation of definitions, axioms, and principles that describe a perfectly arranged society or constellation of some sort. It starts, that is, with a description of an ideal arrangement. A non-ideal theory such as care theory begins with things as they are and, building on what we have, know, feel, and desire, works its way toward a better life—that 'better' under constant analysis and revision. In this regard, it is closely aligned with John Dewey's (1960) form of pragmatism.

It is important to distinguish between caring-for and caring-about. As pointed out earlier, caring-for is relational; it requires the participation of both carer and cared-for. Caring-about is more nearly synonymous with concern. We all 'care about' the victims of natural disasters, children living in poverty, and a host of other events and situations common to contemporary life. Hearing of a disaster, some of us contribute to relief funds and some, lacking resources, express concern but are unable to help. Both care-about people in need of help. Should those who give money or physical help be credited with *caring-for*?

Those who give physical help have probably received handshakes and smiles of gratitude; they have been part of a caring relation. Giving money to help disaster victims seems at first glance to be an example of caring-for, but unless we have evidence that people did indeed receive help—that, in fact, they have acknowledged the help—we may be deceiving ourselves. That is why those who make charitable contributions should make it a point to learn something about the organizations to which they give. Affirmative knowledge brings the caring-about of givers close to genuine caring-for. Perhaps the most salient evidence in this respect comes from accounts on the spot. When receivers of care can point to the work of specific individuals sponsored by an organization to which we have contributed, we are persuaded that caring-for has taken place. This is perhaps as close as we can get to caring-for at a distance in absentia. It provides an excellent example of why non-government agencies (NGOs) are often more highly appreciated than government aid programs; the NGO's put workers on-site to help those in need. Caring relations are actually established. Virtue theory would credit us for caring when, with the best intentions, we give to a charitable organization. Care theory is a bit reluctant to do this. It can grant only that we wanted to care. To credit us with caring, it requires evidence that caring relations have been established.

CARING AND CRITICAL THINKING

Care theory follows David Hume (1983) in arguing that feeling (emotion), not reason, motivates moral response. But reason must guide that response. If we react to another's expressed need with a feeling of 'I must' do something, we have to think about what to do and how it should be done. Thus, critical thinking is an essential element in care theory; it addresses questions concerning how we should respond to the expressed needs of others. Care theory emphasizes *understanding*, not winning arguments, as the main aim of critical thinking. From the earliest years of schooling, a basic aim is to understand what is said, what is read, and—as nearly as possible—what others feel and think (Noddings & Brooks 2017). This emphasis contributes strongly to both intellectual and social growth in our school children. In the moral domain, it concentrates on how we should respond to the expressed needs of particular others.

We should ask, then, whether care theory can give us any help in the public social domain. Can it provide any help in reducing the current highly antagonistic class divisions we observe or hear about every day? It may not be able to cure, or even accurately describe, the current problem, but it can reduce the associated pain and alienation.

Consider a claim made recently by President Trump that there were "good people" on both sides of the conflict in Charlottesville. How might care theory help us to understand this? Let's suppose that the organizing group—one that clearly embraced racist beliefs—might include 'good' people. What could we mean by this? Suppose one of your neighbors clearly has racist views. If you were to collapse on your front walk, would he come running to help you? If the answer to this is yes—and it certainly would be in my neighborhood—we might grant that this is a 'good', if imperfect person. He might even come running to help a black person injured in the street. That does not excuse his racism, but his racism *by itself* does not totally eliminate his goodness.

A question asked by care theorists is this: "Can we find a way to talk to people as individuals even though we strongly disagree on social/political/moral issues"? To combat a morally obnoxious set of beliefs—racism—must we condemn the individuals we hold to be racist? Or is there a way to keep open the avenues of communication while standing firmly against racism? In other words, must both the racist and the racism be condemned? This question arises—or should arise—as we consider what to do with the statues of past 'heroes' who were racists. Is there something admirable for which they might be remembered? If so, why not tell the whole story as nearly as we can with a statue and textual placard? The story should provide a warning as well as a tribute. Care theory may provide some support for those who recommend 'contextualizing' statues instead of removing them.

Fundamentally, care theory reminds us to see people as individuals, not merely as representatives or symbols of an ideology. We should hate and stand against certain ideologies, but can we find a way to separate the ideology from a person espousing it? Care theorists would like to take aside a member of the swastika-waving crowd and invite a genuine conversation. Is not this what we would do as teachers if we found such a student in our classroom? But it is almost unthinkable to suggest that we call out to a member of an opposing protest group, "Hey there! Let's talk!" A protest is simply not the right setting for such conversation. That conversation is needed to prevent protests.

A large part of the peace-making conversational task must fall to our universities where people are supposed to engage in free speech and learn how to listen to both sides.

John Stuart Mill (1993) insisted that government has no business restraining argument, nor should we as citizens try to shut down speeches with which we disagree. Rather, we should assess each individual case:

> ... condemning every one, on whichever side of the argument he places himself, in whose mode of advocacy either want of candor, or malignity, bigotry, or intolerance of feeling manifest themselves; but not inferring these vices from the side which a person takes, though it be the contrary side of the question to our own: and giving merited honor to everyone, whatever opinion he may hold, who has calmness to see and honesty to state what his opponents and their opinions really are, exaggerating nothing to their discredit, keeping nothing back which tells ... in their favor. This is the real morality of public discussion.
>
> (1993/1859, p. 63)

Today, ignoring Mill's advice, many of our colleges and universities would prefer to exclude controversial speakers and or to provide 'trigger warnings' on topics that might offend some listeners. Not only do students fail to hear both sides of an argument; many insist that they should not be forced even to listen to topics they find offensive. Arguing for Mill's stand on open discussion and civility, Timothy Garton Ash reminds us: 'But the university is the last place on earth where the individual, subjective "I'm offended" veto, the assassin's veto, or the heckler's veto should ever be allowed to prevail' (2016, p. 157).

Care theory supports Garton Ash in defending open exploration of contentious, sometimes offensive ideas. In support of palliative intellectual care, we want to reduce the pain induced by anger and lack of understanding. We urge thoughtful people to fight bad ideas and beliefs, not the people who hold them. Isaiah Berlin admired Mill and his defense of open argumentation as the best road to truth, but he forced himself to question his own devotion to that road, asking himself whether it has the power to ensure moral ends. He asked:

> Is it so clear that we must permit opinions advocating, say, race hatred to be uttered freely ...? Are demagogues and liars, scoundrels and blind fanatics, always, in liberal societies, stopped in time, or refuted in the end? How high a price is it right to pay for the great boon of freedom of discussion?
>
> (Berlin 1969, p. 187)

Here, Berlin is questioning his own commitment to free speech, acknowledging that he might be wrong—that, perhaps, one must sometimes act with more than verbal force to stop objectionable verbal behavior.

Accepting that human social knowledge is never complete, that there is no final truth in this area, he nevertheless stood firmly against the evils he allowed to be discussed and defended publicly. He was, in the words of Garton Ash: 'one of the most eloquent, consistent defenders of a liberalism which creates and defends the spaces in which people subscribing to different values, holding incompatible views, pursuing irreconcilable political projects ... can battle it out in freedom, without violence' (2016 p. 275).

In my own teaching and writing, I refer to Berlin and Mill as 'heroes of civility'.

We may not be morally obligated to adopt an affective–receptive mode aimed at understanding in all intellectual matters, but we should do so on many topics that affect the health and well-being of relations among those for whom we care. Both we and they should profit from a deeper understanding of the problems that face us in working to relieve physical, emotional, and mental pain. The example discussed above—working to relieve the social pain caused by current political contentiousness—is meant to illustrate the power of care ethics across the full range of human affairs. Fiona Robinson comments on this possibility:

> I argue that it is indeed the case that an "orthodox" reading of care ethics may be an untenable basis on which to construct an approach to moral relations for the contemporary global context. What is required, instead, is what I call a "critical ethics of care," which is characterized by a relational ontology—that is, it starts from the premise that people live in and perceive the world within social relationships; moreover, this approach recognizes that these relationships are both a source of moral motivation and moral responsiveness and a basis for the construction and expression of power and knowledge.
>
> (1999, p. 2)

CONCLUSION

Care ethics is relational; it concentrates on the quality of relations between individual human beings and how that affects the well-being of the individuals involved and, beyond them, how further relations with others may be affected. It does not ignore virtues and rules of justice, but it analyzes and assesses them in the process of responding to the expressed needs of those for whom we care. The best nurses, doctors, and teachers do far more than follow the rules. In responding to expressed needs, carers adopt an affective–receptive mode of being that is central to care ethics. However, we noted that such a mode is also vital in the intellectual domain and that it may be useful at the global as well as the individual level.

REFERENCES

Berlin, I. (1969) *Four Essays on Liberty*. Oxford: Oxford University Press.

Bishop, A. H. and Scudder, J. R. (1996) *Nursing Ethics: Therapeutic Caring Presence*. Sudbury, MA: Jones & Bartlett Publishers.

Buber, M. (1970) *I and Thou*. Trans. Walter Kaufmann. New York: Charles Scribner's Sons.

Butler, S. (1944) *The Way of All Flesh*. New York: Doubleday.

Candib, L. (1995) *Medicine and the Family: A Feminist Perspective*. New York: Basic Books.

Dewey, J. (1960) *The Quest for Certainty*. New York: G. P. Putnam's Sons.

Freire, P. (1970) *Pedagogy of the Oppressed*. Trans. Myra Bergman Ramos. New York: Herder & Herder.

Garton Ash, T. (2016) *Free Speech: Ten Principles for a Connected World*. New Haven & London: Yale University Press.

Gordon, S., Benner, P. and Noddings, N. Editors. (1996) *Caregiving*. Philadelphia, PN: University of Pennsylvania Press.

Held, V. (2006) *The Ethics of Care: Personal, Political, and Global*. Oxford: Oxford University Press.

Hoffman, M. (2000) *Empathy and Moral Development: Implications for Caring and Justice*. New York: Cambridge University Press.

Hume, D. (1983) *An Enquiry Concerning the Principles of Morals*. Cambridge, MA: Hackett.

Mayseless, O. (2016) *The Caring Motivation: An Integrated Theory.* Oxford: Oxford University Press.

Mill, J. S. (1993) *On Liberty* and *Utilitarianism.* New York: Bantam Books.

Noddings, N. (2013) *Caring: A Relational Approach to Ethics and Moral Education.* Berkeley, CA: University of California Press.

Noddings, N. and Brooks, L. (2017) *Teaching Controversial Issues.* New York: Teachers College Press.

Orwell, G. (1958) *The Road to Wigan Pier.* San Diego: Harcourt.

Rawls, J. (1971) *A Theory of Justice.* Cambridge, MA: Harvard University Press.

Robinson, F. (1999) *Globalizing Care.* Boulder, CO: Westview Press.

Walzer, M. (2015) *The Paradox of Liberation: Secular Revolutions and Religious Counterrevolutions.* New Haven: Yale University Press.

Weil, S. (1977) *Simone Weil Reader,* editor. George A. Panichas. Mt. Kisco, NY: Moyer Bell Limited.

To Learn More

Berlin, I. (1969) *Four Essays on Liberty.* Oxford: Oxford University Press.

Held, V. (2006) *The Ethics of Care: Personal, Political, and Global.* Oxford: Oxford University Press.

Mayseless, O. (2016) *The Caring Motivation: An Integrated Theory.* Oxford: Oxford University Press.

Noddings, N. and Brooks, L. (2017) *Teaching Controversial Issues.* New York: Teachers College Press.

CHAPTER 4

Research and Ethics

Tony Warne and Sue McAndrew

INTRODUCTION

Professional practice should always be undertaken against a backcloth of a comprehensive and contemporary evidence base. Using such evidence in undertaking practice should involve a deliberate and explicit approach on the part of the practitioner, an approach tailored to the needs of each individual for whom care is being provided (Sackett et al. 1996). Evidence can take many forms, as can the research that provides such knowledge. The value and authenticity of research is often measured by the methodology employed. In medicine, a hierarchy of research methods still prevails, albeit this was first described some 20 years ago. This hierarchy places systematic reviews and meta-analysis at its top and case studies at the bottom, with all other approaches accorded a place in between, weighted in terms of validity and reliability (Guyatt et al. 1995). Whilst the research hierarchy has been criticised for its quantitative bias, and as a hierarchy its narrow contextual focus, it is useful in providing a framework of methodological norms that can be tested and recognised.

The choice of methodology is determined by the research question being addressed. When a research method is described, perhaps in an application for funding or in a paper disseminating findings, readers can make a judgement as to its appropriateness and fidelity to the theory underpinning it. The same judgements can be employed when applications to undertake research include the seeking of ethical approval. Not all research requires ethical approval, but much research undertaken in the fields of health and social care will almost certainly require such approval to be gained before a study can be undertaken.

This chapter will consider the nuances inherent in undertaking research with vulnerable people and, in particular, those who experience mental health problems. In particular it will use the lens of mental health care to consider the processes involved in undertaking ethical research and the degree of congruence with mental health care practice itself.

KEY POINT 4.1

Our ability to identify and respond to the ethical questions arising in undertaking mental health research depend on our willingness to self-reflect and to harness the intuitions and theoretical constructs that we develop through both clinical practice and research activities.

The chapter acknowledges the often-parallel processes between therapeutic encounters and the research encounter. Across both, the point of connection for the researcher and the therapist is the endeavour of making sense of, and understanding the world of another (Moodley 2001).

BACKGROUND

Research informed practice is integral to the provision of effective mental health and social care. Indeed, it has been argued that the boundaries between innovative clinical practices and research-related experimentation are becoming increasingly difficult to distinguish, as are the roles between mental health practitioners, clinical researchers and basic scientists (Roberts 2002). Research provides the evidence base that can both shape and inform practice, enhance the care delivered to those who need it, and can be used in identifying the gaps in services and how these might best be met. Whilst research informed practice should be the norm for all mental health practitioners, not all mental health practitioners are equipped to actually undertake research using recognised methodologies.

KEY POINT 4.2

Research methodologies can be divided into two paradigms: quantitative and qualitative, the former acknowledging one truth, the latter accepting multiple realities.

Whilst researchers have often dichotomised these paradigms, depending on the nature of the research question being asked, one approach can often compliment the other. For example, epidemiological studies can inform and provide information of the scale and scope of a situation, for example, the prevalence of depression among the general population, with randomised control trials identifying whether cognitive behaviour therapy is more effective in treating depression than 'treatment as usual'. However, what is missing from this scenario is the person's experience of depression and what it was about the actual treatment that they found most helpful. Through hearing the individual's account of their lived experience in the context of their social world, an understanding can be gained of how each person locates self in relation to their internal and external worlds. For some (McKim 2015) using mixed methods, bringing together both quantitative and qualitative approaches, adding value to the research process. Likewise, Lacan (2003) further urged the need to take account of the subjectivity (of both researcher and participant) that focuses on lived experience being structured in accordance with cultural forces, as this might provide insight into the way in which those forces operate within the individual's life.

SELF-ASSESSMENT EXERCISE 4.1

Time: 5 minutes
What do you understand by the term ethical integrity?

KEY POINT 4.3

Regardless of the methods chosen, implicit in all research is its ethical integrity.

Ethical integrity is critical to mental health research. In its widest sense, ethical integrity supports notions of knowledge, truth, trustworthiness and the minimising of error in making claims arising from research. Such notions are also important for those engaging in undertaking research; collaborative working predicated upon trust and fairness; how data is collected, stored and made available to others, where the intellectual property ownership lies and who should be credited in terms of their involvement when research findings are published and disseminated (Roberts and Roberts 1999).

SELF-ASSESSMENT EXERCISE 4.2

Time: 10 minutes
Can you think of what moral and social values can be protected by ethical integrity?

Ethical integrity can also protect the funders of research, particularly where studies are funded by public money. In so doing, ethical integrity can help promote other important moral and social values such as human rights, protection of the public, animal welfare and compliance with prevailing legalisation. Where ethical integrity is not strong, significant harm may be the result. For example, in 1998, research undertaken into the Measles Mumps and Rubella (MMR) vaccination was said to be linked to an increased risk of autism and some bowel disorders in children. The research sparked an international reduction in the uptake of the MMR vaccination with thousands of children being placed at risk from the serious, and sometimes fatal complications of meningitis, encephalitis and of deafness. However, the original research involved just 12 children and was undertaken by someone being paid by a legal firm seeking to find evidence they could use against the vaccine manufacturers, leaving the integrity of the study open to serious questioning. The research study and its findings have long been discredited with much better and more reliable research showing there is no link and that the MMR vaccination is safe. In this example, the 'participants' were children and should have been much better protected than they were. Likewise, there are a number of other individuals who, for the purpose of research participation, would be considered vulnerable and are equally deserving of similar protection. People are often considered vulnerable because of their health status, social position or dependence on others for health and welfare services, those with mental health problems being one such group. Additionally, topics of study may create vulnerability. For example, research asking women about their experiences of female genital mutilation (FGM) would have the potential to trigger previous traumatic events. In this instance, care, on the part of the researcher, must be taken to ensure relevant support structures are in place immediately following their participation and in the longer term if required.

Researchers and ethics committees need to pay scrupulous attention to the identification and amelioration of risks to participants. Indeed, most health and social care professions will be bound by a code of ethics pertinent to their particular profession.

For example, the Declaration of Helsinki (2017), introduced by the World Medical Association, is widely regarded as the cornerstone document for ethical research involving human beings. The Royal College of Nursing (2011) require the following areas to be addressed prior to human research being initiated:

1. Informed consent
2. Confidentiality
3. Data protection
4. Right to withdraw (v's) potential benefits
5. Potential harms.

Other codes include British Psychological Society's (BSP) Code of Human Research Ethics (2014) and British Association of Counselling and Psychotherapy (BACP): Ethical Framework (2012). When applying for ethics approval the applicant is often expected to identify which code they will be following throughout their study. Where there is a lack of professional guidance, the Declaration of Helsinki (2013) is often adopted.

SELF-ASSESSMENT EXERCISE 4.3

Time: 50 minutes

- First, find out what the guidance is for ethical research within your own profession.
- Second, consider how you would address each of the principles outlined in the guidance.
  - For example, what steps might you take to ensure confidentiality?
  - What parameters might you use to enable a participant to withdraw?
  - What aspects of a study might come under data protection?

- Finally, if you are considering a specific piece of research try and identify any conflicts of interest between the study you are thinking of undertaking and the code of ethics by which you are professionally bound.

PARTICIPANTS

Good research governance should always be predicated upon the careful identification and mitigation of risks to those who choose to become research participants. Research is considered ethically acceptable only when the potential benefits of the research out-weigh the carefully assessed risks (National Health and Medical Research Council – NHMRC 2007). Any potential harm, discomfort or inconvenience of becoming involved in any research study must be clearly explained to potential participants from the outset. It is only in so doing that informed consent (to participate) can be gained.

However, the benefits of research participation can often be overshadowed by a preoccupation with the potential risks associated with working with 'vulnerable' people. Paradoxically, it is often a focus on protecting participants from harm and cushioning vulnerable people that violates the important ethical principles of autonomy and justice. The consequence can be that potential participants may be withdrawn from research studies, excluded, or their viewpoints rendered irrelevant (Rogers 2004). Alternatively, others have mounted strong arguments suggesting that competent individuals should be enabled to participate in research that poses risks (Edwards, Kirchin and Huxtable 2004) with consistent challenges to the assumptions underpinning paternalistic decisions in relation to research participation (Appelbaum et al. 1999; Koivisto et al. 2001; Tee and Lathlean 2004). Wherever possible, competent individuals should be able to choose to participate after weighing potential benefits and harms that might be involved. It is the absolute responsibility of the researcher to express these in lay terms, using language that is jargon free and easy to understand.

SELF-ASSESSMENT EXERCISE 4.4

> **Time: 50 minutes**
> Under the title 'What Will I Have To Do If I Take Part' write a brief description (no more than 300 words) of what a 14-year-old person would have to do to be involved in your research project. This needs to be written in a language they can understand. Once you have done this ask someone in this age group (12–16) to read it and feed back what they understand (or don't) regarding what they will have to do. Given their feedback, rewrite the information.

PARTICIPATION

People may agree to participate in research studies for many reasons. The research study might be thought of as interesting or connect with the individual's own interests; the belief that the research is benefiting the individual or it could benefit others in a similar situation; and or for monetary reasons, or some other reward.

It has been argued that the altruistic desire to assist others is a powerful motivator to participate in research (Fry & Dwyer 2001). Likewise, Yalom (1995) identified altruism as being one of the 12 factors associated with participation in therapeutic groups, perhaps an observation that accurately describes many encounters between researcher and participant(s). However, whilst engaging with others in anticipation of personal benefits is not altruism in the truest sense, acting with the intent to help others appears to be beneficial or therapeutic regardless of what other benefits might accrue (Grant 2002). Other studies (Schwartz et al. 2003) have found that being involved in acts intended to help others was seen to be more beneficial to people's mental health than being the recipient of help.

> **KEY POINT 4.4**
>
> There is considerable empirical evidence for the 'helper-therapy' principle, that is, people who act with the intention of helping, benefit in therapeutic ways, sometimes regardless of whether the act itself actually helped another (Reissman 1993; Grant & Sugarman 2004).

VULNERABILITY

Whilst for many people choosing to take part in research will be a positive experience (Finn, Bishop & Sparrow 2007), for some people it may be experienced as a daunting process. Whether they are to engage in a Random Controlled Trial (RCT), whereby they are unaware of being in either the intervention or the control group, or participating in a qualitative study and being given the opportunity to freely express their story in a non-therapeutic setting, both can be a frightening experience and might set in motion defensive processes (Warne & McAndrew 2010). With regard to the latter, the process of narration often involves an emotional labour on the part of both story-teller and researcher. In order to counterbalance the potential for this engagement being experienced as threatening, the researcher needs to create a safe place in which emotions can be safely contained. This is paramount, not only for the well-being of the participants, but also for the integrity of the research. It is entirely reasonable to anticipate that telling a story about a painful experience might be difficult or stressful. Many people will find it a challenging experience when previously undisclosed experiences are shared and emotions re-experienced. However, although challenging for some, emotional situations, which could not or were not handled in the past, can offer an opportunity to be more effectively addressed in their re-telling as part of a research study or in therapy (De Haene, Hans & Karine 2010).

For the mental health researcher, the ethical issue that arises is not so much who else to refer a distressed participant to, but rather to consider, prior to data collection, if they have the personal capacity to deal with the immediacy of the situation and what strategies they can put in place to enable them to create an emotionally containing space (Bowlby 1969). It has been argued that in providing a containing environment the researcher will be required to use self in demonstrating maturity, perceptiveness and open-mindedness, particularly throughout the interview process (Gadd 2004). Importantly, this may require the researcher to draw on their own personal and professional experiences. Kvale (1999) noted that mental health practitioners undertaking research should be open to the research potential inherent in their own therapeutic practice, although care is required in order to ensure those who might be vulnerable are protected. In demonstrating a capacity for empathic engagement, they should be aware of their emotional experiences within the moment and have a sense of the current dynamics taking place in the encounter (Mackenzie, McDowell & Pittaway 2007; Warne & McAndrew 2010). Central to achieving this is having the capacity to stay with the participant and the ability to pick out the latent content of the person's story, whilst at the same time implicitly accepting their story (Roberts & Roberts 1999; Mackenzie, McDowell & Pittaway 2007).

REFECTIVE PRACTICE EXERCISE 4.1

> **Time: 15 minutes**
> The process of clinical supervision is widely acknowledged and valued for mental health professionals. Reflect on how this could be beneficial for the researcher.

Just as there might be vulnerability on the part of the participant, such feelings can also be experienced by the researcher. Integral to mental health practice is clinical supervision, helping to facilitate understanding of what is happening within therapeutic encounters with the person receiving help. Central to mental health practice is the psychotherapeutic relationship, encompassing an emotional human interaction where there is a reciprocal involvement. Whilst the unconscious cannot be empirically observed, its effects can be explored through the way in which the individual repetitiously re-enacts aspects of experience that occurred in the past with significant others, for example parents.

As discussed above, such re-enactments of emotions and attitudes that belonged to important relationships can be transferred onto the therapist/researcher (Kvale 1999).

KEY POINT 4.5

The process of clinical supervision allows the 'therapist' to explore transference and counter-transference with a person external to the therapeutic encounter.

This practice can equally be of benefit to the researcher, as it has the potential to facilitate the processing of emotionally laden data, while at the same time provides a further dimension to the analytic process.

THE RESEARCH/THERAPY BOUNDARY

It is possible that some participants in a mental health orientated study might become aware of unresolved or painful issues. Indeed, the research focus may explicitly draw attention to an emotionally painful experience. However, the evidence that talking of one's experiences will produce uncomfortable emotions or exacerbate distress is equivocal (Munhall 2001; Alderson 2007). It is more often the case that participants experience positive emotional experiences and outcomes as a result of participation (Jorm, Kelly & Morgan 2007).

KEY POINT 4.6

Where people sometimes do experience distressing emotions when reliving negative experiences, they can often be transitory in nature; not necessarily undesired or overwhelming; and seen as understandable rather than harmful (Draucker, Martsolf & Poole 2009).

There has been ongoing debate regarding the distinction between therapy and research, particularly within the context of mental health. Hollway and Jefferson (2000) clarify the difference as being that the therapeutic encounter is one in which the clinician interprets during the encounter, whilst the research encounter is one in which interpretations are outwith the encounter. They stipulate that these differences in approach should be clearly articulated to the participants. Others (Hunt 1989; Whitelaw 1999) believe that whilst the process of research, particularly qualitative research, has parallels with psychoanalysis, not least with the dynamics of the interpersonal encounter between participant and researcher, it is important that a distinction is made between interviews that are therapy-based, as opposed to an interview that is research-based. It is suggested that the former has a responsibility to lead to new insights and or emotional change, but it would be unethical for the latter to deliberately instigate new self interpretations or emotional change (Kvale 1999).

However, in both the research and therapeutic encounter neither the researcher nor the therapist has control over the effects of the intervention (in this context an interview/conversation/focus group) on the participant or the person receiving therapy. Just like the therapeutic encounter, in-depth research interviews can stir the emotional self and or the conflicted self and this should be acknowledged rather than avoided (Hunt 1989; Ackerman & Hilsenroth 2003). In both settings, the overarching ethic for the researcher and therapist is that of 'doing no harm'. However, for the researcher, therapist, participant and person receiving therapy, the encounter is likely to be imbued with both conscious and unconscious processes, all of which play a part in the construction of our own reality. In turn, these are processes that determine our perception of others and the meanings we attribute to the encounter and may be played out within the research/therapeutic encounter (Clarke 1999; Warne & McAndrew 2010).

As was noted in the introduction, in acknowledging the parallel processes between the therapeutic encounter and the research encounter the point of connection for the researcher and the therapist is the concept of 'searching'. In both contexts, this is a concept aimed at making sense of, and better understanding the world of another (Moodley 2001). Drawing on their therapeutic skills and knowledge, and being aware of the interpersonal dynamics at play during the encounter, the researcher will be able to contextualise a person's lived experience, extrapolate relevant data for interpretation and demonstrate understanding in the immediacy of the encounter. For the participant, through the telling of their story, their self-esteem and sense of personal continuity is promoted and supported (Dijksterhuis 2006). Indeed, Hollway and Jefferson (2000) acknowledge that the process of retelling distressing life events can be therapeutic, particularly in a safe context. In demonstrating understanding and attunement within the research process the interview can often be found to have dual purpose, that of therapy and research, and may be particularly pertinent when exploring sensitive topics (Bourdeau 2000). As with those receiving therapy, for some participants the experience of being listened to and having their life experiences acknowledged may be therapeutic in itself and have the potential to bring about new understandings and meanings and thus promote a process of change within the person (Ackerman & Hilsenroth 2003).

The debate as to whether or not research interviews are therapeutic is arbitrary given that what, as researchers, we have little control over, is whether those people deciding to engage in research as participants would experience the process as being in anyway therapeutic. Just as an individual opts to engage in therapy to address a specific problem and or explore certain aspects of their life, it could be argued that choosing to participate in the research process is done for any number of personal reasons and therefore it has the potential to result in a similar activity. The verbalising and or repeating of a story, particularly one that encompasses trauma (*See* Chapter 11) and attached emotionality, can be a cathartic process as the events gradually become divested of what has previously been experienced as their overwhelming emotionality. Indeed, it has been noted that the therapeutic value of the interview emerges from its clarifying, constructing and cathartic functions (Isay 2006).

CONCLUSION

Within this chapter, rather than focusing on some of the more practical aspects of attaining ethics approval, we have considered more of the nuances inherent in undertaking research with vulnerable people and, in particular, those who experience mental health problems. Most professional bodies have their own ethics guidance and applicants applying to ethics approval panels will be expected to identify which set of principles they will be adhering to throughout the life of their research project. Within higher education institutions and national organisations, such as the National Health Service UK, application forms will be predicated on professional guidance/principles. In the less pragmatic domain of that of participants, participation and vulnerability, more complex issues were considered in the hope of future researchers being more prepared to attend to these before embarking on their research project.

In the concluding section of this chapter we outlined the therapy/research dichotomy, often evident in the field of mental health. While debate exists, it is important to understand the boundaries surrounding these two distinct activities. However, it must also be acknowledged that, as mental health professionals, we do have knowledge and skills that are pertinent to the requirements of being a good researcher and as such must use these to enhance participant experience. We have no control as to whether or not participants experience their involvement in research as therapeutic. What we are able to do is ensure the benefits gained through their participation outweigh any disadvantages and their contribution to the study is appreciated and valued.

Research Case Study 4.1 – Guide to Developing Your Own Research Proposal

Study Title

Exploring the perception of young people regarding their self-harming behaviour and the facilitators and barriers to them using locally available mental health services.

Rationale for the Research Case Study

Epidemiological studies show that there has been a global increase in the incidence of adolescent self-harm during the last decade (Scoliers et al. 2009) It is suggested that around two-thirds of children and adolescents presenting with self-harm are likely to experience depressive disorders, whilst those demonstrating suicidal intent and who have chronic recurrent affective illness are at increased risk of repetition (Harrington et al. 1998; Spirito et al. 2003; Green et al. 2011). While many of the studies have focused on those who attended Accident and Emergency (A & E – Emergency Room) following acts of self-harm, community studies show that large numbers of adolescents using such behaviour do not receive or seek out medical attention (Hawton et al. 2002; Madge et al. 2011). With regard to suicidal intent, a number of studies using a variety of questionnaires agree that the one common motivation is that of intrapersonal reasons (Skögman & Jehagen 2003; Holden & Delisle 2006; Dimmock et al. 2009). However, in the main, many of the studies examining issues of self-harm and suicidality have explored the underlying reasons for the behaviour and the implications for services (Dow et al. 2004; Mental Health Foundation 2006), with only a limited number of studies focusing on provision of services from a service user perspective. However, many of these studies present the views of adult service users rather than the experiences of young people (Palmer et al. 2007; Tatiana et al. 2009) with only one study being found that reports on barriers to help seeking for self-harm from an adolescent perspective (Fortune et al. 2005). Therefore, it is the intention of this research to address this gap in the available to evidence.

continued . . .

Aim

Write down an overall aim for the study.

Objectives

Write down three to five objectives for the study that will allow you to achieve the overall aim.

Now think about how you will carry out the study. Consider the following aspects:

Methodology

The main research paradigm you will use – qualitative, quantitative of a mixed methods study. Give you reasons for the choice made.

Once you established the above consider what particular approach/approaches you will use. For example, cross-sectional survey, experimental design, phenomenology, narrative.

Recruitment

➤ Given this might be considered a sensitive topic how will get people interested in the study?
➤ What organisations might you approach?
➤ Do they have their own ethical procedures?
➤ What information will you need to make available if someone shows interest?

Participants

➤ What inclusion/exclusion criteria will you have for those wishing to participate in the study?
➤ How many people do you want to include – what is this number based on?
➤ What strategy will you put in place if you do not recruit the required number or if too many people want to participate?
➤ Will you offer any incentive to participate?

Informed Consent

➤ How will you gain informed consent from potential participants?
➤ What information will you need to give them and in what format?
➤ How will you ascertain each participant has understood the purpose of the research:
  – what they will be expected to do in order to participate
  – their rights during and after their involvement
  – what will happen to the information they give you
  – how their anonymity and confidentiality will be protected and when the latter will be broken.

➤ Consider the age range of potential participants. If considering involving those under 16 refer to Gillick competence and Frazer guidance (2017) and how these will be incorporated into your project.

Data Collection

➤ What is the most appropriate way to collect data to meet the research aim?

continued . . .

> Where will you undertake your data collection?
> If you decide to use interviews and/or focus groups how will you record the data you collect?
> Will any other people be involved in the process (for example, guardian of young person, colleague who might assist with a focus group)?
> How long will the process of data collection take for each participant?
> Will you be collecting any other information? (for example, demographic information)?
> During data collection how will you attempt to ensure anonymity?
> What will you do if the participant wishes to take a break and or changes their mind about participating?
> What will you do with the data collected up to that point?

Data Analysis

> Depending on how you have chosen to collect data, what will you now do with the data by way of starting the process of analysis?
> Given your chosen methodology what is the framework for analysis?
> How will you ensure all participants' data are included in your analysis?

Presentation of Results

> Where will you present your results? Try and think of at least three ways in which you could disseminate your findings. It is important to present your findings as this validates participants' involvement in your study.
> Who will you acknowledge when presenting your findings?

Code of Conduct/Research Governance

Specify which code you will be adhering to throughout the research.

Data Protection

> Where will data be kept – consider electronic and hard data?
> How long will it be kept for?
> Who will have access to it?
> Will data be used for any other studies?
> If so what have you put in place to ensure the participant is agreeable to this?
> How will you ensure the data is anonymised? If in the UK please refer to the Data Protection Act (2018).

Other Ethical Issues

> Consider the study you have just outlined and think about what other ethics issues might occur when undertaking this research for yourself and for those participating.
> Outline each one you think about and describe how you intend to reduce risk/harm to both yourself as a researcher and the participants in your study.

Patient and Public Involvement

Within the UK there is an impetus to involve the individual, family and or the general public in developing research proposals. This is particularly pertinent when applying for funding

continued . . .

for research, for example National Institute of Health Research (NIHR) grants. It might be worth considering how you would go about involving people in the development of your research proposal.

➤ Consider who you might approach to get this level of involvement.

➤ Where you might meet with people and when?

➤ Will they be reimbursed for their involvement?

➤ How will you ensure this is meaningful involvement?

While there are no fixed answers to the above, working through the questions and giving thought to each section should help you to familiarize yourself with ethics principles required for all research projects.

References

Input supporting references in full here in organisation style.

REFERENCES

Ackerman, S. and Hilsenroth, M. (2003) 'A review of therapist characteristics and techniques positively impacting the therapeutic alliance', *Clinical Psychology Review*, 23, pp. 1–33.

Alderson, P. (2007) 'Competent children? Minors' consent to health care treatment and research', *Social Science and Medicine*, 65, pp. 2272–83.

Appelbaum, P. S., Grisso, T., Frank, E., O'Donnell, S. and Kupfer, D. J. (1999) 'Competence of depressed patients for consent to research', *American Journal of Psychiatry*, 156, pp. 1380–4.

Bowlby, J. (1969) *Attachment and Loss*. Volume 1. London: Hogarth Press.

Bourdeau, B. (2000) 'Dual relationships in qualitative research', *The Qualitative Report*, 4, pp. 3–4.

British Association of Counselling and psychotherapy (2012) Available at: www.itsgoodtotalk.org.uk/assets/docs/BACP-Ethical-Framework-for-Good-Practice-in-Counselling-and-Psychotherapy_1360076878.pdf (Accessed 14 June 2017)

British Psychological Society (2014) Available at: www.bps.org.uk/sites/default/files/documents/code_of_human_research_ethics.pdf (Accessed 14 June 2017)

Clarke, S. (1999) 'Splitting difference: psychoanalysis, hatred and exclusion', *Journal for the Theory of Social Behaviour*, 29, pp. 121–35.

Data Protection Act (1998) Available at: www.gov.uk/data-protection/the-data-protection-act (Accessed 14 June 2017).

Declaration of Helsinki. (2017) Available at: www.wma.net/policies-post/wma-declaration-of-helsinki-ethical-principles-for-medical-research-involving-human-subjects/ (Accessed 14 June 2017)

De Haene, L., Hans, G. and Karine, V. (2010) 'Holding harm: narrative methods in mental health research on trauma', *Qualitative Health Research*, 20, pp. 1664–76.

Dijksterhuis, A. (2006) 'The emergence of implicit self esteem', *Netherlands Journal of Psychology*, 62, pp. 19–25.

Draucker, C. B., Martsolf, D. S. and Poole, C. (2009) 'Developing distress protocols for research on sensitive topics', *Archives of Psychiatric Nursing*, 23, pp. 343–50.

Edwards, S. J. L., Kirchin, S. and Huxtable, R. (2004) 'Research ethics committees and paternalism', *Journal of Medical Ethics*, 30, pp. 88–91.

Finn, L. D., Bishop, B. and Sparrow, N. H. (2007) 'Mutual help groups: an important gateway to wellbeing and mental health', *Australian Health Review*, 31, pp. 246–55.

Fry, C. and Dwyer, R. (2001) 'For love or money? An exploratory study of why injecting drug users participate in research', *Addiction*, 9 (9), pp. 1319–25.

Gadd, D. (2004). 'Making sense of interviewee-interviewer dynamics in narratives about violence in intimate relationships', *International Journal of Social Research Methodology*, 7, pp. 383–401.

Gillick Competence/Fraser Guidelines (2017) Available at: www.nspcc.org.uk/preventing-abuse/child-protection-system/legal-definition-child-rights-law/gillick-competency-fraser-guidelines/ (Accessed 14 June 2017)

Grant, R. (2002) 'The ethics of incentives: historical origins and contemporary understanding', *Economics and Philosophy*, 18, pp. 111–39.

Grant, R. and Sugarman, J. (2004) 'Ethics in human subjects research: do incentives matter'? *Journal of Medicine and Philosophy*, 29, pp. 717–38.

Guyatt, G., Sackett, D., Sinclair, J., Hayward, R., Cook, D. and Cook, R. (1995) 'Users' guides to the medical literature. IX. A method for grading health care recommendations', *Journal of the American Medical Association*, 274, pp. 1800–4.

Hollway, W. and Jefferson, T. (2000) *Doing Qualitative Research Differently: Free Association, Narrative and the Interview Method.* London: Sage.

Hunt, J. C. (1989) *Psychoanalytic Aspects of Fieldwork.* University Paper Series on Qualitative Research Methods, volume 18, Newbury Park, CA: Sage.

Isay, R. A. (2006) *Commitment and Healing: Gay Men and the Need for Romantic Love.* New Jersey: Wiley.

Jorm, A. F., Kelly, C. M. and Morgan, A. J. (2007) 'Participant distress in psychiatric research: a systematic review', *Psychological Medicine*, 37, pp. 917–26.

Koivisto, K., Janhonen, S., Latvala, E. and Väisänen, L. (2001) 'Applying ethical guidelines in nursing research on people with mental illness', *Nursing Ethics*, 8, pp. 328–39.

Kvale, S. (1999) 'The psychoanalytical interview as qualitative research', *Qualitative Inquiry*, 5, pp. 87–113.

Lacan, J. (2003) *Lacan. Ecrits: A Selection.* (Translated by Alan Sheridan). London: Routledge Classics.

Mackenzie, C., McDowell, C. and Pittaway, E. (2007) 'Beyond 'Do no harm': the challenge of constructing ethical relationships in refugee research', *Journal of Refugee Studies* 20, pp. 299–319.

McKim, C. (2015) 'The value of mixed methods research: a mixed methods study', *Journal of Mixed Methods Research*, 11, pp. 202–22.

Moodley, R. (2001) '(Re)Searching for a client in two different worlds: mind the research-practice gap', *Counselling and Psychotherapy Research*, 1, pp. 18–23.

Munhall, P. L. (2001) 'Institutional review of qualitative proposals', in: Munhall, P. L. (ed.). *Nursing Research: A Qualitative Perspective*, 4th edition. Sudbury, MA: Jones and Bartlett, pp. 515–28.

National Health and Medical Research Council (NHMRC – 2007) *National Statement on Ethical Conduct in Human Research.* Canberra, ACT: National Health and Medical Research Council. Available at: www.deakin.edu.au/__data/assets/pdf_file/0004/559669/e72_national_statement_may_2015_150514_a.pdf (Accessed: 24 May 2017)

Riessman, C. K. (1993) *Narrative Analysis.* Newbury Park, CA: Sage.

Roberts, L. (2002) 'Ethics and mental illness research', *Psychiatric Clinics of North America*, 25, pp. 525–45.

Roberts, L. and Roberts, B. (1999) 'Psychiatric research ethics: an overview of evolving guidelines and current ethical dilemmas in the study of mental illness', *Biological Psychiatry*, 46, pp. 1025–38.

Rogers, W. A. (2004) 'Evidence based medicine and justice: a framework for looking at the impact of EBM upon vulnerable or disadvantaged groups', *Journal of Medical Ethics*, 30, pp. 141–5.

Royal College of Nursing. (2011) Available at: www.rcn.org.uk/professional-development/publications/pub-003138 (Accessed 14 June 2017)

Sackett, D., Rosenberg, W., Gray, J., Haynes, R. and Richardson, W. (1996) 'Evidence based medicine: what it is and what it isn't', *British Medical Journal*, 312, p. 7023.

Schwartz, C., Meisenhelder, J. B., Ma, Y. and Reed, G. (2003) 'Altruistic social interest behaviours are associated with better mental health', *Psychosomatic Medicine*, 65, pp. 778–85.

Tee, S. R. and Lathlean, J. A. (2004) 'The ethics of conducting a co-operative inquiry with vulnerable people', *Journal of Advanced Nursing*, 47, pp. 536–43.

Warne, T. and McAndrew, S. (2010) 'Re-searching for therapy: the ethics of using what we are skilled in', *Journal of Psychiatric and Mental Health Nursing*, 17, pp. 503–9.

Whitelaw, A. (1999) 'What researchers can learn from psychotherapists', *Psychology and Psychotherapy*, 17, pp. 304–14.

Yalom, I. D. (1995) *The Theory and Practice of Group Psychotherapy*. 4th ed. New York: Basic Books.

To Learn More

Barker, P. and Davidson, B. eds (1998) *Psychiatric Nursing: Ethical Strife*. London: Arnold. A useful text for understanding the nuances of working with those who experience mental health problems, and raising awareness of what, as a researcher, you might need to consider.

De Haan, E. (2004) *The Consulting Process as Drama: Learning from King Lear*. London: Karnac. This book explores a core theme of responsibility. The five phases of the consulting process, as outlined in the book, will be familiar to the practitioner and easily transposed to the research encounter.

Hawkins, P., Shohet, R., Ryde, J. and Wilmot, J. (2012) *Supervision in the Helping Professions*. Buckingham: McGraw-Hill Education (UK). This book provides a model of supervision that can provide support for practitioner/researcher alike, and also give insight into the analytic process inherent in qualitative research.

Yalom, I. D. (1989) *Love's Executioner and Other Tales of Psychotherapy*. London: Penguin Books. A good book demonstrating how knowing oneself enables one to better understand others.

CHAPTER 5

Understanding Severe Persistent Mental Health Problems and Disorders

Michael Hazelton

> The assumption that a person diagnosed with [severe persistent mental health problems and disorders] is globally incompetent affects the amount of clinical information that a health professional might share with them, and often results in the person not being involved in their own end-of-life care decisions ... people with [severe persistent mental health problems and disorders] have the capacity to make decisions about end-of-life care and participate in advance care planning when their symptoms are in remission.
>
> (Butler & O'Brien 2017, p. 3)

INTRODUCTION

Mental health problems and disorders affect a large number of people in all countries. The impact of mental disorders has been estimated to comprise 7.4 per cent of the world's measurable burden of disease (Murray et al. 2012) and to have accounted for 183.9 million Disability Adjusted Life Years (DALYs) and 8.6 million Years of Life Lost (YLLs) in 2010 (Whiteford et al. 2015). Schizophrenia is associated with a greater burden of long-term disability than any other mental disorder (Galletly et al. 2016).

There is no doubt that the human and economic cost of mental health problems and disorders is high. In Australia, a country with one of the most highly developed health care systems in the world, 1 in 5 people aged 16 to 85 will reach diagnostic requirements for at least one mental disorder in any year, with only 1 in 3 of these receiving any form of professional help for their ill-health (Australian Bureau of Statistics 2008). The economic impact of mental ill-health is now counted in the billions of dollars. In Australia, the direct costs and lost productivity related to schizophrenia alone, which is a low prevalence disorder but ranks among the leading causes of disability worldwide (Carr et al. 2012; Galletly et al. 2016), has been estimated at Aus$2.5 billion annually (Schizophrenia Research Institute 2015).

While the mental health of the population poses considerable challenges for policy makers and health professionals in high-income countries such as Australia, the UK and the United States, in low and middle-income countries the extent of mental health unmet need can be much greater and mental health services much less developed (Jacob et al. 2007; Ae-Ngibise et al. 2010). Indeed, the failure to adequately address the needs of people experiencing mental health problems and disorders, especially in low and middle-income countries has caused prominent commentators to view global mental health as a 'failure of humanity' (Kleinman 2009) and a 'global tragedy' (Becker & Kleinman 2013).

'SEVERE PERSISTENT MENTAL HEALTH PROBLEMS AND DISORDERS'

This worrying backdrop provides a starting point for understanding severe persistent mental health problems and disorders. The terms 'serious enduring mental ill-health', 'severe enduring mental ill-health' and 'severe persistent mental ill-health' have often been used interchangeably and sometimes without definition. For instance, Gournay (1995) used both 'serious and enduring mental ill-health' and 'severe and enduring mental ill-health' without defining either. Even when definitions have been offered these have often been contested (Barr & Cotterill 1999). More recently the terms 'severe persistent mental illness' or 'severe and persistent mental health problems and disorders' have been used widely (Trachsel et al. 2016; Galletly et al. 2016; Butler & O'Brien 2017). In general, however, what is being referred to when these terms are used is the experience of schizophrenia, major depressive disorder or bipolar disorder, of people aged 18 and older, where the ill-health is accompanied by prolonged recurrent symptoms and impaired functioning requiring long-term treatment. Personality disorder, post-traumatic stress disorder and anorexia nervosa have sometimes been included (Woods et al. 2008).

There is a high prevalence of physical ill-health in people experiencing severe persistent mental health problems and disorders. The more serious psychiatric symptoms are associated with medical comorbidity and poor physical health status and outcomes. People experiencing severe persistent mental health problems and disorders are at much greater risk of dying from natural causes at any age compared to the general population; areas of particular risk include death from neoplasms, respiratory and gastrointestinal ill-health, and also injury, suicide and homicide (Woods et al. 2008; Butler & O'Brien 2017).

SCHIZOPHRENIA AND RELATED DISORDERS

The psychiatric diagnosis most often associated with severe persistent mental health problems and disorders is schizophrenia. Schizophrenia is a complex disorder with a high degree of variation in presenting symptoms. The fifth edition of the *Diagnostic and Statistical Manual of Mental Disorders (DSM-5)* (American Psychiatric Association 2013) identifies a number of essential features for a diagnosis of schizophrenia to be made. These include that the person must present with a combination of symptoms, including delusions, hallucinations, disorganised speech/behaviour, reduced emotion, limited speech or low motivation; they must not have received treatment for at least a month. Self-care, work and social life must have been adversely affected and the symptoms must have been evident for months.

KEY POINT 5.1

Other possible explanations for the symptoms, such as mania, depression, substance ingestion, medical problems or disability, must also have been ruled out.

Schizophrenia is diagnosed by identifying signs and symptoms (*See* Chapter 9) including delusional beliefs, hallucinations, disorganised thinking and speech, cognitive impairment, abnormal behaviour and negative symptoms such as loss of pleasure, reduced motivation and apathy (Galletly et al. 2016). It should be noted that over time the word 'schizophrenia' has taken on negative connotations and is now under challenge within psychiatry and that terms such as 'psychotic spectrum disorder' have been proposed as alternatives (Henderson & Mahli 2014).

Schizophrenia disrupts cognitive, emotional and behavioural functioning and affects approximately 1 in 100 people during their lifetime. The incidence of schizophrenia is higher in men than in women, with a ratio of 1.4 to 1. Some migrant groups have substantially higher risks of schizophrenia and people born and raised in urban areas are more at risk of developing schizophrenia than those born and raised in rural locations (Galletly et al. 2016). Onset usually occurs between the mid teenage years and the early 30s; diagnosis occurs most frequently in the early 20s for men and late 20s for women (Carr et al. 2012). There is also variability in the progression of schizophrenia. For some people ill-health is experienced as episodic, with periods in which the symptoms are very severe while at other times being much less intense. For other people, ill-health takes a continuously deteriorating course. The Australian Survey of High Impact Psychosis found that the episodic form of ill-health occurred in approximately 70 per cent of cases with the remainder following the course of continuous deterioration (Carr et al. 2012).

The symptoms of schizophrenia are often described as being 'positive', 'negative' and 'cognitive'. Positive symptoms are considered to represent an excess or distortion of normal functioning and negative symptoms are considered deficits in functioning. Hallucinations (false sensory experiences such as hearing voices) and delusions (false beliefs such as believing one is being controlled by a computer) are examples of positive symptoms. Examples of negative symptoms include significantly reduced emotional responsiveness (flat affect), brief, empty verbal responses (alogia), reduced motivation (avolition) and anhedonia (inability to experience pleasure). Cognitive symptoms include deficits in memory, attention and executive functioning (Galletly et al. 2016). People experiencing schizophrenia are often highly reactive to environmental factors and social marginalisation is often accompanied by disability, low self-esteem and apathy. Functional limitations may be intensified by social circumstances, resulting in loss of peer support, meaningful goals, role fulfilment, living skills and the lowering of expectations (Galletly et al. 2016).

Variation in symptom presentation can have important implications for treatment choices and longer-term outcomes for people experiencing severe persistent disorders such as schizophrenia. The currently available neuroleptic medications used to treat schizophrenia are reasonably effective in controlling positive symptoms. However, negative symptoms have proven to be much more difficult to treat (Galletly et al. 2016). In addition, all the medications used to treat disorders such as schizophrenia are accompanied by often distressing and in some cases, potentially life-threatening side effects. Indeed, some of the side effects are very similar to the negative symptoms discussed above.

In the last few decades, the introduction of newer antipsychotic medications, referred to as 'atypical' or 'second generation antipsychotics', has contributed to more effective control of positive symptoms (and possibly some improvement in negative symptoms although this is unclear). However, this has been accompanied by a significant increase in the occurrence of certain types of side effects, the most serious of which has been rapid weight gain. This contributes to a large number of people being treated with antipsychotic medication, meeting criteria for serious physical health problems such as metabolic syndrome – a group of conditions characterised by increased blood pressure, hyperglycaemia, excess of body fat around the waist and abnormal cholesterol and triglyceride levels. Taken together these significantly increase the risk of heart disease, stroke and diabetes (Galletly et al. 2016; Butler & O'Brien 2017).

For many people, experiencing severe persistent mental health problems and disorders, the cost of more effective treatment for symptoms has been significantly reduced physical health status. In the Second Australian National Survey of Psychosis, 53 per cent of participants aged 18–64 met criteria for metabolic syndrome. About one-quarter were at high risk of a cardiovascular event in the next five years. However, less than half of those with known hypertension or elevated cholesterol were receiving medication for these conditions (Galletly et al. 2016). Other factors that have been identified as contributing to increased rates of physical health comorbidities among people experiencing severe persistent mental health problems and disorders include high levels of tobacco smoking, unhealthy dietary behaviours, little or no exercise, and harmful alcohol and drug use (*See* Chapter 17 and 21) (Butler & O'Brien, 2017). This, of course, has implications for palliative care in this population.

Recent research has highlighted variations in the course and outcomes of schizophrenia, with a small percentage of people affected experiencing a single episode followed by a good recovery; about 50 per cent experiencing multiple episodes and good to partial recovery; and almost 40 per cent experiencing an unremitting course with deterioration (Morgan et al. 2014). It has been estimated that worldwide, about one in seven people who would meet diagnostic thresholds for schizophrenia will reach complete or near complete recovery. Factors predicting recovery include higher levels of premorbid occupational attainment and social competence, lower likelihood of substance use, better insight and a sense of being in control of personal circumstances (Galletly et al. 2016).

A STAGING APPROACH TO SEVERE PERSISTENT MENTAL HEALTH PROBLEMS AND DISORDERS

Better understanding of variations in the course and outcomes of disorders such as schizophrenia has been accompanied by the development of a staging model that considers the course of ill-health as a continuum. An important assumption of this way of thinking about mental health problems and disorders is that treatments provided earlier during ill-health are likely be safer, more acceptable and more cost-effective than those used at a later stage. As Galletly et al. (2016) point out, the key to effective clinical care in all stages is the therapeutic relationship: 'Time must be spent building trust and good communication. This is just as important for people with unremitting illness, as it is for those early in the course of the disorder. It is essential to take a respectful approach, provide accurate information and address the person's questions and concerns (Galletly et al. 2016, p. 416).

The application of a staging model for clinical care in schizophrenia and related disorders has resulted in the development of a four-stage approach as follows (Galletly et al. 2016):

1. Stage 1 involves the pre-psychotic or prodromal stage and is typified by an often-extended period of sub-clinical positive symptoms and rising disability. While such

symptoms do not meet thresholds for a diagnosis of schizophrenia, emerging functional deficits are evident.

2. Stage 2 entails first episode psychosis and is characterised as one week or more of positive symptoms meeting requirements for positive symptoms such as delusions and hallucinations. In recent decades first episode psychosis has become a focus for intensive early intervention designed to ensure the safety of the person being treated, to reduce the period in which psychotic symptoms are untreated and to maintain and restore functioning using a combination of psychotropic medication and psychosocial interventions.

3. In Stage 3 ill-health has become established and is persistent. A high number of people experiencing a first episode of psychosis go on to have further episodes with continuing disability. As many as half of those experiencing first episode psychosis relapse within three years; failure to take antipsychotic medications as prescribed contributes greatly to relapse during this stage of ill-health.

4. Stage 4 involves severe persistent or unremitted ill-health. A substantial minority of people experiencing schizophrenia experience distressing and disabling symptoms that persist. Within the context of developing and maintaining an effective thera-peutic relationship with a person experiencing severe persistent or unremitting psychosis, the engaged health professional works to manage treatable factors such as unrecognised mood problems, sub-optimal medication treatment, inadequate psychosocial rehabilitation, poor treatment adherence, substance use, medication side effects and drug interactions.

Galletly et al. (2016, p. 422) outline two key considerations in the management of people experiencing severe persistent or unremitted ill-health:

1. Secure, safe housing and income support are key priorities for people experiencing severe persistent ill-health.

2. Suboptimal care for people experiencing severe persistent or unremitting ill-health increases their risk of developing physical ill-health, social isolation and marginal-isation.

THE LIVED EXPERIENCE OF SEVERE PERSISTENT MENTAL HEALTH PROBLEMS AND DISORDERS

Trachsel et al. (2016, p. 4) have identified people experiencing severe persistent mental health problems and disorders as 'a particularly vulnerable population, at risk of either therapeutic neglect or overly aggressive care' (p. 4).

People in this population face many challenges; while a number of these relate directly to the experience of symptoms of disorders such as schizophrenia, others are more connected to ill-health-related life circumstances. For instance, the findings of studies such as the Survey of High Impact Psychosis (SHIP) in Australia point to the extent to which people experiencing psychotic ill-health experience significant educational and employment disadvantage and are heavy users of alcohol and illicit drugs; many live what can best be described as marginal lives characterised by social isolation and uncertain access to income and accommodation (Morgan et al. 2012). The extent of the impact of psychosis on the lives of people experiencing psychotic disorders such as schizo-phrenia can be gauged from items in the SHIP study that asked about challenges expected to be faced in the coming year. In rank order participants listed financial matters, loneliness/social isolation, lack of employment and poor physical health ahead of uncontrolled symptoms of mental ill-health. Perhaps surprisingly, concerns over stable/suitable housing and stigma/discrimination were ranked further down the list (Carr et al. 2012). Concerns such as those listed above point to the need for a comprehensive system of mental health treatment, rehabilitation, housing and support services, especially for people experiencing severe persistent mental health problems and disorders (Hazelton & Rossiter 2016).

The identification of poor physical health as a main concern in the coming year by SHIP study participants (Morgan et al. 2012; Carr et al. 2012) is in line with the findings of research into the physical health status of people experiencing mental ill-health. People experiencing severe persistent mental health problems and disorders such as schizophrenia are known to have poor physical health and much-reduced life expectancy compared to the general population. Reduced life expectancy has been estimated to be 18.7 years for men and 16.3 years for women experiencing schizophrenia, with the leading causes of early death in this population being cardio-metabolic disease, suicide and accidents (Bradshaw & Pedley 2012; Galletly et al. 2016).

To some extent the high occurrence of metabolic ill-health can be attributed to the prevalence of high risk behaviours such as tobacco smoking amongst people experiencing schizophrenia – estimated to be as high as 72.2 per cent in men and 59.7 per cent in women; more than three times higher than for the general population in Australia. Another important contributing factor, weight gain, can be attributed to a combination of the symptoms of ill-health (e.g. low motivation, fatigue), poor diet and the side effects of antipsychotic medication. The findings of the SHIP study indicated that more than half of those experiencing psychotic ill-health met the requirements for metabolic syndrome, which as we have seen consists of a group of risk factors that increase the likelihood of a person developing coronary heart disease and other health problems such as diabetes and stroke (Morgan et al. 2012).

Woods et al. (2008) conducted a review of the literature on the palliative care needs of people experiencing severe persistent mental health problems and disorders, with the purpose of informing clinical practice, research and education. While people experiencing severe persistent mental health problems and disorders are vulnerable, often have multiple comorbidities and higher-than-average mortality rates, there is scant knowledge regarding their palliative care experiences or needs (Woods et al. 2008). The 68 articles included in the study by Woods et al. (2008) comprised 11 empirical papers and 57 theoretical papers. The analysis of this material identified four main themes:
1. decision-making capacity and advanced care planning
2. access to care
3. provision of care
4. and vulnerability.

1. Decision-making Capacity and Advanced Care Planning

There is a tendency for discussions about end-of-life care to by-pass people experiencing severe persistent mental health problems and disorders because of assumed global incompetence and concern that such discussions may be emotionally and cognitively destabilising (Woods et al. 2008; Butler & O'Brien 2017). Left out of discussions, especially if lacking others who care for them, people experiencing severe persistent mental health problems and disorders may have decisions made 'in their best interests'; such decisions may not be in accord with their wishes (*See* Chapter 8). With so little known about the preferences of people experiencing severe persistent mental ill-health there is a high risk of them receiving care they do not want (Woods et al. 2008).

2. Access to Care

People experiencing severe persistent mental health problems and disorders may struggle to access health care that is timely and appropriate. One area of particular concern is the high burden of medical comorbidity and social problems such as substance use problems and homelessness. Medical comorbidity is often complex and serious health problems can go unrecognised and untreated even when medical help is sought. Such problems intensify in circumstances where individuals have lost contact with their families and have little or no access to social support networks (Woods et al. 2008).

3. Provision of Care

Issues surrounding provision of care can be differentiated based on being ill-health related or health care provider related. People experiencing severe persistent mental health problems and disorders may present with behaviours that make engagement difficult, posing challenges to conducting assessments, building therapeutic relationships, care plan decision-making, and providing palliative care. In general, such difficulties are likely to be more manageable if the person experiencing severe persistent mental health problems and disorders is known to the health care practitioner. However, lack of prior contact can intensify difficulties in the provision of care. The extent of practitioner experience of and comfort in working alongside people experiencing severe persistent mental health problems and disorders are also important considerations. These challenges are especially likely to be intensified in health care practitioners who lack experience of working alongside people experiencing severe persistent mental health problems and disorders and/or caring for people at the end-of-life (Woods et al. 2008).

4. Vulnerability

In many instances the susceptibilities associated with experiencing severe persistent mental health problems and disorders can be expected to amplify the knowledge and power differentials that underscore the relationship between health care professionals and people with lived experience of mental ill-health. Such vulnerabilities can involve disorders of:

- thought and mood
- cognitive deficits
- altered abstract reasoning
- limited health care choices
- estrangement from family and supporting social networks
- and in some cases, homelessness.

(Woods et al. 2008)

Based on the outcomes of their review Woods et al. (2008) identify a number of clinical implications for health professionals working alongside people experiencing severe persistent mental health problems and disorders.

KEY POINT 5.2

First, palliative care must be centred on the needs of people experiencing severe persistent mental health problems and disorders; a relationship based on respect, dignity, hope and non-abandonment is of critical importance.

Second, in anticipation that a significant minority of people experiencing severe persistent mental health problems and disorders will need palliative care at some point, principles of hospice palliative care should be integrated into end-of-life care for people in this population. On this basis the provision of cross training in palliative care and mental health care is warranted.

Third, access is needed to a system that integrates people experiencing severe persistent mental health problems and disorders, families, mental health care, palliative care, family health services and social supportive services (Woods et al. 2008).

When the extent of morbidity and mortality associated with people experiencing severe persistent mental health problems and disorders are taken into account there is clearly a high need for end-of-life care. However, as Butler and O'Brien (2017, p. 3) have recently argued the 'level of need is not matched by access to palliative care services' (p. 3).

REFLECTIVE PRACTICE EXERCISE 5.1

Time: 20 minutes
Consider this statement. In your place of work, and thinking laterally, how might you organise a change in practice, to offer a palliative care approach to those within your care? Consider how palliative care could translate to your area of healthcare.

EVIDENCE-BASED PRACTICE AND RECOVERY-ORIENTED MENTAL HEALTH CARE

Health professionals are typically eclectic and pragmatic in deciding the information they will use in working alongside a person experiencing mental ill-health; they draw upon various sources of information and are practical in applying these clinically. Two important areas of consideration that have emerged to guide the work of health professionals in recent decades are evidence based practice (EBP) and recovery oriented mental health practice. Both are enshrined in the national mental health policies of many countries and are increasingly evident in the discourses used by mental health professionals in their day-to-day work.

The main intention driving evidence based practice is where possible to choose intervention strategies based on scientific evidence about their effectiveness in a population of people experiencing a health problem. It is important to note that the primacy of EBP has not gone uncontested. For instance, concerns have been expressed regarding the influence of the pharmaceutical industry on the conduct of medical science and health professional practice (and thus evidence-based practice) (Boyce & Mahli 2012; Smith 2012). In addition, the emergence of the recovery movement has meant that decisions regarding what works best in mental health treatments must be balanced against what the person experiencing mental ill-health prefers. The lived experience context of recovery has become an (if not the most) important aspect of mental health thought and practice; increasingly this has extended to considerations of the types of research that are consistent with the principles of recovery-oriented mental health practice (Gordon & Ellis 2013).

In mental health, recovery refers to living a fulfilling life while facing the challenges posed by experiencing mental health problems and disorders. Several approaches have been proposed for understanding the main characteristics of recovery. One influential approach has suggested that the experience of recovery involves at the least the following:

➤ Refusing to define self-worth by the experience of a mental health problem or disorder
➤ Participating in the community as a family member, worker, neighbour, friend and citizen
➤ Accepting responsibility for and making decisions about one's own life
➤ Engaging with a personal and social support network beyond the mental health system
➤ Celebrating the strengths and capabilities gained from experiencing and recovering from a mental health problem or disorder
➤ Maintaining hope and optimism for the future.

(Leamy et al. 2011)

Recovery-oriented mental health practice places great importance on the lived experience and the perspective of the person experiencing a mental health problem or disorder. Distinctions have been made between clinical recovery (reduction of symptoms), functional recovery and personal recovery (Galletly et al. 2016). Understood as a process of individual change in attitudes, values, feelings, goals, skills and or roles, personal recovery involves living a satisfying, hopeful and contributing life despite the limitations of ill-health. Personal recovery goals may include gaining knowledge about the ill-health and available treatments, developing ill-health management and self-care skills, and taking responsibility for one's own treatment. Recovery-oriented practice emphasises peer relationships, social networks, person centred and strengths-based assessment and collaborative care planning (Galletly et al. 2016).

Recovery ideas and practices can be applied at all stages of ill-health and can be used to guide a range of interventions including providing effective support for the people experiencing a mental health problem or disorder, timely response to requests for help, collaborative care-planning and decision-making, listening to and addressing the needs of family members, facilitating connections with peer support networks, helping people to secure suitable accommodation (Galletly et al. 2016). A recently published clinical practice guideline for the clinical management of schizophrenia has recommended the following in relation to recovery-oriented practice:

➤ Recovery training should be mandatory for all practitioners working in mental health
➤ People experiencing mental health problems and disorders should be treated in an appropriate, caring and respectful environment that promotes a collaborative relationship between the individual and practitioners

➤ A recovery plan developed in partnership with a person experiencing a mental health problem or disorder should guide mental health care
➤ Psychoeducation should be available
➤ Peer specialist workers should be employed to assist with counselling, support and psychoeducation for people experiencing schizophrenia, provide advice to practitioners and help plan and audit services
➤ Clinicians and mental health services should work in partnership with the individual, their carers, the non-government sector and relevant support organizations.

(Galletly et al. 2016)

In addition to the above recommendations, it is also suggested that health professionals undertake training to address the values and practical aspects of the recovery model with a view to developing understanding of mental ill-health, treatments and recovery in a variety of cultural contexts (*See* Chapter 6). There should be a focus on respectful communication, consumer strengths and the impact of stigma and social exclusion (Galletly et al. 2016).

Despite the considerable efforts to prevent mental ill-health, and in cases where it develops to promote and support recovery, a proportion of people affected will develop severe persistent mental ill-health.

KEY POINT 5.3

People within this group are an especially vulnerable population that risk (perhaps ironically) either therapeutic neglect or very aggressive intervention.

MENTAL HEALTH CARE AND PALLIATIVE CARE

In a number of ways mental health care and palliative care are similar. Both are now specialised areas of health care, are heavily invested in the biopsychosocial model and provide services that are multi-professional in nature. While in recent decades there has been increasing cross-over between the fields of mental health and palliative care, the latter has not been readily available for people experiencing mental health problems and disorders except when this was provided in relation to physical ill-health.

Between one fifth and one third of people experiencing schizophrenia worldwide (approximately 4 to 7 million people) suffer from severe treatment-resistant schizophrenia. These people may experience a high level of negative symptoms, leading to impaired quality of life and social functioning. The needs of this very vulnerable population are often overlooked by mental health services, resulting in inadequate treatment or even abandonment. As Trachsel et al. (2016, p. 200) comment, there

is no consensus on best practice, nor are there specialised services. Eventually some of these patients receive palliative care and die in a medical setting ... Patients themselves may be unable to press for a more palliative approach to their mental ill-health by virtue of their impaired decision-making capacity.

(p. 200)

This treatment gap for people experiencing severe persistent mental ill-health has caused some commentators to call for a specialised service within psychiatry, which would place emphasis on quality of life rather than aggressive symptom management, increasing the possibility of an individual concerned staying in regular contact with their mental health care providers (Trachsel et al. 2016). This new paradigm for the management of severe persistent mental ill-health, which would have its own conceptual framework and clinical approach, has been referred to as 'palliative psychiatry'.

DEFINITION AND FEATURES OF PALLIATIVE PSYCHIATRY

Palliative psychiatry is an approach that improves the quality of life of individuals and their families in dealing with the problems associated with life-threatening severe persistent mental health problems and disorders.

KEY POINT 5.4

The focus of palliative psychiatry is on the prevention and relief of suffering by means of timely assessment and treatment of associated physical, mental, social and spiritual needs.

There is an explicit emphasis on harm reduction and avoidance of burdensome psychiatric interventions with questionable impact (Trachsel et al. 2016).

The main features of palliative psychiatry are that it:

➤ provides support in coping with and acceptance of distressing mental symptoms
➤ affirms life but acknowledges that severe persistent mental health problems and disorders can be incurable
➤ intends neither to hasten nor to postpone death
➤ integrates the physical, psychological, social and spiritual aspects of the individual's care
➤ offers a support system to help people experiencing severe persistent mental health problems and disorders to live as actively as possible until death
➤ offers a support system to help family members to cope while supporting a loved one experiencing severe persistent mental health problems and disorders
➤ uses a team approach to address the needs of people experiencing severe persistent mental health problems and disorders and their families
➤ will enhance quality of life and may also positively influence the course of severe persistent mental health problems and disorders
➤ is applicable in conjunction with other therapies oriented towards prevention, curation, rehabilitation or recovery.

(Trachsel et al. 2016)

It has been proposed that palliative psychiatry be limited to people experiencing severe persistent mental health problems and disorders with multiple comorbidities and high mortality rates. However, this ought not to be interpreted as a form of 'terminal ill-health'; instead, palliative psychiatry implies that an ill-health cannot be treated using a curative approach.

KEY POINT 5.5

The main techniques of palliative psychiatry thus involve ongoing communication of psychiatric diagnosis and prognosis, symptom assessment and management, support for advanced (mental health) care planning, assessment of caregiver needs and referral to specialised services.

Overall, the approach ought to involve an awareness of the limited functional capacity and lifespan of the person receiving the care (Trachsel et al. 2016).

A number of risks have been associated with adopting a palliative psychiatry approach. First, given a lack of consensus regarding what constitutes 'futility' in the treatment of severe persistent mental ill-health, it is not yet clear when a palliative approach is warranted (See Chapter 18). Trachsel et al. (2016) point to the following criteria for 'treatment futility' in psychiatry proposed by Lopez, Yager and Feinstein (2010): poor prognosis, unresponsiveness to competent treatment, continuing physiological and psychological decline, and the appearance of an inexorable and terminal course, suggesting that these could be further developed to include a staging model similar to that used in cancer care. They lament, however, that so far, such an approach is lacking within the context of mental ill-health.

A second area of concern is that palliative psychiatry may be understood as standing in opposition to the concept of recovery in mental health care. While the former involves ideas surrounding remission as an improvement in symptoms and functional capacity with the aim of improving mental stability and psychosocial functioning, the focus of the latter is on personal development, growth, regaining control and meaning in life despite experiencing mental health problems and disorders. Palliative psychiatry could play a role – in conjunction with other services – in supporting a person experiencing severe persistent mental health problem or disorder to reach recovery goals through self-determination and autonomy, dignity and acceptance.

A third area of concern is that so far in palliative psychiatry there has been very little development of the kind of service model and skills outlined by Trachsel et al. (2016). There are few training opportunities for mental health professionals and the term palliative psychiatry is largely absent from professional curricula and textbooks (See To Learn More p. 64).

'PROTECTIVE EMPOWERING'

One of the challenges to be faced when working alongside people with lived experience of severe persistent mental health problems and disorders is how to balance protection-related needs with individual preferences in a highly vulnerable population (Woods et al. 2008; Trachsel et al. 2016). Chiovitti (2011) has proposed an approach to balancing safety concerns with a person's choices, which she refers to as 'protective empowering'. The ideas informing protective empowering may be usefully applied to the provision of palliative care for people experiencing severe persistent mental health problems and disorders. Depending upon the needs of the person concerned and or the health care situation faced, protective and empowering dimensions of caring are emphasised in varying degrees through:

> ➤ respecting the person
> ➤ not taking their behaviour personally
> ➤ maintaining safety
> ➤ encouraging and supporting health promoting behaviours
> ➤ authentic relating
> ➤ and interactive teaching.

(Chiovitti 2011)

As Chiovitti (2011) explains, the application of protective empowering, respecting the individual and not taking their behaviours personally are key values and actions necessary for care to occur.

KEY POINT 5.6

Respect is the guiding value for how professionals seek to establish a meaningful connection with people experiencing mental health problems and disorders.

Not taking the person's behaviour personally assists in gaining therapeutic perspective in situations in which safety concerns and individual preferences may not align. Encouraging health-promoting behaviours, authentic relating and seeking opportunities for interactive teaching are used when opportunities present, both in relation to the safety related actions of the health professional and in supporting the choices of the person experiencing a mental health problem or disorder.

Following Chiovitti (2011), mental health professionals must develop the capacity to balance the degree of liberty extended to people experiencing mental health problems and disorders with the requirements for managing risk and providing effective care. Getting the balance right is especially challenging when working with highly vulnerable groups such as people experiencing severe persistent mental health problems and disorders. There is no doubt that risk is a central concern for professionals regardless of experience and disciplinary background. Undergraduate health professional students such as those studying nursing will often discuss risk and security prior to undertaking mental practicum placements – it would perhaps be surprising if they did not do so. Safety concerns are stressed from the moment a new graduate enters the mental health workforce (Hazelton & Rossiter 2016). At the same time university studies also emphasise the ethical and human rights concerns associated with vulnerable populations such as people experiencing severe persistent mental health problems and disorders. Concepts such as 'person with lived experience of mental health problems and disorders', 'least restrictive environment', 'recovery oriented mental health practice', imply what might be thought of as 'soft' professional authority, to safeguard the behaviours of vulnerable and distressed individuals (Hazelton & Rossiter 2016). There is, however, an ever-present threat that risk concerns will overshadow therapeutic concerns.

The dictum that relationships 'are the heart and soul of mental health care' (Wright et al. 2011, p. 171) holds true when working alongside people experiencing severe persistent mental health problems and disorders. It has been suggested that when health care professionals work in ways that support the autonomy, dignity and complexity of individuals, they are fostering humanization (Todres, Galvin & Holloway 2009). Historically, the caring values of mental health treatment have often been secondary to restrictive and even punitive treatments designed to achieve broader social aims for the control of people experiencing mental health problems and disorders (Beresford, Nettle & Perring 2010). In the absence of a carefully thought out caring framework to guide practice – such as that provided by Chiovitti's (2011) notion of 'protective empowerment', restrictive practice will often undermine therapeutic considerations (*See* Chapter 9). This is especially likely to be the case with vulnerable populations such as people experiencing severe persistent mental health problems and disorders.

Hazelton and Rossiter (2016) have recently outlined suggestions for working alongside vulnerable people experiencing mental health problems and disorders who are considered to be treatment resistant.

➤ First, they advocate the use of evidence-based therapeutic practices focusing on challenging stigma-laden narratives and practices when these are encountered in mental health work.

➤ Second, the risk-bound nature of mental health work requires that professionals have opportunities to regularly engage in conversations addressing the moral and ethical implications of practice.

➤ Third, health professionals who regularly engage in reflective practices, self-awareness and mindfulness, are likely to be better equipped to resist inclinations to misuse the power inherent in their work roles.

➤ Fourth, adopting therapeutic assumptions such as 'the person is doing the best that they can' supports a focus on working alongside people experiencing mental health problems and disorders in a person-centred manner.

➤ Finally, abiding by the 'golden rule' to 'treat others as you would wish to be treated' and 'practicing what you preach' is likely to assist practitioners to see the person experiencing severe persistent mental health problems and disorders as a fellow human.

There is no doubt that evidence based practice is fundamental to improving the care provided to people experiencing severe persistent mental health problems and disorders. However, it may be that morals-based practice is even more important when working alongside people experiencing mental health problems.

REFERENCES

Ae-Ngibise, K., Cooper, S., Adiibokah, E., Bright, A., Crick, L., Doku, V. and The MHaPP Research Programme Consortium. (2010) 'Whether you like it or not people with mental health problems are going to go to them': A qualitative exploration into the widespread use of traditional and faith healers in the provision of mental health care of Ghana', *International Review of Psychiatry*, 22, pp. 558–67.

American Psychiatric Association (2013) *Diagnostic and Statistical Manual of Mental Disorders. 5th edition.* Arlington, VA: American Psychiatric Publishing.

Australian Bureau of Statistics (2008) *2007 National Survey of Mental Health and Wellbeing: Summary of Results.* (Document 4326.0) Canberra: Australian Bureau of Statistics.

Barr, W. and Cotterill, L. (1999) 'Registering concern: The case of primary care registers for people with severe enduring mental illness', *Health and Social Care in the Community*, 7, pp. 427–33.

Becker, A. and Kleinman, A. (2013) 'Mental health and the global agenda', *The New England Journal of Medicine*, 369, pp. 66–73.

Beresford, P., Nettle, M. and Perring, R. (2010) *Towards a Social Model of Madness and Distress? Exploring What Service Users Say*. York: Joseph Rowntree Foundation.

Boyce, P. and Malhi, G. (2012) 'Supping with the devil? The dangers of liaisons between pharma and our profession', *Australian and New Zealand Journal of Psychiatry*, 46, pp. 493–4.

Bradshaw, T. and Pedley, R. (2012) 'Evolving role of mental health nurses in the physical health care of people with serious mental health illness', *International Journal of Mental Health Nursing*, 21, pp. 266–73.

Butler, H. and O'Brien, A. (2017) 'Access to specialist palliative care services by people with severe and persistent mental illness: A retrospective cohort study', *International Journal of Mental Health Nursing*. Available at: DOI:10.1111/inm.12360 (Accessed: 2 December 2017)

Carr, V., Whiteford, H., Groves, A., McGorry, P. and Shepherd, A. (2012) 'Policy and service development implications of the second Australian National Survey of High Impact Psychosis', *Australian & New Zealand Journal of Psychiatry*, 46, pp. 708–18.

Chiovitti, R. (2011) 'Theory of protective empowering for balancing patient safety and choices', *Nursing Ethics*, 18, pp. 88–101.

Galletly, C., Castle, D., Dark, F., Humberstone, V., Jablensky, A. et al. (2016) 'Royal Australian and New Zealand College of Psychiatrists clinical practice guidelines for the management of schizophrenia and related disorders', *Australian & New Zealand Journal of Psychiatry*, 50, pp. 410–72.

Gordon, S. and Ellis, P. M. (2013) 'Recovery of evidence-based practice', *International Journal of Mental Health Nursing*, 22, pp. 3–14.

Gournay, K. (1995) 'Mental health nurses working purposefully with people with serious and enduring mental illness – an international perspective', *International Journal of Nursing Studies*, 32, pp. 341–52.

Hazelton, M. and Rossiter, R. (2016) ' "Talk about trouble": practitioner discourses on service users who are judged to be resisting, contesting, or evading treatment', in O'Reilly, M. and Lester, J. (eds) *The Palgrave Handbook of Adult Mental Health*. Houndmills: Palgrave Macmillan, pp. 419–40.

Henderson, S. and Mahli, G. (2014) 'Swan song for schizophrenia?', *Australian & New Zealand Journal of Psychiatry*, 48, pp. 302–5.

Jacob, K., Sharan, P., Mirza, I., Garrido-Cumbrera, M., Seedat, S., et al. (2007) 'Mental health systems in countries: where are we now?', *The Lancet*, 370, pp. 1061–77.

Kleinman, A. (2009) 'Global mental health: A failure of humanity', *The Lancet*, 374, pp. 603–4.

Leamy, M., Bird, V., Le Boutillier, C., Williams, J. and Slade, M. (2011) 'Conceptual framework for personal recovery in mental health: Systematic review and narrative synthesis', *British Journal of Psychiatry*, 199, pp. 445–51.

Lopez, A., Yager, J. and Feinstein, R. (2010) 'Medical futility and psychiatry: Palliative care and hospice care as a last resort in the treatment of refractory anorexia nervosa', *International Journal of Eating Disorders*, 43, pp. 372–7.

Morgan, V., Wattereus, A., Jablensky, A., Mackinnon, A., McGrath, J., et al. (2012) 'People living with psychotic illness in 2010: The second Australian national survey of psychosis', *Australian & New Zealand Journal of Psychiatry*, 46, pp. 735–52.

Morgan, V., McGrath, J., Jablensky, A., Badcock, J., Wattereus, A., et al. (2014) 'Psychosis prevalence and physical, metabolic and cognitive co-morbidity: data from the second Australian national survey of psychosis', *Psychological Medicine*, 44, pp. 2163–76.

Murray, C., Vos, T., Lozano, R., Naghavi, M., Flaxman, A. D., et al. (2012) 'Disability-adjusted life years (DALYs for 291 diseases and injuries in 21 regions, 1990–2010: A systematic analysis for the Global Burden of Disease Study 2010', *Lancet*, 380, pp. 2197–3223.

Schizophrenia Research Institute (2015) *About schizophrenia.* Available at: www.schizophreniaresearch. org.au/schizophrenia/about-schizophrenia/ (Accessed: 4 December 2017)

Smith, G. P. (2012) 'For richer, for poorer, in sickness and in health: The entanglement of Science and marketing', *Australian and New Zealand Journal of Psychiatry*, 46, pp. 498–500.

Todres, L., Galvin, K. and Holloway, I. (2009) 'The humanization of healthcare: A value framework for qualitative research', *International Journal of Qualitative Studies on Health and Wellbeing*, 4, pp. 66–77.

Trachsel, M., Irwin, S., Biller-Andorno, N., Hoff, P. and Riese, F. (2016) 'Palliative psychiatry for severe persistent mental illness as a new approach to psychiatry? Definition, scope, benefits, and risks', *BMC Psychiatry*, 16, pp. 260. Available at: https://bmcpsychiatry.biomedcentral.com/articles/ 10.1186/s12888-016-0970-y (Accessed: 2 December 2017)

Whiteford, H., Ferrari, A., Dengenhardt, L., Feigin, T. and Vos, T. (2015) 'The global burden of mental, neurological and substance use disorders: An analysis form the Global Burden of Disease Study 2010', *Plos One*, 10, pp. 1–11. Available at: http://journals.plos.org/plosone/article?id=10. 1371/journal.pone.0116820 (Accessed: 2 December 2017)

Woods, A., Willison, K., Kington, C. and Gavin, A. (2008) 'Palliative care for people with severe persistent mental illness: A review of the literature', *The Canadian Journal of Psychiatry*, 53, pp. 725–35.

Wright, D., Lavoie-Tremblay, M., Drevniok, U., Racine, H. and Savignac, H. (2011) 'Relational dimensions of a positive integration of experience for new graduate mental health nurses', *Archives of Psychiatric Nursing*, 25, pp. 164–173.

To Learn More

Palliative Psychiatry

Trachsel, M., Irwin, S., Biller-Andorno, N., Hoff, P. and Riese, F. (2016) 'Palliative psychiatry for severe persistent mental illness as a new approach to psychiatry? Definition, scope, benefits, and risks', *BMC Psychiatry*, 16, p. 260. https://bmcpsychiatry.biomedcentral.com/articles/10.1186/ s12888-016-0970-y

Palliative Care Services for People with Severe Persistent Mental Health Problems and Disorders

Butler, H. and O'Brien, A. (2017) 'Access to specialist palliative care services by people with severe and persistent mental illness: A retrospective cohort study', *International Journal of Mental Health Nursing*, http://onlinelibrary.wiley.com/doi/10.1111/inm.12360/abstract.

Cooper, D. B. and Cooper, J. (2012) *Palliative Care within Mental Health: Principles and Philosophy.* New York: CRC Press.

Cooper, D. B. and Cooper, J. (2014) *Palliative Care within Mental Health: Care and Practice.* New York: CRC Press.

Protective Empowerment

Chiovitti, R. (2011) 'Theory of protective empowering for balancing patient safety and choices', *Nursing Ethics*, 18, pp. 88–101.

CHAPTER 6

Culture and Cultural Awareness

Roxanne Amerson

INTRODUCTION

> Culture is the collective programming of the mind that distinguishes the members
> of one group or category of people from others.
>
> (Hofstede 2011, p. 3)

While culture is a collective phenomenon associated with groups of people, great variety
may exist among the individuals of the group. Culture reflects every aspect of one's
life; thus, education, politics, economics, historical factors, family relationships, time,
communication, and human biological variations influence culture. Furthermore, culture
is defined as 'the totality of socially transmitted behavioral patterns, arts, beliefs, values,
customs, lifeways, and all other products of human work' (Purnell 2013, p. 6). Caring
for an individual's cultural needs goes beyond simply being aware of religious or spiritual
needs.

The work of Madeleine Leininger forever changed the professional practice of
healthcare through her development of the field of transcultural nursing. In the 1950s,
Leininger recognized differences in the ways parents from different ethnicities cared
for their children (Leininger & McFarland 2002; Leininger & McFarland 2006). This
led to her seminal work on the culture of caring and the universality of caring practices
of diverse people. This chapter will:

➤ examine key culture theories and models, which provide a foundation for cultural
  awareness
➤ distinguish between individualistic and collectivistic cultures
➤ identify cultural beliefs and practices among specific ethnicities, which have potential
  influence for palliative care in mental health.

Becoming culturally aware is the first step in providing culturally appropriate care for
all people.

CULTURAL THEORY AND MODELS

The Culture Care Theory

Madeleine Leininger developed the Culture Care Theory in the 1960s and published her
first book in 1970 (Leininger 2002). Her work was unique as it sought to combine the

caring practice of nursing and the research-based comparative view of cultures from anthropology. The Culture Care Theory provided a broad, holistic framework to discover the universalities (commonalities) and diversities (differences) of cultural groups. This theory is based on the central premise of caring.

KEY POINT 6.1

Caring must be present for curing to occur and curing cannot occur without caring. Caring when curing does not occur is a concept essential to the practice of palliative care.

Furthermore, the theoretical premise explains, 'culturally based care (caring) is essential to the individual's well-being, health, survival, or death' (Leininger 2002, p. 192). Professionals providing palliative care must recognize the influence of culture on an individual's response to injury, sickness, and even death.

The Sunrise Enabler by Leininger provides a visual representation of the factors that influence culture care according to the Theory of Cultural Care Diversity and Universality (Leininger & McFarland 2006). According to this enabler, cultural and social structure dimensions influence many factors (education, politics, economics, kinship, religion, technology, and cultural beliefs), which in turn influence the individual's or people's practices or beliefs during health, ill-health, and eventually death. During health, ill-health, or in preparation for death, two forms of nursing care exist: professional care and generic (folk) care. Doctors, nurses, or other health-related disciplines provide professional care. Generic (folk) care is provided by families or in the home setting and is heavily influenced by traditions passed from one generation to another. Health professionals seeking to provide culturally congruent care are encouraged to adapt treatments according to the three culturally based action and decision modes (Leininger & McFarland 2006):

1. Culture Care Preservation – this mode seeks to preserve and maintain practices that are helpful and do not provide any harm
2. Culture Care Accommodation – this mode seeks to accommodate or negotiate practices that may be helpful, but have the potential to be harmful
3. Culture Care Repatterning – this mode seeks to repattern or restructure harmful practices.

Choosing the appropriate mode of care will help to ensure the provision of culturally congruent care for health, well-being, and death.

THE PROCESS OF CULTURAL COMPETENCE IN THE DELIVERY OF HEALTHCARE SERVICES

Josepha Campinha-Bacote developed her model during the years shortly after Madeleine Leininger introduced the Theory of Culture Care. Campinha-Bacote (2002) sought to expand the transcultural nursing work of Leininger through the introduction of multicultural counseling techniques. This model focused on cultural competence as a process, not a final product.

KEY POINT 6.2

Health professionals must recognize that no one person can ever become completely competent in the field of transcultural care. Professionals are constantly evolving and learning about new cultures through a variety of experiences.

SELF-ASSESSMENT EXERCISE 6.1

Time: 15 minutes
Consider – personal attitudes or values needed to maintain competency in the field of transcultural care?

According to Campinha-Bacote (2002), her model consists of five cultural constructs:
1. Awareness – awareness is a process of self-reflection whereby the individual considers his or her own biases, prejudices, and values
2. Knowledge – knowledge is the cognitive process of learning about health beliefs, disease incidence, and treatments associated with specific cultural groups
3. Skill – skill is the ability to collect cultural information while performing a physical assessment
4. Encounters – encounters is the action of working alongside individuals or groups from diverse cultural backgrounds
5. Desire – desire is the willingness and attitude to become culturally aware and to provide culturally congruent care.

Campinha-Bacote's earlier work identified desire as the 'key and pivotal component' for the process of cultural competence with this component providing the motivation to engage in the process (2003, p. 14). Amerson (2009) postulates that encounters may be equally, if not more, influential in the process than desire, as health professionals may develop desire based on an encounter with someone from a different culture. A 25-item instrument, 'The Inventory for Assessing the Process of Cultural Competence – Revised', developed by Campinha-Bacote (2002) has been used to measure the constructs of the model among healthcare professionals (Bentley & Ellison 2007; Kardong-Edgren et al. 2010; Noble, Noble & Hand 2009).

SELF-ASSESSMENT EXERCISE 6.2

Time: 30 minutes
1. What are my personal experiences with end-of-life (EOL) care?
2. How do I expect to be medically treated or not treated when I am no longer able to care for myself physically or mentally?
3. What are my biases regarding curing when quality of life is negatively impacted?
4. What potential areas of conflict may arise between my personal beliefs and an individual for whom I am assigned to provide care?

THE PURNELL MODEL FOR CULTURAL COMPETENCE

Larry Purnell began his model as a framework for assisting nursing students to conduct cultural assessments (2002). His model posits 19 assumptions associated with providing culturally competent care including similar concepts derived from Leininger's work (e.g. all cultures have similarities and differences, culture influences the response to healthcare, cultural information must be incorporated in the nursing process to ensure culturally appropriate care). Collecting cultural information from 12 different domains:

1. overview of heritage
2. communication
3. family roles
4. workforce issues
5. biocultural ecology
6. high-risk behaviors
7. nutrition
8. pregnancy and childbearing practices
9. death rituals
10. spirituality
11. healthcare practices
12. healthcare practitioners.

… allows for a thorough understanding of cultural phenomena, which influences the individual's state of health. His model further emphasizes that health professionals may range from unconsciously incompetent, consciously incompetent, consciously competent, to unconsciously competent. Heath professionals must diligently work to become knowledgeable and competent in delivering cultural care. Purnell's recent work (2013) provides a collection of data for more than 30 different cultural-specific groups. Each group is analyzed based on the 12 domains for assessment of the individual, family, or group. Thus, providing an excellent resource for health professionals to learn about various cultural groups.

THE GIGER AND DAVIDHIZAR TRANSCULTURAL ASSESSMENT MODEL

This cultural assessment model addresses the six areas of cultural phenomena as presented by Giger and Davidhizar (2002). According to this model, health professionals should assess each area of phenomena to determine the unique aspects that will influence an individual's self-care as well as an individual's response to professional care. Cultural phenomena include:

1. Communication – language, dialect, paralanguage, body movements, and eye contact function as mechanisms for communication. Variation in communication patterns is associated with different ethnic and cultural groups. The health professional must be cognizant of his or her own communication patterns and how these patterns may facilitate or impede communication with an individual. Misunderstandings related to communication commonly occur due to cultural differences.
2. Space – the distance that is considered appropriate for intimate, personal, or public relationships varies greatly. Intimate space (0–18 inches) may be reserved for family or very close friends. Personal space is considered reserved for close friends or extended family, while public space is commonly associated with general friends

or colleagues. The health professional should be aware of differences in perceived 'appropriate' space among cultures. The use of touch varies widely; thus, it is important to ask permission before touching individuals.

3. Social organization – the recognition of family status and the roles of family members are based on cultural norms. Family members may include individuals who are not blood relatives. It is essential to clarify with individuals, whom do they consider family? Individuals that are more traditional tend to recognize a much larger, extended family compared to less traditional individuals who may associate with a more nuclear family unit.

4. Time – individuals may be past, present, or future-oriented. Past-oriented refers to cultures who rely on traditional beliefs to guide current thinking and actions. Present-oriented cultures tend to focus on the day-to-day routine of life, with less emphasis placed on future considerations. Future-oriented cultures are looking to the future and may be more open to preventative healthcare practices.

5. Environmental Control – control remains outside of the individual. Individuals may exhibit an internal or external locus of control. A common belief doctrine, fatalism, recognizes a higher power that controls the outcome of events. Individuals with a fatalistic view may fail to follow health advice because the long-term consequences of health are pre-determined by their higher power. This area of phenomenon may also include physical environmental factors that influence health.

6. Biological variations – physiological differences do exist between ethnic groups that may influence their response to medications. Disease susceptibility varies among ethnic groups as well. Nutritional variations exist and may lead to health problems or interactions with medications.

It is the responsibility of the health professional to be willing to take the time to assess these phenomena and adapt a plan of care to accommodate these variations. Adherence to a plan of care will be greatly influenced by the individual's unique beliefs and physiological state.

MULTICULTURAL COUNSELING AND THERAPY

Sue and Torino (as cited in Sue & Sue 2008, p. 42) define multicultural counseling and therapy (MCT) as:

> both a helping role and process that uses modalities and defines goals consistent with the life experiences and cultural values of clients, recognizes client identities to include individual, group, and universal dimensions, advocates the use of universal and culture-specific strategies and roles in the healing process, and balances the importance of individualism and collectivism in the assessment, diagnosis, and treatment of client and client systems.

This view of counseling closely parallels the work of Leininger by recognizing the importance of universal and diverse dimensions of cultural care. Sue and Sue (2008) further expand the concept of culturally competent care by focusing on the unique aspects of this model, which include broader roles for counselors, deliberate use of life experiences and cultural values, culture-specific strategies during therapy, individualistic and collectivistic approaches, and an appropriate systems approach. Individuals of diverse ethnicities may experience mental health issues that result from system-initiated prejudice, bias, and racism.

Similar to the work of Campinha-Bacote, Sue and Sue (2008) suggest three competencies for providing cultural competence. The first competency is to increase awareness of one's own prejudice and biases. The second competency focuses on knowledge and understanding of the worldview of the individual, which may conflict with the view of the health provider. The third competency addresses the development of appropriate interventions based on culture-specific knowledge. In addition, competencies are divided into the three learning domains of attitudes, knowledge, and skills. Therefore, they posit a multidimensional model of cultural competence in counseling with three dimensions:

1. group-specific worldviews (specific ethnic groups)
2. components of cultural competence (attitudes, knowledge, skills)
3. foci of therapeutic interventions (individual, professional, organizational, and societal).

One clear distinction between MCT and the traditional counseling roles is the helping role. Differences in worldviews of individuals may require the health provider to function as a consultant, change agent, teacher, or advocate in mental health situations.

INDIVIDUALISM AND COLLECTIVISM

Health professionals working alongside individuals and families must be cognizant of the cultural dimensions of individualism and collectivism, which determine how individuals respond within groups and independently of others. While many researchers have viewed these cultural dimensions through the lens of social systems, economic development, cultural patterns, and self-concept (Powers 2013); the consensus among cultural experts is that individualism focuses on the independence of the individual, while collectivism focuses on the shared needs of the group (Triandis 2001). Understanding this concept is crucial to working effectively with an individual and with the individual as a member of a group.

Individualistic cultures have historically developed from hunter – gatherer societies where the individual relies on his or her own skills to meet the needs of survival, whereas collectivistic cultures tend to have origins in agrarian societies where members must rely on help to plant, tend, and harvest fields to sustain the needs of the group (Powers 2013). Furthermore, individualistic cultures tend to have smaller, more nuclear families as compared with collectivistic cultures with large, extended families. The collective needs of the family are considered paramount to the needs of the individual. Even the distribution of wealth and the level of education may be linked to this cultural dimension. Researchers have found that as economic resources increase, an individual may have the means to act more independently with less reliance on family or group support. Younger and more highly educated individuals also tend to display more characteristics of individualism than older, less educated individuals who may be more dependent on the resources of the family.

Individualistic cultures encourage the individual to be independent and responsible for their own actions, decisions, and consequences with less regard for input from

Table 6.1 Examples of individualistic and collectivistic cultures (Purnell 2013, p. 9)

Individualistic	Collectivistic
European American	Arabic
British	Amish
Canadian	Chinese
German	Filipino
Norwegian	Korean
Swedish	Japanese
	Latin American
	Mexican American
	American Indians
	Thai
	Vietnamese

others. Individualistic cultures tend to have individually oriented goals (Powers 2013). In contrast, collectivistic cultures encourage decisions and actions that value the group needs over the individual. Therefore, the consequences of actions must benefit the needs of the group. Even individualism influences emotions, with individuals commonly displaying egocentric behaviors and collectivistic cultures tending to display more empathy for the needs of others within the group. Of importance are the differences in values between individualism and collectivism. A sense of adventure, willingness to take a risk, self-pleasure, uniqueness, privacy, creativity, and self-reliance are associated with individualism (Powers 2013; Triandis 2001). Conformity, harmony, equality, shared information, reliability, and interdependence are associated with collectivism (Powers 2013; Triandis 2001). It must be acknowledged that an individual or a cultural group do not adhere to these values consistently at all times. An individual or group will exist on a continuum with circumstances that allow the person or group to display the tendencies appropriate for the situation (Triandis 2001). For example, the potential for individualistic behavior increases in situations when others are making individual decisions, the person sees himself distinct from others, the action is competitive, or the situation is public. An individual will tend more toward collectivistic behavior when others are working collaboratively, the individual comes from a collectivistic family or culture, the focus is on members with similarities, or the action is cooperative (Powers 2013). Understanding this cultural dimension can prove instrumental in developing an approach for working alongside the individual experiencing mental health problems, or the individual's family (*See* Table 6.1).

Specific ethnic groups have been identified as more likely to be individualistic compared to collectivistic. East Asian cultures commonly display behaviors or values that demonstrate a higher esteem for their group members than the individual self (Heine & Buchtel 2009). Their behavior depends upon their audience and is commonly adjusted to reflect the expectations of the audience. The need to save face for the group may even facilitate deceit, because morality is based on what the group expects or needs (Triandis 2001). In contrast, western cultures such as the citizens of the United

States (US) tend to be more likely to act independently with less concern for the expectations of the audience. Western cultures tend to engage in more self-esteem and self-enhancing behaviors as they act more independently. Asians may engage in less self-enhancing behaviors as they rely more on the regard of the group in which they are interdependent. East Asian cultures tend to be more concerned with maintaining harmony in their interpersonal relationships, than a positive self-image. Clearly, this cultural implication has relevance for working alongside individuals experiencing chronic depression or dysphoria.

Relational mobility refers to the ability to form new relationships. American college students display a higher level of relational mobility as they are constantly forming new relationships and meeting new individuals. In Japanese societies, a lower level of relational mobility is observed as individuals tend to belong to, and remain in groups, with limited movement outside the established group (Heine & Buchtel 2009). Understanding the propensity for relational mobility may enhance or limit therapies that require group therapy with individualistic or collectivistic groups.

Communication is influenced by individualism and collectivism as well (Triandis 2001).

KEY POINT 6.3

Individualistic cultures tend to use low context communication, meaning the specific words or content of the message is most important. In collectivistic cultures, high context communication is valued. High context communication focuses heavily on voice volume, tone, body posture, eye contact; therefore, 'how' something is said is more important than 'what' is said (Purnell 2013; Triandis 2001).

Respect and high priority for maintaining harmony in collectivistic cultures also influences the communication process. An individual from a collectivistic culture is less likely to disagree openly with the health professional and may simply nod his or her head, 'yes', in order to maintain harmony, rather than create conflict (Purnell 2013). Subsequently, the cultural implications of these communication styles will influence the response and veracity of counseling sessions in mental health.

Developing an appreciation of the important aspects of individualistic and collectivistic cultures is essential for working alongside individuals and families in mental health. Collectivistic cultures are more likely to expect family members to participate in care and decision-making, especially in end-of-life (EOL) situations. Individuals will decide what is best for the group or respond in a manner that is expected by the family or group. The health professional must be in tune to this and be flexible to accommodate group expectations, rather than focus solely on the individual. Conversely, the individualistic family may choose to leave all decisions to the affected individual and take the stance, 'Whatever he or she wants is best'. In all situations, the optimal approach is to explore how decisions are commonly made within the family or group. This will provide the best direction for the health professional to determine where the individual resides along the continuum from individualism to collectivism.

SELF-REFLECTIVE EXERCISE 6.3

Time: 45 minutes

> **Case Study 6.1**
>
> You have been assigned to care for Rosa Morales. She is an 84-year-old, Guatemalan woman with a recent diagnosis of late-stage Alzheimer's disease. She is bedridden, requires total care, and has recently begun choking on foods and fluids. Until recently, her family has been providing all the care for Mrs. Morales in the family home. The family physician has ordered a consult for placement of a gastrostomy tube to begin feedings. Large numbers of family members have arrived at the hospital and are waiting in the hospital room and hallways. This has become a distraction for the staff and other patients. The remainder of Mrs. Morales's children are expected to arrive from Guatemala in the next day or two. A decision for the care of their mother will not be made until the oldest son has arrived from Guatemala City.

- How do you accommodate the large number of family members, while maintaining a restful environment for other individuals on your unit?
- Several staff members have expressed frustration in waiting for one son when at least two of Mrs. Morales's daughters are here and could give consent. How do you address the frustration of the staff?
- Several of the family members have made comments that this 'new feeding tube' will make their mother well again. It is clear that they do not have a realistic understanding that the feeding tube will not restore Mrs. Morales's previous condition. How do you help them to understand the intent of the feeding tube?

CULTURAL BELIEFS AND PRACTICES

Health professionals delivering palliative and mental health care need to explore and seek to understand the cultural beliefs associated with mental health, death, dying, and EOL care issues among specific ethnic groups. It is important to reflect on the work of Campinha-Bacote and Purnell related to this section. Cultural competence is a process and health professionals never become fully competent (Campinha-Bacote 2002). As the health professional seeks knowledge of various ethnic groups, it allows movement along a continuum of becoming more culturally competent (Purnell 2013). The following section serves as a starting point to understanding the differences in cultural beliefs and is not meant to be all-inclusive. Readers are encouraged to learn about the unique communities in which they serve. Commonalities do exist among specific groups of people, but it is crucial to confirm with individuals and their families their unique beliefs and values that deviate from the overall group.

BELIEFS ASSOCIATED WITH MENTAL ILL-HEALTH

Health professionals should begin care with an understanding of what the individual believes contributed to the origin of mental health disorders. Cultures who prescribe to a biomedical perspective are most likely to understand that mental health disorders stem from physiological processes or psychosocial trauma among other things. In more traditional cultures or indigenous cultures, individuals may attribute mental ill-health to supernatural forces. A multiethnic study with Whites, Latinos, African-Americans, and Asian-Americans found significant differences in cultural attitudes about mental ill-health among older adults (Jimenez et al. 2012). In this study, African-Americans contributed mental ill-health to stress and loss compared with Asian-Americans who contributed mental ill-health to family issues, medical problems, and cultural differences. Beliefs about the etiology of the mental ill-health strongly influenced the preference for help-seeking behaviors and the type of health professional to consult. African-Americans were more likely to seek spiritual help from family or friends and less likely to consult a psychologist or psychiatrist. Asian-Americans were less likely to consult any type of professional, while Latinos were less likely to consult a medical doctor. The researchers acknowledge that Asian-Americans represent an ethnic group with vast differences depending on the country of origin, but this finding is consistent with the considerable stigma of mental ill-health that contributes to loss of face among Filipino cultures (Tuliao 2014). Kleinman, Eisenberg and Good (1978) recommend that health professionals begin care by inquiring with the following questions:

➤ What caused the problem?
➤ When did the problem begin?
➤ How does the problem affect you?
➤ How do you think the problem should be treated?

Asking these questions will allow the health professional to understand the individual's beliefs regarding the causes of mental ill-health and the most appropriate treatment. This helps to establish trust and respect that the individual's beliefs are valued, even if the beliefs conflict with the recognized etiology and treatment plan of the health professional. This provides a foundation to work toward a mutually agreed care plan.

STIGMA AND MENTAL ILL-HEALTH

Researchers have identified stigma associated with mental ill-health (Al-Alawi et al. 2017; Tawiah, Adongo & Aikins 2015; Tuliao 2014) Stigma may be perceived or enacted (Tawiah, Adongo & Aikins 2015), meaning that perceived stigma may be imagined while enacted stigma results in acts of discrimination. Mental health disorders affect the individual's ability to cope with life stresses and to manage daily activities for a satisfying life within a community. When stigma occurs, either real or imagined, it negatively influences the willingness of the individual to seek treatment, to share the diagnosis, and contributes to feelings of isolation or hopelessness. While stigma is documented in all regions of the world, it may be more prominent in certain cultures. In Oman, researchers identified a clear trend of negative attitudes associated with people experiencing mental ill-health (Al-Alawi et al. 2017). Younger generations reflected more negative attitudes than older age groups, which may be associated with the collectivistic mind set of older Omanis. Collectivistic cultures are more likely to support each other and promote social cohesion. Moreover, negative attitudes were found to be more prevalent in rural communities than urban settings, where people have learned to be more tolerant of others in confined spaces. A review of literature associated with mental health among Filipinos found significant evidence of public and private stigma contributing to an unwillingness to seek professional help, as the stigma of mental ill-health was associated with shame and embarrassment (Tuliao 2014). In this cultural group, the 'loss of face' (shame or embarrassment) may affect social standing within the community. Additionally, people experiencing mental health disorders are more likely to seek the treatment of lay providers or folk healers from the community, rather than a health professional who is an 'outsider' to the community. Filipinos may prefer online counseling as an alternative to face-to-face counseling to reduce the loss of face.

Stigma associated with mental ill-health transcends geographical boundaries. In Latin America, Mascayano et al. (2016) noted that individuals experiencing mental ill-health expressed feelings of stigma from mental health professionals and felt significant social distance when diagnosed with schizophrenia. Fear associated with working alongside or being around individuals experiencing mental ill-health contributed to a decreased quality of life and lower self-esteem for the individual experiencing a mental health disorder. Stigma generated from the family toward the individual experiencing mental ill-health was common and frequently resulted from a lack of knowledge about the diagnosis. Stigma increases when individuals display behaviors that deviate from social norms or appear odd. Thus, increasing the social isolation and decreasing the social support that is needed when mental health disorders exacerbate. This critical period of increasing dysfunction may benefit the most from palliative care measures.

Furthermore, stigma can lead to economic, social, and psychological consequences (Shrivastava, Johnston & Bureau 2012). Individuals experiencing mental ill-health may be reluctant to allow employers information about a diagnosis, yet the diagnosis may affect job performance and result in unemployment. This further complicates the situation as a loss of employment may lead to a loss of insurance; thereby resulting in the inability to pay for treatment or medications. The economic consequences then continue, psychological consequences are precipitated by treatment delays and medication non-compliance. The increasing psychological dysfunction further influences social support from families or the community. Family responses may represent one of the most significant sources of discrimination resulting from the stigma of mental ill-health (Mascayano et al. 2106). The stigma of mental ill-health perpetuates a vicious cycle resulting in hopelessness and further isolation.

Mental ill-health represents a significant burden of disease in low-to-middle-income countries (LMICs) as compared to high income countries (Mascayano, Armijo & Yang 2015). Governments in LMICs spend the least on mental health services with most care provided in psychiatric institutions, if care is even available. It is estimated that approximately 75 percent of individuals experiencing mental ill-health do not receive care in LMICs. Individuals coming from LMICs are more reluctant to seek care based on their previous experiences in their home countries where quality care is severely lacking, even when quality care is available. The stigma of mental ill-health is particularly strong in LMICs and affects the most vulnerable populations, such as the poor, women, and indigenous populations. In Latin American cultures, women are expected to fulfill their duties to the family, even when personal physical and mental health present challenges. A woman who is unable to fulfill her obligation to the family will experience even greater stigma within the family (Mascayano et al. 2016). It is important for health professionals to understand the cultural implications of mental health stigma when caring for immigrants and refugees who may need palliative care.

BELIEFS RELATED TO DEATH AND DYING

Palliative care focuses on improving the quality of life, regardless of the stage of ill-health, in contrast to hospice care, which generally focuses on the last six months of life. Yet, every health professional working in palliative care or using a palliative care approach must deal with death, dying, and end-of-life (EOL) care issues. Therefore, it is essential to recognize the cultural implications associated with these concepts. A study conducted in Australia with a multicultural cohort, including Anglo-Celtic, Mediterranean, Eastern European, and Asia/Pacific, found significant differences in beliefs regarding death, dying, truth telling, and advance directives (Ohr, Jeong & Saul 2016). Approximately 50 percent of participants believed death should be avoided at all costs, although Eastern Europeans and Asia/Pacific participants most often indicated this belief. Almost 75 percent of the participants wanted to be informed by their doctor if they were dying, but this preference was slightly higher in Anglo-Celtics. Yet, only 27 percent of participants had actually talked with their doctor about any form of advance directive. Furthermore, 80 percent wanted to die free of pain, which was more important than prolonging life and 60 percent wanted to die at home. Of particular interest, 60 percent of Asia/Pacific participants preferred to be in the hospital or to go to the emergency department at the time of death. Clearly, different preferences for EOL care exist among cultural groups.

Not only do individuals and families have different preferences for EOL care, but the cultural values of the health professional have the potential to influence the plan of care. Culture influences perceptions of certain diseases, such as cancer. In Chinese cultures, health professionals give a higher priority to allowing the family to make the decision whether to inform the individual of a terminal diagnosis. In Western cultures, health professionals place a higher priority on the autonomy of the individual and usually insist on informing the individual of the terminal diagnosis. This clearly represents an ethical dilemma in palliative care settings. In Chinese culture, maintaining hope for the dying individual is paramount (Dong et al. 2016). Traditional Chinese tradition dictates that death should not be discussed with the dying patient and to do so will diminish hope. A similar belief is common in traditional African cultures, where talk of death is taboo, and individuals do not prepare advance directives (Ekore & Lanre-Abass 2016). Health professionals in China may go as far as avoiding terms such as 'cancer' or 'tumor' and instead refer to 'the disease'. In the study by Dong et al. (2016), physical contact was important to express concern for the individual and as well as providing 'false hope' to help individuals continue to live well until the moment of death. Pain management was a high priority for the dying individual. Communicating with the family of the dying individual to ensure appropriate decision-making, treatment, and arrangements after death necessitated highly developed communication skills among health professionals.

Even death itself represents a concept with wide variation among cultures. How does one define a 'good death'? Health professionals commonly associate pain management, symptom control, autonomy for advance directives, and a sense of peace as components required for a good death. In a study with American Indians of South Dakota, dying alone or being abandoned was a significant fear (Schrader, Nelson & Eidsness 2009). For this group, dying at home and preparing for death by reviewing life events with family would lead to a good death. A multiyear, qualitative study initiated in 1997 and continued through 2007 examined the perceptions of a good death for cancer patients enrolled in palliative care (Kastbom, Milberg & Karisson 2017). Participants in this Swedish study described the importance of preparing for death, which required knowledge of their impending death. Furthermore, independence and autonomy were highly valued. These values are far different from the cultural expectation previously discussed related to traditional Chinese culture. Swedish individuals preferred to prepare for death by saying goodbye to loved ones and family. Independence equated with acts of autonomy regarding decision-making about the events surrounding the time of death. One similarity with the Chinese culture surfaced as health professionals expressed the need for strong communication skills to help families with the approaching death and the loss of hope. The researchers suggest asking individuals directly (Kastbom, Milberg & Karisson 2017, p. 937), 'Have you ever experienced the illness and death of a family member or friend'? This question may open the door to conversations that allow the health professional to understand what the individual or family expects or wants in the context of a good death.

CONCLUSION

The specific cultural examples presented here represent only a small glimpse into the vast realm of cultural beliefs surrounding mental health and palliative care. The value of conducting a cultural assessment of individual beliefs cannot be overly emphasized.

KEY POINT 6.4

Recognition of cultural beliefs that are common among groups of people is the foundation upon which to build and identification of individual variations is crucial.

The following key points (6.5) are recommended to provide culturally appropriate care.

KEY POINT 6.5

➤ Understand that help-seeking behaviors are influenced by past experiences with racism, discrimination, and violations of social justice and may need to be addressed before moving forward with a treatment plan (Tuliao 2014).

➤ Support the family strength and social networks among collectivistic cultures to mitigate the stigma and isolation associated with mental ill-health when possible (Mascayano et al. 2016).

➤ Seek out successful anti-stigma programs developed in LMICs to help migrants or refugees cope with the stigma of mental ill-health, to increase self-esteem, and to increase care-giving by families (Mascayano, Armijo & Yang 2015).

➤ Identify high-context communication cues to communicate with individuals and facilitate true agreement on interventions (Tuliao 2014).

➤ Recognize that establishing a personal relationship with individuals may be required to gain the trust of individuals from cultures where 'losing face' is highly regarded (Tuliao 2014). The personal relationship allows the health professional to move from stranger to trusted friend (Leininger 2002).

➤ Incorporate non-detrimental, traditional mental healthcare practices into the treatment plan along with Western biomedical treatments based on the preferences of the individual (Leininger 2012; Leininger & McFarland 2006; Mascayano, Armijo & Yang 2015).

➤ Recognize that the health professional's preferences for a good death may vary from the preferences of the individual (Kastbom, Milberg & Karisson 2017).

➤ Recognize that culture and religion will affect preferences for EOL care directives and truth telling (Ohr, Jeong & Saul 2016).

➤ Inquire about EOL care preferences before documenting advance care directives (Ohr, Jeong & Saul 2016).

➤ Provide education about palliative or hospice programs that are available and the benefits of pain management and medications to complement other measures for a good death (Schrader, Nelson & Eidsness 2009).

REFERENCES

Al-Alawi, M., Al-Sinawi, H., Al-Adawi, S., Jeyaseelan, L. and Murthi, S. (2017) 'Public perception of mental illness in Oman: a cross sectional study', *International Journal of Culture and Mental Health*, 10, pp. 389–99. Available at: 10.1080/17542863.2017.1325916 (Accessed: 22 November 2017)

Amerson, R. (2009) *The influence of international service-learning on cultural competence in baccalaureate nursing graduates and their subsequent nursing practice* (Doctoral dissertation, Clemson University). Available at: http://tigerprints.clemson.edu/cgi/viewcontent.cgi?article=1457&context=all_dissertations (Accessed: 22 November 2017).

Bentley, R. and Ellison, K. (2007) 'Increasing cultural competence in nursing through international service-learning experiences', *Nurse Educator*, 32, pp. 207–11. Available at: 10.1097/01.NNE.0000289385.14007.b4 (Accessed: 22 November 2017)

Campinha-Bacote, J. (2002) 'The process of cultural competence in the delivery of healthcare services: a model of care', *Journal of Transcultural Nursing*, 13, pp. 181–4. Available at: 10.1177/10459602013003003 (Accessed: 22 November 2017)

Campinha-Bacote, J. (2003) *The Process of Cultural Competence in the Delivery of Healthcare: A Culturally Competent Model of Care.* Cincinnati, OH: Transcultural C.A.R.E. Associates.

Dong, F., Zheng, R., Chen, X., Wang, Y., Zhou, H. and Sun, R. (2016) 'Caring for dying cancer patients in the Chinese cultural context: A qualitative study form the perspectives of physicians and nurses', *European Journal of Oncology Nursing*, 21, pp. 189–96. Available at: 10.1016/j.ejon.2015.10.003 (Accessed: 22 November 2017)

Ekore, R. and Lanre-Abass, B. (2016) 'African cultural concept of death and the idea of advance care directives', *Indian Journal of Palliative Care*, 22, pp. 369–72. Available at: 10.4103/0973–1075.191741 (Accessed: 22 November 2017)

Giger, J. and Davidhizar, R. (2002) 'The Giger and Davidhizar transcultural assessment model', *Journal of Transcultural Nursing*, 13, pp. 185–8. Available at: 10.1177/10459602013003004 (Accessed: 22 November 2017)

Heine, S. J. and Buchtel, E. (2009) 'Personality: the universal and the cultural specific', *Annual Review of Psychology*, 60, pp. 169–94. Available at: 10.1146/annurev.psych.60.110707.163655 (Accessed: 22 November 2017)

Hofstede, G. (2011) 'Dimesionalizing cultures: the Hofstede model in context', *Online Readings in Psychology and Culture*, 2. Available at: https://doi.org/10.9707/2307–0919.1014 Accessed: 22 November 2017)

Jimenez, D., Bartels, S., Cardenas, V., Daliwal, S. and Alegria, M. (2012) 'Cultural beliefs and mental health treatment preferences of ethnically diverse older adult consumers in primary care', *American*

Journal of Geriatric Psychiatry, 20(6), pp. 533–542. [Online] DOI: 10.1097/JGP.0b013e318227f876 (Accessed: 31 October 2017)

Kardong-Edgren, S., Cason, C., Brennan, A., Reifsnider, E., Hummel, F., Mancini, M. and Griffin, C. (2010) 'Cultural competency: graduating BSN students', *Nursing Education Perspectives*, 31, pp. 278–85.

Kastbom, L., Milberg, A. and Karisson, M. (2017) 'A good death from the perspective of palliative cancer patients', *Support Care Cancer*, 25, pp. 933–9. Available at: 10.1007/s00520-016-3483-9 (Accessed: 22 November 2017)

Kleinman, A., Eisenberg, L. and Good, B. (1978) 'Culture, illness, and care: clinical lessons from anthropologic and cross-cultural research', *Annals of Internal Medicine*, 88, pp. 251–8.

Leininger, M. (2002) 'Culture care theory: a major contribution to advance transcultural nursing and practices', *Journal of Transcultural Nursing*, 13, pp. 189–92. Available at: 10.1177/104596020130 03005 (Accessed: 22 November 2017)

Leininger, M. and McFarland, M. (2002) *Transcultural Nursing: Concepts, Theories, Research & Practice.* 3rd edition. New York, NY: McGraw-Hill Companies, Inc.

Leininger, M. and McFarland, M. (2006) *Culture Care Diversity and Universality: A Worldwide Nursing Theory.* 2nd edition. Sudbury, MA: Jones and Bartlett.

Mascayano, F., Armijo, J. and Yang, L. (2015) 'Addressing stigma relating to mental illness in low- and middle-income countries', *Frontiers in Psychiatry*, 8, pp. 1–4. Available at: 10.3389/fpsyt.2015. 00038 (Accessed: 22 November 2017)

Mascayano, F., Tapia, T., Schilling, S., Alvarado, R., Tapia, E., et al. (2016) 'Stigma toward mental illness in Latin America and the Caribbean: a systemic review. *Revista Brasileira de Psiquiatria*, 38, pp. 73–85. Available at: 10.1590/1516–4446–2015–1652 (Accessed: 22 November 2017)

Noble, L., Noble, A. and Hand, I. (2009) 'Cultural competence of healthcare professionals caring for breastfeeding mothers in urban areas', *Breastfeeding Medicine*, 4, pp. 221–4. Available at: 10.1089/ bfm.2009.0020 (Accessed: 22 November 2017)

Ohr, S., Jeong, S. and Saul, P. (2016) 'Cultural and –religious beliefs and values, and their impact on preferences for end-of-life care among four ethnic groups of community-dwelling older persons', *Journal of Clinical Nursing*, 26, pp. 1681–9. Available at: 10.1111/jocn.13572 (Accessed: 22 November 2017)

Power, S. (2013) 'Implications of individualism and collectivism on the individual's social identity', CMC Senior Thesis, Paper 658. http://scholarship.claremont.edu/cmc_theses/658.

Purnell, L. (2002) 'The Purnell Model for cultural competence', *Journal of Transcultural Nursing*, 13, pp. 193–6. Available at: 10.1177/10459602013003006 (Accessed: 22 November 2017)

Purnell, L. (2013) *Transcultural Health Care: A Culturally Competent Approach.* 4th edition. Philadelphia, PA: F.A. Davis Company.

Schrader, S., Nelson, M. and Eidsness, L. (2009) 'Reflections on end of life: Comparison of American Indian and Non-Indian peoples of South Dakota', *American Indian Culture and Research Journal*, 33, pp. 67–87. Available at: 10.17953/aicr.33.2.j4528878vk615j7g (Accessed: 22 November 2017)

Shrivastava, A., Johnston, M. and Bureau, Y. (2012) 'Stigma of mental illness-1: Clinical reflections,' *Mens Sana Monographs*, 10, pp. 70–84. Available at: 10.4103/0973–1229.90181 (Accessed: 22 November 2017)

Sue, D. W. and Sue, D. (2008) *Counseling the Culturally Diverse: Theory and Practice.* 5th edition. Hoboken, NJ: John Wiley & Sons, Inc.

Tawiah, P., Adongo, P. and Aikins, M. (2015) 'Mental health-related stigma and discrimination in Ghana: Experience of patients and their caregivers', *Ghana Medical Journal*, 49, pp. 30–6.

Triandis, H. (2001) 'Individualism-collectivism and personality', *Journal of Personality*, 69, pp. 907–24. Available at: 10.1111/1467-6494.696169 (Accessed: 22 November 2017)

Tuliao, A. (2014) 'Mental health help seeking among Filipinos: A review of the literature', *Asia Pacific Journal of Counseling and Psychotherapy*, 5, pp. 124–36. Available at: 10.1080/21507686.2014.913641 (Accessed: 22 November 2017)

To Learn More

AMCD Multicultural Counseling Competencies (n.d.) www.counseling.org/Resources/Competencies/Multcultural_Competencies.pdf.

Dimensions of Culture: Cross-Cultural Communication for Healthcare Professionals (n.d.) www.dimensionsofculture.com/2010/11/cultural-aspects-of-death-and-dying/.

Multicultural care at the time of death and dying. (n.d.) www.alfredicu.org.au/assets/Documents/ICU-Guidelines/DeathAndDying/CALDMulticulturalCareDeathDying.pdf.

CHAPTER 7

Sex, Gender, and Sexuality

Lyn Merryfeather

THEORETICAL FRAMEWORK

In his book, *I and Thou*, Martin Buber (1970) describes the difference between relationships that are reciprocal and ones that are simply experiences. Experience, he says, is remoteness that creates an *I-it*, and only as I step into relationship do I know *I-you*. He describes people encountered this way as: 'no longer He or She, limited by other Hes and Shes, a dot in the world grid of space and time, nor a condition that can be experienced and described, a loose bundle of named qualities. Neighborless and seamless, he is You and fills the firmament' (p. 59).

Buber (1970) believed that beholding others (and sometimes things) as *you* rather than *it* 'is the cradle of actual life' (p. 60).

Buber's (1970) ideas were personified for me in the movie *Avatar* (Cameron 2009). In this movie, a soldier inhabits an avatar that looks like one of the native people on the planet his army had destined for invasion. He enters the world of the Na'vi people intending an *I-it* experience but discovers a relational *I-you* with the people and with his own avatar. He falls in love with a Na'vi woman who eventually discovers he is not actually one of her own, but rather a small and unattractive man (compared to her people) who is paralyzed from the waist down. One of the sayings the native people have in relating to one another is 'I see you' and this woman truly sees him through the eyes of love. She rescues him and helps him to inhabit his avatar permanently, since that is who he knows himself to be. This was fresh in my mind as I took up my new head nurse position in a small facility dedicated to caring for physically challenged older adults.

I met a man there in his 60s who liked to dress in women's clothing in the privacy of his room. The staff were aware of his preference but it was not general knowledge to management or the other residents. This person had sustained a head injury in childhood that resulted in blindness and poor impulse control but in all other respects was competent to make his own decisions. Because he was blind, he needed help from the care staff in choosing clothes that suited him. The staff were very supportive when he decided he would like to wear women's clothes full time. At this point I became involved and asked him if he wanted to use a feminine name and be addressed in feminine pronouns. He said this was something he had wanted for a long time but was afraid his family would disapprove. He felt like a woman and wanted to try living as one, and chose the name Susan (a pseudonym). I called a staff meeting and gained the understanding and cooperation of everyone. The chosen name, the pronouns, the clothing all were easily managed and the resident was happier than many had seen her for years. She was finally seen for whom she felt she always was. Her brother and his family lived in another town and rarely visited. However, when they did visit after the changes were put into place, they were furious. The family demanded that management instruct me and the care staff to call their sibling by a masculine name, remove all the feminine clothing, and revert to treating them (used in the singular) as a man.

The treatment of this resident left the staff and me with serious ethical questions. We engaged her in an *I-you* relationship and embraced her and her choices as we would any other resident. The family not only related to this person in an *I-it* experience, but also tried to force the staff to their way of thinking. They didn't really see any of us and our best intentions for their family member, nor did they see her as a person who could make choices for herself. Unfortunately, this is not an unusual occurrence anywhere for people who express a gender that is different from the sex they were declared at birth, but it is especially so for those who live in a situation where they are cared for by others.

The answer to providing culturally safe care for everyone is to enter into an *I-you* relationship with them and 'see' people for who they believe they are. This way of encountering others is foundational to all of what I am about to illustrate in the rest of the chapter.

VOCABULARY

It is like visiting a foreign country for many of us in learning about gender, sex, and sexuality that is expressed differently or on a continuum from what we have been taught by our culture. It is important to know a few key words in the language of this land in order to relate to the inhabitants in a respectful manner.

SEX

Sex refers to the identification made at birth based on external genitalia. If there is a penis, the child is declared male and every attempt is made to raise it as a boy. If there is something 'wrong' with the penis or there isn't one, the child is identified as female and raised as a girl. Until fairly recently ambiguity in this sexing was considered an emergency and steps were taken quickly and sometimes without the parents' consent to correct the genitals so the child could be designated as male or female (Davis & Murphy 2013). Male and female are often presented as the only two viable choices. In truth, there are several choices for designating sex. Along with male or female, there is intersex, neither, or both. In any case, sex can be unapparent or hidden.

GENDER

If 'sex' is about the physical body's parts, 'gender' is about soul expression written on the body. Gender is what we read on a person's body, or struggle to identify, when we first meet. It is an expression or a performance of belief in whom we really are. The soldier in *Avatar*, even though he was born human, saw himself as a Na'vi, and that is who he became. Some people are born with female genitalia and are declared girls at birth but see themselves and believe in themselves as male. They might never be able to erase or deny their chromosomes but they can identify as male and dress and behave in masculine ways. They can even alter their bodies to conform more closely to their chosen gender. On the other hand, some people do not identify as masculine or feminine. They prefer the pronoun 'they' used in the singular as their designation.

Recently, the Global Citizen, a webpage devoted to alternative news, told the story of a Canadian baby born to a person whose gender is fluid who has been issued a genderless health card (Marchildon 2017). The parent uses 'they' for themselves and says of their baby: 'I'm raising Searyl in such a way that until they have the sense of self and command of vocabulary to tell me who they are, I'm recognizing them as a baby and trying to give them all the love and support to be the most whole person that they can be outside of the restrictions that come with the boy box and the girl box' (Para 8).

SEXUALITY

Sexuality is quite apart from sex or gender but is often conflated with them. For example, it is often assumed that a man who expresses himself in more feminine behaviors is sexually attracted to other men and masculine women are lesbians. This is frequently a mistaken idea. As I have shown above, gender does not follow sex, just as sexuality does not follow gender presentation. Both men who express themselves in feminine ways and women who seem more masculine can be solidly heterosexual while 'manly' men and 'girly' women can be attracted to same-sex partners.

LESBIAN, GAY, BISEXUAL, TRANSGENDER, QUESTIONING, INTERSEX (LGBTQI)

This combination of letters encompasses both sexuality and gender. Lesbian, gay, and bisexual, indicate sexuality. Lesbian and gay also usually indicate sex in that lesbians are usually women and gays are frequently men, although some use this last term as an all-encompassing one denoting non-heterosexuality. However, people born male who express their gender as feminine can be lesbians and vice versa. Bisexual is not a gendered term and can be applied to any gender and indicates someone whose sexual attraction is not confined to only certain genders. Intersex can refer to a person born with either ambiguous genitalia or genitals of both male and female sexes or any combination of genitalia. A person who identifies as intersex might express their gender in various ways. The letter Q indicates questioning and usually means sexuality but it could also apply to other areas of questioning. Transgender is a blanket term that can apply to those who express their gender differently from the sex assigned at birth and can also include transsexual to indicate people who have altered their bodies to more closely conform to their chosen sex.

A ROSE BY ANY OTHER NAME

What difference can a name make? And isn't using the correct pronoun just a matter of semantics? In her classic book *Gender Outlaw* (1994), Kate Bornstein writes about her experience of being called by the wrong pronoun. She says: 'All the joy sucked out of my life in that instant, and every moment I'd ever fucked up crashed down on my head' (p. 126).

In later discussions of this event Bornstein discovered that all three participants were very aware of the mistake yet each one chose to ignore it, to brush it under the rug as an insignificant slip. Maya Angelou says: 'Words are things. You must be careful, careful about calling people out of their names, using racial pejoratives and sexual pejoratives and all that ignorance. Don't do that. Some day we'll be able to measure the power of words. I think they are things. They get on the walls. They get in your wallpaper. They get in your rugs, in your upholstery, and your clothes, and finally in to you' (Angelou 2017, p. 24).

In the famous line from Romeo and Juliet, 'What's in a name? That which we call a rose . . . by any other name would smell as sweet' (Literary Devices 2017), Shakespeare seems to have Juliet saying that the fact that Romeo was a Montague rather than a Capulet made no difference. In fact, it made the difference between life and death for these lovers. And so, it does for anyone who identifies outside the normative male female dichotomy. Judith Butler (2006) puts it this way:

> Since justice not only or exclusively is a matter of how persons are treated, how societies are constituted, but also emerges in quite consequential decisions about what a person is, what social norms must be honored and expressed for personhood to become allocated, how we do or do not recognize animate others as persons depending on whether or not we recognize a certain norm manifested in and by the body of that other.
>
> (Butler 2006, p. 184)

She goes on to show that persons who are not recognized for who they are, not called by their preferred name or pronoun, are effectively rendered not human.

Elizabeth (a pseudonym) was over six feet tall, wore size ten shoes, and was going bald above her long blond hair. I met her when she came to live at a facility where I worked. Her arms were heavily tattooed from her days as a naval officer and underneath her short pink dressing gown, she possessed male anatomy. She was a brittle diabetic and because of this deemed a poor candidate to venture into any other ways to live her life as a woman other than her clothing and choice of name and pronoun. She also identified as a lesbian. Many of the older people who lived in the facility were religious people of the Christian faith and struggled with many aspects of how Elizabeth presented. She was flamboyant and exuberant. She flounced around the facility and frequently shocked the more sedate of the other residents with her immodesty. If you think this sounds like a recipe for disaster, I would have agreed. However, until the very end of her life, Elizabeth was loved and respected by staff and other residents alike. I organized workshops on gender, sex, and sexuality. Some of the senior women, both staff and residents, amazed me with their questions and willingness to learn. Elizabeth was able to live out her days happily, being seen for who she was. It was only upon her death that her sister, who lived out of town and was not close to her, reverted to Elizabeth's original name and gender, but we all knew who she really was.

Compare this heartwarming story of recognition to what I heard when I met with nurses who had cared for Elizabeth at her previous facility. As I spoke of Elizabeth as feminine, these nurses became angry and accused me of supporting the whim of a manipulative person. According to them, if a person has male genitalia, then they must have a masculine name and behave in the culturally sanctioned ways of men. They effectively erased Elizabeth as a person of value and made her into a freak who refused to behave in the expected way. They made her an 'it', inhuman, and invisible as a real person. And, as in the story of Susan, sadly, this is not unusual behavior among care workers.

Gerald (a pseudonym), who identifies as a female-to-male (FTM) transsexual, was admitted to hospital for surgery quite unrelated to his gender. When he arrived on the ward he learned that his records had preceded him and he was called by his previous feminine name and the feminine pronouns. This was devastating to him and eventually interfered with his healing process. He had asked the operating room nurse if she would make sure he was covered during the surgery but later he found himself the centre of attention that seemed close to voyeurism. Gerald took great pains to cover his genitals during dressing changes and examinations but heard one nurse gasp as she saw he lacked a penis. After discharge, the wound became infected and the physician he saw, who was not the surgeon, asked if he could see his genitals because he had never seen a transsexual before. This request was rightly denied as inappropriate. The dressing had to be changed on a daily basis and home-care nurses went to Gerald's house to perform these. Frequently the nurses were not aware of Gerald's transsexual status and were puzzled to find him positioned carefully to protect his privacy. This meant he had to call out to them to come in when they arrived. He lost what little trust he had of health care institutions and this affected him for years to come because he avoided seeking care until the situation went beyond serious.

NURSING ETHICS

Nursing colleges and governing bodies all over the world have mandated ethical care of patients. I will draw from the United States, Great Britain, and Canada. In the United States, the American Nurses Association's Code of ethics for nurses (ANA 2017), revised in 2015, makes very clear statements about the sanctity and worth of those for whom nurses provide care. Provision 1 mentions dignity and self-determination, provision 2 speaks of the 'primacy of the patients' interests' (p. iii), and provision 3 makes clear the need to respect persons' privacy and confidentiality. In Great Britain, The Nursing and Midwifery Council's Code for Nurses and Midwives (NMC 2016) was also revised in 2015. The first section in this document, which is 'not negotiable or discretionary' (para 2), is called 'Prioritize people' (para 8). Under this section, nurses are called upon to '. . . put the interests of people . . . first'. [They are to] 'make their care and safety' [the] 'main concern and make sure that their dignity is preserved and their needs are recognized, assessed and responded to', '. . . make sure that those receiving care are treated with respect, that their rights are upheld and that any discriminatory attitudes and behaviours towards those receiving care are challenged' (para 8). Further, under the heading 'Preserving safety' (para 22) nurses are admonished to 'Raise concerns immediately if you believe a person is vulnerable or at risk and needs extra support and protection' (para 27).

In Canada, similar sentiments are expressed in the Code of Ethics for Registered Nurses: 2008 Centennial edition (Canadian Nurses Association – CNA 2008). On page 17, nurses are encouraged to 'uphold principles of justice by safeguarding human rights, equity and fairness . . .'

The ways to do this are described as not discriminating based on a number of categories that include 'gender, sexual orientation . . . lifestyle . . . or any other attribute'. As well, nurses are not to judge, label, demean, stigmatize, or humiliate those in their care. It is clear, although there are legislated ways for nurses to treat people, some are exempted because of our culturally mediated beliefs about who counts as human and worthy of this protection. Shelley, in his book *Transpeople* (2008), calls this exemption 'repudiation', which he describes as: 'to reject, refuse, condemn, repel, disown, renounce and back away from that which engenders repulsion' (p. 37).

This repudiation can lead to poor self-esteem, violence, substance use, self-harm, and suicide (pp. 59–61).

A discussion of multiculturalism might seem odd at this juncture, but I believe it will show some of the political sources of repudiation. Canada, in 1971, became the first country in the world to officially embrace multiculturalism (Government of Canada 2012). It was claimed that: 'Canada affirmed the value and dignity of all Canadian citizens regardless of their racial or ethnic origins, their language, or their religious affiliation' (para 1).

The goals were lofty and well-meaning and soon other countries followed with similar policies. Since then, much has been said to illustrate that the results of these policies have not been as intended. Malik (2015) said:

> As a political tool, multiculturalism has functioned as not merely a response to diversity but also a means of constraining it. And that insight reveals a paradox. Multicultural policies accept as a given that societies are diverse, yet they implicitly assume that such diversity ends at the edges of minority communities. They seek to institutionalize diversity by putting people into ethnic and cultural boxes – into a singular, homogeneous Muslim community, for example – and defining their needs and rights accordingly. Such policies, in other words, have helped create the very divisions they were meant to manage.
>
> (Malik 2015, para 4 – *See* Chapter 6)

I would agree completely. People who identify with some of the LGBTQI labels are, within those categories, diverse. There is no such thing as a category where all the people so labelled are the same, and some are not even remotely similar. Toward the end of the same paper, Malik has this to say: 'An ideal policy would marry multiculturalism's embrace of actual diversity, rather than its tendency to institutionalize differences, and assimilationism's resolve to treat everyone as citizens, rather than its tendency to construct a national identity by characterizing certain groups as alien to the nation' (Malik 2015, para 50).

I would suggest that those certain groups thought to be alien would include sexual minorities.

So, let us go back to the first story I told about Susan. Because she had a history of head trauma it was assumed by her family that she was incapable of making her own decisions or even knowing what she really wanted. The direct care staff rose to the task brilliantly and supported Susan's decision to live as a woman. Their care exemplified the requirements of ethical treatment. Management, who initially supported the staff and me in helping Susan to live as she wished, bowed to family pressure, with the result that Susan was shamed, chastised, and forced to return to living as a man. This effectively made what she thought of as her true self invisible, repudiated, and rendered non-human. Because she was not allowed to be seen, she was not validated. All of the ethics statements I mentioned earlier included sections on treating one another, as well as those in care, ethically. In this story, the staff were also repudiated.

Elizabeth's story is largely a happy one and I think a lot of the reason for that was her buoyant personality. It is, however, full of inconsistencies, shame, and outright unethical behavior. Her physician, who was well known by the staff, refused to call Elizabeth by her feminine name or to use the appropriate pronouns. I had previously discussed end-of-life choices with Elizabeth and recorded that she wanted to be resuscitated in the event of cardiac arrest. On his first visit the physician ripped up that agreement (a legal document) and forced her to sign what he had decided appropriate, which was not to resuscitate. When I learned this, I consulted with my manager who supported me in tearing up that document, which didn't represent Elizabeth's choices, getting her to sign a new document, and sending it to the physician, telling him this was her choice and his job was to support her choice. He signed but wasn't happy about it.

The other residents, who were mostly older church women, struggled with their outrage over Elizabeth's way of being in the world. We explained to Elizabeth that some proprieties had to be observed, such as coming to meals dressed, as all residents were asked to do. She was also asked to wear a longer housecoat or adequate underwear under her short one because she had not developed some so-called feminine behaviors like keeping her knees together. She was more than willing to comply and asked that we help her to remember or to point out behavior that might bother others. One older woman worried that Elizabeth was attracted to her, as some women do when they encounter lesbianism for the first time. Elizabeth toned down her 'friendliness' to that woman, and I took the risk of telling the other woman that it might be sexual attraction, but more likely it was because she was so smartly dressed and groomed that Elizabeth was probably wanting to emulate her. That resulted in a heartwarming change of attitude from fear to mentoring. Some staff also struggled with homophobia and transphobia but gradually came to understand that they must put those fears aside to provide ethical care to Elizabeth. Staff and residents attended a workshop provided by a well-known trans activist and asked excellent questions for how to best relate to Elizabeth and other people like her.

The nurses at the other facility who flatly repudiated Elizabeth left me feeling stunned and saddened. I wondered when they had last read their profession's ethical guidelines. It made me wonder who else they discriminated against. Did they disallow same-sex partners to visit or be named next-of-kin? What about people identified as having substance use problems? Did they refuse to give them adequate pain relief? I was deeply troubled. I was very appreciative that my management rose to the occasion and supported a person who was 'different' and surmised that those nurses who did not must have had management who were unaware or unconcerned with ethical treatment.

There is not much to recommend Gerald's story. He sought care for an issue unrelated to his status as an FTM and was treated unethically and inhumanely from a variety of care givers. To begin, he clearly identified himself as a trans man. Regardless of his previous records, his new status should have been entered into all his records at the time. Ethics takes precedence over policy, and if it was not policy to change names and genders on admission documents, then the policy must change to fit the ethical concerns. It was clear that word had spread quickly through the hospital about his status and care providers demonstrated a prurient interest in him that had nothing to do with his surgery. The physician who asked to see his genitalia showed a gross disrespect to his patient. The outcome of the story is that Gerald lost all trust in what he might expect from care providers. He could have helped to educate the staff in the hospital and the nurses who came to his house, but he was too traumatized to do anything but hide and protect himself from what he thought of as their prying eyes. He felt like an 'it' and was invisible to all who cared for him as himself. Instead, he was 'that FTM'.

HOW TO CHANGE THE WORLD: I AND THOU

One of my favorite nursing theorists, Rosemarie Parse, suggested approaching people as a 'not knowing stranger' (Parse 1997, p. 173). This is putting our professional knowing (as in, the health care professional knows best) aside and instead find out what the person who needs care wants. She also used the expression 'true presence' and this is explained as 'a non-routinized, non-mechanical way of "being with" in which the nurse is authentic and attentive to moment-by-moment changes in meaning for the person . . .' (Martin et al. 1992, p. 83). This is similar to what happened to the soldier in *Avatar*. His job, at the outset, was to learn about the Na'vi people so the army could discover their weaknesses. As he came to admire their way of life he could say to them 'I see you' and mean it. And, as Martin Buber (1970) encouraged, both Parse and the soldier entered 'I-You' relationships. This is the way to change the world, but how do we do it, exactly? What are the requirements to meet this challenge?

The first requirement is to be present. This means dropping assumptions, being aware of our own prejudices as they arise, and looking at the person with fresh eyes. The best words to admit to oneself, without shame, are 'I don't know'.

The next is to ask questions. Most people, upon meeting someone whose gender is not clear, will struggle with the not-knowing. We were all taught from infancy to wonder 'Is it a boy or a girl'? Ask the person's name. Sometimes that solves the problem since it might be clearly a feminine or masculine name. However, many people who present androgynously choose names that are also genderless. In this case, the best approach is to ask the person what pronoun they want you to use. Contrary to what we often feel, that this is an unwanted invasion, many people who are asked this respectfully appreciate the effort.

Next, it is imperative to lose the mindset and language of pathology: deviant, confused, homosexual, perverted and other such labels.

The World Professional Association for Transgender Health (WPATH 2011) has devised standards of care for all who present in a gender that is non-conformist. In this lengthy document, they list their core principles as:

> ➤ exhibit respect for patients with nonconforming gender identities (do not pathologize differences in gender identity or expression)
> ➤ provide care (or refer to knowledgeable colleagues) that affirms patients' gender identities and reduces the distress of gender dysphoria, when present
> ➤ become knowledgeable about the health care needs of transsexual, transgender, and gender nonconforming people, including the benefits and risks of treatment options for gender dysphoria
> ➤ match the treatment approach to the specific needs of patients, particularly their goals for gender expression and need for relief from gender dysphoria
> ➤ facilitate access to appropriate care
> ➤ seek patients' informed consent before providing treatment
> ➤ offer continuity of care
> ➤ and be prepared to support and advocate for patients within their families and communities (schools, workplaces, and other settings).
>   (WPATH 2011, p. 3)

What would change in the scenarios provided if this kind of approach were used?

The management of the facility where Susan lived could gently explain to her family that she is competent to make her own decisions and the facility stands by her choices.

It is not only the person in care who needs ethical compassionate care; their families have the same needs. Some teaching could be offered, or perhaps just a listening ear.

Elizabeth's physician would be directed that, while he is in her home, he will use Elizabeth's preferred name and pronoun. Once family moves the body for its final destination, it is, of course, out of the facility's hands. But before then Elizabeth's sister could be approached with stories of Elizabeth and her happiness living as a woman.

There are many teaching opportunities in the story of Gerald. At the time of his surgery, Gerald did not have a physician sensitive to his gender needs. All care providers need education to bring them in line with current understanding of gender and transgender issues. It should be a requirement, when meeting a person whose needs are unfamiliar, that all care givers learn how to respond appropriately. Gerald now has an educated and compassionate doctor. Prior to any hospitalization, the admitting doctor needs to alert the facility to use the correct current names and gender designations regardless of what is on the previous chart. The nursing staff must behave in ways that conform to the standards of care devised by WPATH (2011). When mistakes are made (and there will be mistakes . . . see 'I don't know' above) a sincere apology is in order.

All of this reflects an 'I-Thou' relationship. All of those who are indicated by the initials LGBTQI are, at the base of it all, just like us and deserve the best care we can provide. This mentality will indeed change the world.

SELF-ASSESSMENT EXERCISE 7.1

Time: 55 minutes
- Have you ever seen a person you couldn't 'categorize' as male or female? What happened for you in that experience? Has reading this chapter changed your perspective?
- Is it upsetting for you to encounter a person you would describe as male behaving in a feminine manner? If so, is it more upsetting than meeting a woman who is dressed and behaving in a masculine way? Why?
- Do you think of partners of gay or lesbian people differently than the partners of heterosexual people? Do you assume everyone is heterosexual until you know they are not?
- Have you ever met someone with attributes of both sexes, such as beards and breasts? How has reading this chapter changed the way you would handle such a meeting?
- What is the difference between sex and gender? How does sexuality relate to sex or gender?
- How would you handle colleagues' or friends' prejudicial remarks about people who present differently than what is usually expected?
- In what ways do people who are outside the mainstream of sex, gender, and sexuality contribute to your thinking about what is 'normal'? Is there room for such people in your professional life? What about your private life? What are the benefits of making room?
- How has the idea of an I/You relationship impacted your thoughts on care-giving? Does entering a relationship with a person as a not-knowing stranger resonate for you?

REFERENCES

American Nurses Association (2017) *Code of ethics for nurses with interpretive statements*. Available at: http://nursingworld.org/DocumentVault/Ethics-1/Code-of-Ethics-for-Nurses.html (Accessed: 24 August 2017)

Angelou, M. (2017) *Goodreads*. Available at: www.goodreads.com/quotes/tag/names (Accessed: 24 August 2017)

Bornstein, K. (1994) *Gender Outlaw*. New York: Routledge.

Buber, M. (1970) *I and Thou*. Translated by W. Kaufmann. New York: Charles Scribner's Sons.

Butler, J. (2006) 'Doing justice to someone', in Whittle, S. and Stryker, S. (eds) *The Transgender Studies Reader*. New York: Routledge, pp. 183–93.

Cameron, J. (2009) *Avatar*. Los Angeles: Twentieth Century Fox. DVD.

Canadian Nurses Association. (CNA – 2008) *Code of ethics for registered nurses: 2008 Centennial edition*. Available at: www.nurses.ab.ca/content/dam/carna/pdfs/DocumentList/EndorsedPublications/RN_CNA_Ethics_2008.pdf (Accessed: 24 August 2017)

Davis, G. and Murphy, E. L. (2013) 'Intersex bodies as states of exception: an empirical explanation for unnecessary surgical modification'. *Feminist Formations*, 25, pp. 129–52. *Project MUSE*, doi:10.1353/ff.2013.0022

Government of Canada (2012) *Canadian multiculturalism: An inclusive citizenship*. Available at: www.cic.gc.ca/english/multiculturalism/citizenship.asp (Accessed: 24 August 2017)

Grant, J. M., Mottet, L. A., Tanis, J., Harrison, J., Herman, J. L., and Keisling, M. (2011) *Injustice At Every Turn. A Report of the National Transgender Discrimination Survey* (p. 228). Washington, DC: National Center for Transgender Equality and National Gay and Lesbian Task Force.

Literary Devices. (2017) *A rose by any other name*. Available at: https://literarydevices.net/a-rose-by-any-other-name/ (Accessed: 24 August 2017)

Malik, K. (2015) *The failure of multiculturalism*. Available at https://kenanmalik.wordpress.com/2015/02/17/the-failure-of-multiculturalism/ (Accessed: 24 August 2017)

Marchildon, J. (2017) *A Canadian baby has been issued a genderless ID card*. Available at: www.globalcitizen.org/en/content/canadian-baby-genderless-id/ (Accessed: 24 August 2017)

Martin, M., Forchuk, C., Santopinto, M. and Butcher, H. K. (1992) 'Alternative approaches to nursing practice: Application of Peplau, Rogers, and Parse'. *Nursing Science Quarterly*, 5, pp. 80–5.

Nursing and Midwifery Council (NMC – 2016) *The code for nurses and midwives*. Available at: www.nmc.org.uk/standards/code/ (Accessed: 24 August 2017)

Parse, R. R. (1997) 'Transforming research and practice with the human becoming theory'. *Nursing Science Quarterly*, 10, pp. 171–4.

Shelley, C. A. (2008) *Transpeople: Repudiation, Trauma, Healing*. Toronto, ON: University of Toronto Press.

World Professional Association for Transgender Health (WPATH – 2011) *The standards of care, 7th version*. Available at: www.wpath.org/site_page.cfm?pk_association_webpage_menu=1351 (Accessed 24 August 2017)

To Learn More

Devor, H. (1997) *FTM: Female-to-Male Transsexuals in Society*. Bloomington and Indianapolis, IN: Indiana University Press.

Feinberg, L. (1993) *Stone Butch Blues: A Novel*. Milford, CT: Firebrand Books.

Lev, A. I. (2004) *Transgender Emergence: Therapeutic Guidelines for Working with Gender-Variant People and Their Families*. Binghamton, NY: The Hawthorn Press, Inc.

McCloskey, D. N. (1999) *Crossing: A Memoir*. Chicago & London: University of Chicago Press.

Merryfeather, L. (2016) *You've Changed: An Evocative Autoethnography*. Victoria, BC: Friesen Press.

CHAPTER 8

Human Rights

Scott Macpherson and Dan Warrender

Human rights are the fundamental rights and freedoms that belong to everyone, everywhere throughout their lifespan, by virtue of being human. They apply regardless of a person's thoughts, beliefs or behaviours and cannot be permanently removed ... though there are some circumstances under which they can be restricted, including when a person commits a crime or when they are detained under mental health legislation.

Human rights are based on values such as dignity, respect, equality and autonomy and are enshrined in law.

THE IDEA OF 'RIGHTS'

In all likelihood the concept of 'a right' has likely existed (even if the word did not) for as long as there have been primitive human communities. It is likely that (as is the case today) these populations would have had rules stipulating permissions for certain individuals or groups to perform certain actions and, conversely, rules that others were not permitted to perform such actions. These rules can be used to ascribe rights to people or groups.

In their most basic sense rights can be seen as either negative or positive. Negative rights are entitlements not to be interfered with while positive rights are rights to the provision of certain goods or services.

Generally, when talking about the rights of vulnerable people we are talking about passive rights (claim-rights and immunity-rights in Hohfeldian terms – Hohfeld 1919). Claim-rights entitle their holders to freedom from physical interference or close observation of others, or to be free of undesirable conditions such as fear. For example, a person living with dementia in a nursing home has the claim-right to not be physically assaulted by the staff of the home. Immunity-rights entitle their holders to be free of the authority of others. For example, a person who has informal status in a mental health hospital has the immunity-right to not be held there against their will.

When talking about the rights of people in positions of relative power we are generally talking about active rights (privilege-rights and power-rights in Hohfeldian terms), which entitle their holders to act in particular ways. For example, a mental health professional has the privilege-right (the 'freedom to') read the confidential notes of the people in their care. The holders of power-rights have the normative ability to exercise authority in certain ways (Sumner 1987). For example, under particular circumstances, certain mental health professionals have the power-right to restrain a person in their care and administer sedative medication to them against their will.

Dworkin (1984) considered the idea of rights as trumps, with some rights having a higher power or priority over others. As in a game of cards, a king trumps a 9 and a 9 trumps a 6. Mill (1989, p. 20) wrote: 'If all mankind minus one were of one opinion, mankind would be no more justified in silencing that one person than he, if he had the power, would be in silencing mankind'.

In accord with the ideas of Immanuel Kant (1993) [1785] – explored further later in this chapter), consideration should be given to the possibility of any of us being the 'one person', and how we would feel to be powerless against 'all mankind'. Empathy for the person who is on the receiving end of a power right is a necessary step towards balanced discussion on the circumstances in which they can be justified.

The idea of some rights being more important than others is the sort of rationale that is used when justifying the detention of a person who is suicidal 'to protect their right to life'. The justification being that their right to life trumps their right to liberty and security. Even though the person may not value this right themselves, the right is sufficiently valued by society, based on an assumption that reason, rationality and a desire to live will return. In this way, 'mankind minus one' justify the removal of this human right, fully expectant that when the mental state of the 'one person' improves, that the person will be grateful and re-join their ranks.

Following the atrocities and massive loss of life during World War II and the creation of the United Nations, world leaders worked together to produce the Universal Declaration of Human Rights 1948: a guidance document designed to guarantee the rights of everyone, everywhere, regardless of age, race, gender, religion, health status or any other defining characteristic, and thus protect against such atrocities occurring again (Donnelly 2013). Human rights, as set out in the declaration, are interdependent and interrelated, meaning that if one right is fulfilled it supports the fulfilment of others and, conversely, if one right is denied it makes the fulfilment of others more difficult.

Though not a legally binding document in itself, the declaration has inspired over 60 human rights instruments that deal with rights in relation to a wide variety of issues including war crimes, marriage, social welfare, physical and mental health and many more (Office of the United Nations High Commissioner for Human Rights (OHCHR) 2016). Together, these instruments provide a worldwide standard for human rights.

The application of human rights creates obligations through international law for states to respect, protect and fulfil human rights for all. States must not interfere with or remove human rights (respect), they must safeguard both individuals and groups from human rights abuses (protect) and they must be pro-active in enabling the realisation of human rights (fulfil). Whilst everyone is entitled to have their human rights respected, protected and fulfilled, there is also a universal obligation to ensure that peoples' actions or inaction do not infringe the human rights of others.

In Scotland, human rights are protected by the European Convention on Human Rights (ECHR), the UK Human Rights Act 1998 and the Scotland Act 1998.

THE EUROPEAN CONVENTION ON HUMAN RIGHTS (ECHR – 1953)

The ECHR consists of 17 key articles, each of which is a brief explanation of a right along with any exceptions that can apply to it.

REFLECTIVE PRACTICE EXERCISE 8.1.1

> **Time: 40 minutes**
> Consider these key ECHR articles pertaining to the rights of people accessing care for mental health issues and then answer the questions that follow (*See* Reflective Practice Exercise 8.1.2).

Article 2

The right to life. This is an absolute right and can be interpreted as a duty to not take anyone's life and also to take reasonable steps to protect people's lives.

Article 3

The right not to be subjected to torture or to inhuman or degrading treatment or punishment. Degrading treatment can be understood as treatment that is grossly humiliating and undignified.

Article 5

The right to liberty. In mental health treatment people often have their right to liberty (Article 5) restricted in the form of detention when they are assessed as a risk to themselves or others, and further restricted when they are placed on enhanced observations. Barker (2010) suggests that the prevailing use of risk assessments presents a real danger to liberty and human rights since they are founded primarily on subjective judgements, which are set out as clinical judgements and, as such, cannot be challenged in a court of law.

Article 6

The right to a fair trial. The definition here includes other kinds of hearings such as mental health tribunals. When a person is detained under mental health legislation, it is the duty of mental health professionals to ensure that they are aware of their rights to advocacy and legal representation in order that they can challenge any concerns relating to the restriction of their freedom.

Article 8

The right to private and family life. This article is very broad ranging, covering rights to physical, psychological and moral wellbeing, with wellbeing maintained by preserving autonomy, choice and dignity.

Article 9

The right to freedom of thought, conscience and religion. This article allows that people should be free to hold a wide variety of thoughts and beliefs.

Article 14

The right not to be discriminated against. Peoples' human rights should be promoted and protected without discrimination on any basis, including the nine protected characteristics defined by the Equality Act (2010): age, gender reassignment, disability, marriage and civil partnership, sex, sexual orientation, pregnancy and maternity, race and religion or belief.

Article 25

The right to the highest attainable standard of physical and mental health. This includes both a right to healthy living conditions and a right to satisfactory health care. This article sets out that health care should be of good quality and be available, accessible and acceptable to those who need it.

REFLECTIVE PRACTICE EXERCISE 8.1.2

Time: 75 minutes

- Consider 'taking reasonable steps' to protect someone's life as is set out in Article 2. As a professional do you have a duty to do whatever you reasonably can do to prevent a person self-harming or completing suicide?
- How might this interpretation of your role infringe on some of the other ECHR articles? For example: Articles 3, 9 and 10?
- Consider the words 'grossly humiliating and undignified' as they relate to Article 3. Could it be argued that the enhanced observation of people in our care fits under this definition?
- Is the use of force and restraint in the name of mental health treatment 'grossly humiliating and undignified'?
- Could it be argued that focusing on risk in mental health treatment actually creates risk? Have you seen any examples where this may have been the case?
- Are you fully aware of the rights of people you care for in relation to advocacy and legal representation? If not, how will you go about addressing this?
- Is it reasonable to restrict the right to private and family life (Article 8) when it comes to decisions the person might make about the use of particular drugs or whether to self-harm or even take their own life?
- In Article 8 'private life' relates to wherever the person may be not just in their own home. Consider some of the ways in which this right may be infringed when a person is detained in hospital. For instance, how might detention affect a person's right to smoke cigarettes or to meet their sexual needs?
- Staying with Article 8 'family life' should be understood to include relationships not just with family members, but also with friends and communities. Take a minute to think about how much or how little importance mental health professionals give to helping people fulfil this right.
- Also in Article 8 'correspondence' covers all forms of communication including e-communications. Are the restrictions of communications that you may see in practice always fully justifiable?
- In relation to Article 9, consider whether it is the case that, within the field of mental health practice, people are really only allowed to think and believe things within the confines of certain, socially defined norms (which can differ markedly over time and place) and when their thoughts and beliefs breach these norms they can be said to be mentally unwell and treated against their will?
- Consider whether you have seen people discriminated against (Article 14) on the basis of their diagnosis or behaviour e.g. people who use drugs or who have been given a personality disorder diagnosis.

- An important component of Article 25 is that any health care provided should be acceptable to those who need it. Consider whether mental health care is always acceptable to those who are in need of it when a curative approach is taken rather than a palliative approach.

THE UK HUMAN RIGHTS ACT (1998)

The UK Human Rights Act (1998) enshrines the rights set out in the ECHR into UK law. All other UK legislation should be understood and applied in a manner consistent with this Act.

The Scotland Act (1998): This Act was passed to guarantee that parliament only passes laws consistent with human rights and that any laws passed are not in breach of either the ECHR or the UK Human Rights Act (1998).

Also important is the UN Convention on the Rights of Persons with Disabilities (UNCRPD – 2008), which, though technically not part of Scottish law, helps with understanding and interpreting the rights set out in the UK Human Rights Act (1998) in relation to people with disabilities. The Convention specifies the actions that should be taken to remove the obstacles that (among others) people with long-term mental health problems may encounter in realising their human rights.

The UK Human Rights Act (1998) provides the basis upon which the Mental Health (Care and Treatment) (Scotland) Act (2003) is applied. Consequently, both Acts are underpinned by similar principles. The PANEL principles (Scottish Human Rights Commission 2017) are a handy way of breaking down what an approach grounded in human rights should look like in practice:

➤ **P** – participation – people being truly and meaningfully involved in every decision about their care – being not just allowed but actively encouraged to participate in and own decisions affecting their lives
➤ **A** – accountability – there should be effective monitoring of human rights standards, requiring appropriate means to rectify issues in order to secure these
➤ **N** – non-discrimination and equality – prioritising the prohibition, prevention and elimination of all forms of discrimination. This requires prioritising people in the most vulnerable situations who face the greatest obstacles in protecting and fulfilling their rights
➤ **E** – empowerment – ensuring people understand their rights, are able to claim them when necessary and are fully supported to participate meaningfully in the development of policies and procedures that can affect their day-to-day lives
➤ **L** – legality – practicing in a way that ensures the full range of human rights are respected, protected and fulfilled for all, recognising rights as entitlements enforceable by law. Grounding all approaches in human rights law (both domestic and international).

WILL BREXIT AFFECT HUMAN RIGHTS IN THE UK?

The short answer is that our human rights as set out in the ECHR will not be affected by leaving the EU as the ECHR comes from the Council of Europe (which the UK is not leaving). The slightly more complex answer is that currently many of the human rights protections set out in EU law are also written into UK law, however after leaving the EU the government would have the ability to pass laws that repeal or weaken current rights to a standard below that of EU law rights (Equality and Human Rights Commission 2017).

THE MENTAL HEALTH (CARE AND TREATMENT) (SCOTLAND) ACT 2003

While mental health legislation differs across the UK, each country's Mental Health Act is built around similar ethical principles. In Scotland the Scottish Executive Millan Committee (2001) was commissioned by Parliament to make recommendations for a new Mental Health Act including consideration of an ethical underpinning for the compulsory treatment of people experiencing mental disorders. The committee developed a set of principles on which they recommended mental health law should be based. These are now known as the 'Millan Principles':

BOX 8.1 Millan principles

1. Non-discrimination
2. Equality
3. Respect for diversity
4. Reciprocity
5. Informal care
6. Participation
7. Respect for carers
8. Least restrictive alternative
9. Benefit
10. Child welfare

(Scottish Executive Millan Committee 2001)

The Mental Health (Care and Treatment) (Scotland) Act 2003, details when and how people can be treated if they are deemed to have a mental disorder. This includes provision for when people can be treated or detained against their will. The Act also sets out what peoples' rights are and safeguards around these.

Under the Act, a doctor (ideally together with a mental health officer) can issue an Emergency Detention Certificate, which allows a person to be held in hospital for up to 72 hours while their condition is assessed. This allows for emergency treatment to be given to a person. However, other than in an emergency, no treatment should be given to a person against their will under this type of detention. The person must be assessed by a doctor as soon as possible and must have information about their stay in hospital and their rights explained to them. There is no right of appeal against an Emergency Detention Certificate.

In terms of formal detention under the Act, the normal route into hospital should be through a Short-Term Detention, which can only be put in place if recommended by both a doctor and a mental health officer. A psychiatrist must be assigned as the Responsible Medical Officer (RMO) for the person and must speak with them about their wishes and seek to understand and follow their Advance Statement if they have one. An advance statement is written by a person when they are well and witnessed and signed by a health or social care professional. The statement details how a person would like to be treated if they become unwell. In the UK an advance statement is not a guarantee that the person's wishes will be followed. However, it does mean that they will be considered.

Advance Statements are not to be confused with Advance Decisions (Advance Directives in Scotland). This document (also known as a living will) is written by a person when they are well and sets out any treatment they would wish to refuse should they become unwell. This can include any situations where they would or would not wish to refuse such treatment. An Advance Decisions is legally binding as long as it:

➤ Complies with mental capacity legislation
➤ Is valid
➤ Applies to the person's situation.

Note: although it has not been tested in Scottish courts, an Advance Directive is likely to be treated as legally binding if it meets the criteria set out above.

If the RMO decides that the person is likely to require treatment, the person can be detained under a Short-Term Detention Certificate. This allows for the person to be detained for up to 28 days and grants the right to treat the person against their will if this is deemed necessary. Again, the person should be given information about their stay in hospital and have their rights explained to them. They should also be supported to get an independent advocate. The person or their named person has the right to appeal to the Mental Health Tribunal against this type of detention.

A named person is someone chosen by the person to help protect their interests if they are in need of treatment under the Act and unable to make decisions for themselves. The named person will have the right to be consulted about certain aspects of the person's care.

Longer-term detention is possible under the Act through the use of Compulsory Treatment Orders (CTOs). These can last for up to six months initially, followed by a further six month-extension and then for periods of 12 months at a time if necessary. Applications for CTOs need to be made to the Mental Health Tribunal and consist of two medical reports, a mental health officer's report and a proposed care plan. The person also has the right to have their thoughts heard by the tribunal and, if a CTO is put in place, the person or their named person can apply to have it removed only after it has been in place for at least three months.

COMPULSION

If a person is convicted of a crime and the punishment is prison but the person is deemed to require treatment for mental ill-health a decision can be taken to either detain the person in hospital or enforce treatment in the community under a Compulsion Order (CO), rather than detaining them in prison (Mental Welfare Commission for Scotland 2017). Similar to a CTO, a CO lasts for six months, can be followed by a further six-month extension and then further extended by periods of 12 months at a time if necessary. Anyone subject to treatment in the community under a CO will be told by the court where they must go for care and treatment and also where they must live. The court can also add a Restriction Order (RO) to a CO if they think a person poses a serious risk to the general public. Under an RO any move to a different hospital or periods spent out of hospital must be approved by Scottish Ministers. An RO can be in place indefinitely but must be reviewed by the person's psychiatrist, who must submit an annual report to Scottish Ministers. Ministers must refer the person's case to the Mental Health Tribunal if their psychiatrist thinks their order should be changed, or that they should be discharged from hospital. If the Tribunal agrees, the person may be given a 'conditional discharge' meaning that they may leave hospital but must comply with certain restrictions as ordered by Scottish Ministers. This may involve restrictions on where the person may or may not go and on whether the person may use drugs or alcohol.

REFLECTIVE PRACTICE EXERCISE 8.2

Time: 20 minutes

Consider these restrictions on where a person may live, where they must access care and treatment, where they can go and whether they can use alcohol. If you were subject to these restrictions, what might be the impact on your mental health? How might you feel about the status of your own human rights?

The Patient Rights (Scotland) Act (2011) was designed to support optimum health care for all people accessing health services. It is grounded in human rights principles and provides a framework for involving people in decisions about their own health and health care. The Act also grants people the right to give feedback and raise concerns about the care they receive. A requirement of the Act is the publication of a Charter of Patient Rights and Responsibilities (The Scottish Government 2012), which summarises the rights and responsibilities of everyone accessing NHS services in Scotland and details what a person should do if they feel their rights have not been respected. Underpinning The Patient Rights (Scotland) Act (2011) is the right to be treated with respect, dignity and compassion (which comes from Article 8 of the ECHR). There are times in mental health care when this right is restricted (examples may include the removal of possessions, seclusion or enhanced observations). However, while these restrictions may be allowed under certain circumstances by the Mental Health (Care and Treatment) (Scotland) Act (2003) they must be human rights compliant by being proportionate, time limited and kept under review.

REFLECTIVE PRACTICE EXERCISE 8.3

Time: 40 minutes

- Consider the practice of supervised urine sampling for people with substance use disorders who are prescribed substitute medication.
- Can watching a person pass urine be considered a proportionate measure if the risk it is used to mitigate against is that the person might otherwise lie about whether they have used illicit drugs?
- What if the person has sole care of a young child?
- Does illicit drug use itself provide sufficient evidence of risk to the child? This practice is carried out in the name of risk and aligns with a curative, medical model philosophy, that people who are prescribed a substitute medication should have no need to use illicit drugs.

DE FACTO DETENTION

'You are free – to do as we tell you' – Bill Hicks (2005, p. 132).

The right to liberty (Article 5 of the ECHR) can be limited under certain conditions (for example by detention under the Mental Health (Care and Treatment) (Scotland) Act 2003. However, a person who is in hospital informally and wishes to leave must not be placed in a situation where they feel that they must remain in hospital because if they do not stay they will be formally detained under the Act. This unlawful pressure is known as 'de facto detention' and puts restrictions on a person without providing them with the rights they would otherwise have if they were formally detained. The person's belief about the likelihood of them being detained if they don't comply with the wishes of staff is key in deciding whether a de facto detention situation exists, rather than simply whether staff believe that this is the case.

REFLECTIVE PRACTICE EXERCISE 8.4

Time: 30 minutes
Consider a situation where a person who is in hospital informally wishes to leave against medical advice and you are part of a staff team who feel this would not be safe. How could you avoid creating a de facto detention situation?

DEHUMANIZATION

Szasz (1973) argued that psychiatry's deterministic explanations and coercive treatments relieve individuals of their autonomy and moral agency. Szasz viewed psychiatric classification as dehumanising, saying that it involves a 'mechanomorphic' style of thinking that 'thingifies' people and treats them as 'defective machine[s]' (p. 200). Hinshaw and Cicchetti (2000) agree that stigma dehumanises people experiencing mental disorders.

Kelman (1976) talked about the moral dimensions of dehumanisation. Kelman argued that dehumanisation involves denying a person 'identity': a perception of the person 'as an individual, independent and distinguishable from others, capable of making choices' (p. 301), [and 'community': a perception of the other as] 'part of an interconnected network of individuals who care for each other' (p. 301). Kelman said that when people are treated in this way they are deindividuated, lose the capacity to evoke compassion and moral emotions, and may be treated as a means toward vicious ends. Opotow (1990) worked on 'moral exclusion'. This can be understood as the process by which people are placed 'outside the boundary in which moral values, rules, and consideration of fairness apply' (p. 1). Exclusion from the moral community is promoted by social conflict and feelings of unconnectedness and varies in intensity from genocide to indifference to another person's suffering. Dehumanisation can also be seen in the health care context as a mechanism that practitioners use to cope with the empathic distress that comes with working alongside dying people (Schulman-Green 2003).

TOURO COLLEGE LIBRARY

REFLECTIVE PRACTICE EXERCISE 8.5

Time: 30 minutes
Consider the following:

> Ethel is a sweet, 75-year-old lady who loves her daughters and her cat. Ethel
> has a keen sense of humour and enjoys watching crime dramas on television.
> Ethel was admitted to the ward you work on this morning. In addition, Liz,
> experiencing schizophrenia, was admitted to the ward.

- Is there any difference in how you would feel about confiscating a pair of nail scissors
  on safety grounds from either Ethel or Liz?
- How about providing medication against Ethel or Liz's will?
- . . . and restraining Ethel or Liz?

It is likely that it is easier to justify the use of coercion or restraint if we view the subject of these acts as an ill-health or 'defective machine' rather than as a human. It could perhaps even be argued that dehumanisation, in this way, is a necessary condition for carrying out any coercive treatment.

Bar-Tal (2000) discussed 'delegitimizing beliefs'. These are: 'extremely negative characteristics attributed to another group with the purpose of excluding it from acceptable human groups and denying it humanity' (pp. 121–2). These beliefs share extremely negative valence, emotional activation (typically contempt and fear), cultural support and discriminatory rejection of the outgroup. Delegitimising beliefs exist not only around mental health but also within the field of mental health. Commonly these types of beliefs are held about people experiencing substance use issues, suicidal ideation and psychoses.

In contemporary health care a person's subjective experience is often neglected in favour of objective, technologically mediated information and a strong emphasis on interventions/tasks performed on passive individuals whose agency and autonomy are neglected. Student nurses and newly qualified nurses often express a desire to learn the important or common tasks for the area they are working in and value the learning of these tasks in practice over theory in university: 'I learned nothing in university, I learned it all in practice' while also saying 'practice is dangerously understaffed, there's just no time for spending with patients/therapeutic work'. Opotow (1990) described this phenomenon as 'technical orientation'. This can be understood as a focus on means-end efficiency and mechanical routine. The pressure to 'fit in' can mean that new ideas, criticism of existing practice and healthy professional debate are stifled, smothered under the reality or fear of ostracism. Meissner (1986) described a bullying culture in nursing (although it can be assumed that the same can happen within any large professional body), whereby nurses 'eat their young'. In any profession that holds power over vulnerable people, professionals need to have the ability to speak their minds, making balanced ethical decisions based on the interests of people, not fearing the wrath of a comfortable ritualism. Decisions on human rights should never be reduced to tasks, with standardised routine answers.

Human rights would appear to be less a problem of the legal expressions of rights and duties than they are a problem of human classification, of who is counted as a full human being, deserving of the complete range of human rights (Agier 2011). Curra (2014) sees deviance in almost every form as a standard element of human societies and discourages the temptation to equate deviance with disease and abnormality.

Curra gives the example that, just as it would be wrong to conclude that eating dog meat instead of cow meat is an indicator of mental ill-health, so it must be wrong to conclude that people who inhale one kind of substance (for example heroin or marijuana) are more abnormal or mentally ill than those who inhale other substances (for example tobacco). Curra's point is that deviance can be shocking to a person who is alien to it. However, this does not make this difference necessarily abnormal or 'sick' everywhere and across all time.

MENTAL CAPACITY

Every country in the UK has its own legislation in place around mental capacity, with each one based on the principles of justice, autonomy, beneficence and non-maleficence. The Adults with Incapacity (Scotland) Act (2000) is designed to protect the interests of people (age 16 and over) who cannot make some or all decisions for themselves. 'Incapacity' in terms of the Act means being unable to act on, make, communicate, understand or remember decisions due to mental disorder or inability to communicate due to physical disorder. The Act allows certain other relevant and appropriate people to take decisions on their behalf providing that any intervention is:

➤ Necessary and of benefit to the person
➤ The least restrictive option.

Anyone taking decisions for an 'Adult with Incapacity' must:

➤ Encourage the person to use any skills they have to make decisions for themselves and encourage the development of new skills
➤ Consider whether intervention is possible without the use of the Act
➤ Act in keeping with the person's wishes (present and past)
➤ Consult with relevant others.

The Act includes a number of safeguards that are intended to prevent abuse of these powers. These include preventing certain decisions being made on the person's behalf such as giving consent to marriage or the drawing up of a will, having the person admitted to a mental health hospital against their will or consenting to certain medical treatments on their behalf. The Act charges four public bodies with responsibility for the supervision and regulation of people who are authorised to make decisions for people who are deemed to lack capacity: The Mental Welfare Commission for Scotland, The Office of the Public Guardian (Scotland), local authorities and the courts. Variously, they provide advice and support, supervise financial decisions, investigate complaints and restrict or remove decision-making powers.

INFORMED CONSENT

Each of the UK's Acts of Mental Health legislation make provisions for circumstances under which people can be compulsorily treated for a mental disorder without their consent. A person's capacity to consent to treatment can change over time and a lack of capacity to make decisions in one aspect of life does not necessarily mean that a person is incapable of making decisions in other aspects of their life. For these reasons, incapacity must never be presumed and instead must always be assessed with respect to each specific decision and for each given moment in time. Should treatment be provided against the wishes of a person who is capable of consenting this would violate their right to autonomy and can constitute assault.

In relation to consent to mental health treatment 'capacity' means that a person is capable of understanding the nature, implications and consequences of their decisions.

A person can be said to have capacity to consent to treatment if they:

➤ Can understand in simple terms what the treatment is, the purpose of the treatment, its features and why it is being recommended.
➤ Can understand its main advantages, risks and other options and be able to make a choice based on these understandings.
➤ Have a broad understanding of the potential consequences of not having the treatment.
➤ Can remember the information for enough time to enable them to weigh-up the likely outcomes in order to arrive at a decision.
➤ Can communicate that decision to other people.
➤ Can make the same decision consistently – this takes into account people who might have trouble remembering a decision but, given the same information at some other time, make a consistent decision.

There are many factors, both internal and external to the person that can influence a person's capacity to give informed consent such as their environment, the quality and type of information provided, how the information is communicated, any previous health care experience, and current physical or mental health problems.

Relationships can play a considerable role in the decisions people make. It is possible that a person may feel under undue pressure to accept or refuse a particular treatment due to the wishes of their partner, parent, children, carer or health care professional. If professionals ascertain that a person's ability to make an autonomous decision is affected in this way then they should follow adult protection procedures, as set out in the Adult Support and Protection (Scotland) Act (2007).

SELF-ASSESSMENT EXERCISE 8.1

Time: 40 minutes
For each point, consider the multiple perspectives of Magdalena, her family and all involved healthcare professionals.
• Can Magdalena's initial emergency detention be justified?
• Are there any potential consequences of not admitting Magdalena to hospital? If so, what are they?
• Do any potential consequences outweigh the potential consequences of admitting her to hospital without consent?
• Describe the issues that may arise from Hugh's dual role as an agent of both therapeutics and containment. Consider both Magdalena's and Hugh's perspectives.
• Would coercion and forced treatment best fit into curative or palliative philosophies of care?

Case Study 8.1 – Magdalena

Magdalena is a 33-year-old woman, living with her parents and younger sister. She has an established diagnosis of schizophrenia and has been prescribed antipsychotic medication. Against professional advice, Magdalena had stopped taking her medication over a period of a year. Her mental health had deteriorated and was causing her family some concern. She had isolated herself into an annexe of the family home, had stopped tending to her personal care, and had voiced strange ideas, which had led to her sister feeling intimidated. She had spent all of her time painting surrealist images on a large canvas, and was no longer engaging with her family. Her living conditions had become cluttered and untidy, with litter and food-waste collecting over a period of months. She had refused to engage with her consultant psychiatrist, General Practitioner (GP)/Medical Doctor (MD) and mental health officer.

Hugh is a mental health nurse. Magdalena's consultant tells him that he is detaining Magdalena on an emergency detention certificate so that she can be taken into hospital for up to 72 hours, for further assessment and with the aim of being re-established on medication. Alongside a support worker, Hugh has been assigned as a 'hospital escort', with detention papers acting as the legal authority under which Magdalena may be medicated and taken into hospital against her will. Hugh and the support worker attempt to engage with Magdalena, however, she refuses them entry to her annexe. There is an ambulance on hand as transport back to hospital.

Hugh and the support worker then use physical restraint to remove Magdalena from her home. She resists, becoming aggressive, angry and extremely agitated. In order to get her into the ambulance safely, a decision is taken to administer intra-muscular medication to Magdalena to sedate her. Magdalena screams and pleads that she not be injected, saying 'please don't inject me with poison'! She is nonetheless sedated, and restrained until Hugh and the support worker feel she is sufficiently calm and will cooperate with her hospital admission. She enters the ambulance and is driven to hospital without incident. She sleeps for the rest of that day.

The next day, Hugh is on shift and is a named nurse for Magdalena. He asks her to speak with him in an interview room. She does not engage well with Hugh, who she says 'kidnapped' her. She has little insight, and does not share the belief of her consultant or family that she is unwell. After Magdalena is detained for a further 28 days, Hugh continues to act as her nurse, yet is unable to establish a therapeutic relationship. She appears guarded, unwilling to tolerate one to one discussions and never accepting that her mental health has been worthy of concern.

Magdalena begins different courses of antipsychotic medication, and with each new medication claims to have blurred vision. Despite professionals seeing no evidence of this, her subjective experience is accepted. At the end of a six-week period of admission, Magdalena had still not engaged well with professionals or agreed with them regarding her mental state. She was discharged after discussion with her family and sent home with a low dose of antipsychotic medication. Professionals involved in her care found it difficult to assess her due to her reluctance to engage and were not convinced Magdalena would maintain her prescribed medication.

Case Commentary 8.1 – Ethics

Mental health care and treatment has long existed in an ethical grey area, which can be explained as a moral triage of duties, consequences and virtues. The ethics in this case primarily exist in a fray, central to the tug of war between deontological and consequentialist thinking.

Duty

Deontological advocate Immanuel Kant (1993)[1785] asserted that morality was synonymous with rationality, and expressed this through his categorical imperative: 'Act only on that maxim through which you can at the same time will that it should become a universal law' (p. 30).

In Kant's view something such as stealing cannot ever be moral, given the irrationality it would take to look at this through the categorical imperative. Were we to justify stealing, we would also have to accept without complaint that we could be stolen from. This would entail a chaos of moral anarchy where no-one benefits. Moving this argument onto coercion in mental health care is nonetheless problematic due to the relativity of dignity. If we accept that a person who is considered a risk to themselves or others as a result of their mental state may be given treatment against their will, in order that this be moral, we must also accept this same rule for ourselves. The problem then lies in the subjectivity of what can be described as quality of life and dignity. Whilst one may look at Magdalena and describe her as being at risk to herself due to a lack of self-care, this is distinct from Magdalena's reality and may also be for others. Life does not come with a rule book or guideline, and perceptions of what is 'risk' can then be heavily influenced by social norms, which can change over culture and time. The argument can then rapidly become sociological as we ask, who decides on what is the accepted norm? Intervention in this case may be justified as taking a curative approach to mental health, but also sociologically critiqued as a paternalistic and corrective approach to social deviance.

It is clear that despite Kant's claim that morality is rationality, this does not darken or lighten the grey of mental health care into black and white. Duties to respect a person's human rights may be superseded by duties to protect either the human rights of that person or others around them. The subjectivity of life leads to duty being altogether relative and open to interpretation.

Consequences

Deontology is a useful foundation for exploring ethics, yet quickly gets lost as duties compete. Magdalena's detention may violate the duty to respect all people's human rights, although it can perhaps be justified in terms of perceived consequences. Given Magdalena's poor self-care and damaged relationships with family members, professionals may have felt obliged to intervene to prevent a spiral of detrimental effects. The consequentialist argument is utilitarian, which at its core looks for the greatest happiness for the greatest number of people. 'People' in this statement could relate to positive outcomes for not only Magdalena, but also her family. Whilst families and carers are hugely important in terms of supporting people experiencing mental health distress, and as persons themselves, if an action is done

continued . . .

for their benefit it could be viewed as veering away from person-centredness. Ideally the consequences should relate to the person whose human rights have been restricted.

Despite an infringement of human rights, the potential consequences of this may have been positive. Sometimes in the course of coercive treatment, people regain insight, repair interpersonal relationships and are grateful for the intervention they received. The darker side of the consequentialist argument is when we consider whether or not services can do more harm than good. This may be particularly true for people with histories of trauma, with professionals however, unintentionally facilitating an institutional re-traumatisation (Sweeney et al. 2016). In Magdalena's case, there were significant negative experiences for her with tentative benefits if any. In ascribing moral value, this act of involuntary detention would therefore have none. It may be frustrating for all to carry out and experience the removal of human rights, to little or no benefit.

Virtue

As the protectors and breakers of duties, and agents of both positive and negative consequences, it may be of comfort to professionals to know that a third means of moral judgement exists. Virtue ethics describes moral value as being distinct from both duty and consequences and lay in the character and intentions of the moral agent. Therefore, as moral agents, if professionals make decisions or take actions that are intended for the benefit of the persons they relate to, they could be described as moral acts. Whilst this may be a source of comfort for the professional working in the abyss of the ethical grey, it should nonetheless never negate the need to consider both duties and consequences alongside it. Each point of the triage has exploratory and explanatory power yet can be altogether unhelpful in isolation. The three are needed when carefully considering each individual case.

The Application of Ethics to Human Rights

While each point in the triage can be impotent alone, the triage can act as a point of reflection for every professional involved in care that may remove a person's human rights. Some key questions for self-reflection could be:
- Duty
  - What are my duties?
  - Who are these duties to?
  - Do any of these duties clash, and if so, can I justify one duty superseding another?
- Consequences
  - What may be the consequences of restricting/removing human rights?
  - What may be the consequences if there is no treatment?

- Virtues
  - What are the genuine reasons behind my decisions and actions?
  - Are my decisions genuinely for the benefit of the person, or are there other influences?

These questions will not suddenly make every decision easy, however, they will ensure a thoughtful professional, considering all avenues of morality.

CURATIVE/PALLIATIVE APPROACHES

Specifically addressing the core premise of this book, that palliation rather than curative approaches may be most appropriate for mental health care, the restriction of human rights can be examined through the moral triage. Duties to respect human rights can and always will clash with perceived duties to protect and provide care for our most vulnerable. It could be argued that the virtue behind all restriction of human rights may be primarily a beneficent curative intention, not to comfort but to rectify the distress. The argument then rests on whether it is better to harm in the short term to prevent harm in the longer term. This consequentialist tension may be viewed very differently depending on whether the professional has a curative or palliative focus. It certainly seems illogical that a palliative agent would attempt to relieve pain through delivering the pain that comes with human rights violation. Whilst it is clear the weight of consequences would need to be carefully considered, there is certainly an argument to be made that palliation would involve letting people be rather than forcing treatment. This debate will always fall within the context of society and what is deemed reasonable by its people. Palliative philosophy must pay particular attention to the potential institutional re-traumatisation involved in mental health care, and consider whether it may in some cases be of more benefit to do nothing, rather than an iatrogenic something.

SELF-ASSESSMENT EXERCISE 8.2 – ANSWERS ON P. 109

Time: 30 minutes

Using this chapter, address the following multiple-choice questions. Check your answers on p. 109

1. In Hohfeldian terms, a right to be free from another person's authority is a:
   a) Claim-right
   b) Immunity-right
   c) Privilege-right
   d) Power-right

2. The PANEL principles stand for:
   a) Participation, Accountability, Non-discrimination, Equality and Legality
   b) Participation, Access, Non-discrimination, Empowerment and Legality
   c) Participation, Accountability, Non-discrimination, Empowerment and Legality
   d) Power, Access, Non-discrimination, Equality and Legality

3. An Emergency Detention Certificate allows for a person to be detained in hospital while their condition is assessed for a period of up to:
   a) 24 hours
   b) 48 hours
   c) 72 hours
   d) 7 days

4. An Advance Decision is legally binding if it:
   a) Complies with mental capacity legislation, is valid and applies to the person's situation
   b) Was written in Scotland, is signed by an RMO and sets out how the person wishes to be treated if they become unwell
   c) Complies with the ECHR, is proportionate and is ratified by a tribunal

    d) Complies with mental capacity legislation, is proportionate and sets out how the person wishes to be treated if they become unwell

5. A 'de facto detention' scenario is created when:
    a) Staff detain someone using mental health legislation
    b) A person is detained in hospital for a period of up to 28 days
    c) A person is secluded for an unreasonable amount of time
    d) A person believes that if they do not stay in hospital they will be formally detained under mental health legislation

6. If a person is deemed to lack capacity under the Adults with Incapacity (Scotland) Act (2000) certain other relevant and appropriate people can take decisions on their behalf providing that any interventions are:
    a) Necessary and of benefit to the person and the least restrictive option
    b) Necessary and agreed by a mental health officer
    c) Included in a person's Advance Statement and time limited
    d) Compliant with the ECHR and approved by a mental health tribunal

REFERENCES

Adults with Incapacity (Scotland) Act 2000. a.s.p 4. Available at: www.legislation.gov.uk/asp/2000/4/contents (Accessed: 13 January 2018)

Adult Support and Protection (Scotland) Act 2007. a.s.p 10. Available at: www.legislation.gov.uk/asp/2007/10/contents (Accessed: 13 January 2018)

Agier, M. (2011) *Managing the Undesirables: Refugee Camps and Humanitarian Government.* Cambridge: Polity Press.

Barker, P. (2010) *Mental Health Ethics: The Human Context.* Abingdon: Routledge.

Bar-Tal, D. (2000) *Shared Beliefs in a Society: Social Psychological Analysis.* Thousand Oaks, CA: Sage.

Convention for the Protection of Human Rights and Fundamental Freedoms (European Human Rights Convention) (Rome, 4 November 1950; T.S. 71(1953)); Cmd. 8969. Available at: www.echr.coe.int/Documents/Convention_ENG.pdf (Accessed: 24 January 2018)

Curra, J. (2014) *The Relativity of Deviance.* 3rd edition. Los Angeles, CA: Sage.

Donnelly, J. (2013) *Universal Human Rights in Theory and Practice.* 3rd edition. Ithaca, NY: Cornell University Press.

Dworkin, R. (1984) 'Rights as trumps', in Waldron, J. (ed.) *Theories of Rights.* Oxford: Oxford University Press, pp. 153–67.

Equality Act 2010. c. 15. Available at: (Accessed 24 January 2018)

Equality and Human Rights Commission (2017) *What does Brexit mean for equality and human rights in the UK?* Available at: www.equalityhumanrights.com/en/our-human-rights-work/what-does-brexit-mean-equality-and-human-rights-uk (Accessed 24 January 2018)

Finnis, J. (1980) *Natural Law and Natural Right.* Oxford: Clarendon Press.

Hicks, B. (2005) *Love All the People. Letters, Lyrics, Routines.* London: Constable.

Hinshaw, S. P. and Cicchetti, D. (2000) 'Stigma and mental disorder: conceptions of illness, public attitudes, personal disclosure, and social policy', *Development and Psychopathology,* 12, pp. 555–98.

Hohfeld, W. (1919) 'Fundamental legal conceptions', in Cook, W. (ed.) *Fundamental Legal Conceptions.* New Haven, CT: Yale University Press.

Human Rights Act 1998. c. 42. Available at: www.legislation.gov.uk/ukpga/1998/42/contents (Accessed: 24 January 2018)

Kant, I. (1993) [1785] *Grounding for the Metaphysics of Morals.* Translated by Ellington, J. W. (3rd edition.). Cambridge, MA: Hacket Publishing Company Inc.

Kelman, H. C. (1976) 'Violence without restraint: reflections on the dehumanization of victims and victimizers', in Kren, G. M. and Rappoport, L. H. (eds) *Varieties of Psychohistory.* New York: Springer, pp. 282–314.

Meissner, J. E. (1986) 'Nurses: are we eating our young?' *Nursing,* 16, pp. 51–3.

Mental Health (Care and Treatment) (Scotland) Act 2003. a.s.p 13. Available at: www.legislation.gov.uk/asp/2003/13/contents (Accessed: 13 January 2018)

Mental Welfare Commission for Scotland (2017) *Compulsion Order.* Edinburgh: Mental Welfare Commission for Scotland.

Mill, J. (1989) 'On liberty and other essays', in Collini, S. (ed.), *On Liberty and Other Essays,* Cambridge: Cambridge University Press.

Office of the United Nations High Commissioner for Human Rights (OHCHR), (2016) *The International Bill of Human Rights, Fact Sheet No.2 (Rev.1).* Available at: http://www.ohchr.org/Documents/Publications/FactSheet2Rev.1en.pdf (Accessed 23 January 2018)

Opotow, S. (1990) 'Moral exclusion and injustice: an introduction', *Journal of Social Issues,* 46, pp. 1–20.

Schulman-Green, D. (2003) 'Coping mechanisms of physicians who routinely work with dying patients', *OMEGA,* 47, pp. 253–64.

Scotland Act 1998. c. 46. Available at: www.legislation.gov.uk/ukpga/1998/46/contents (Accessed: 13 January 2018)

Scottish Executive Millan Committee (2001) *New Directions: Report on the Review of the Mental Health (Scotland) Act 1984.* (Chairman: Rt. Hon Bruce Millan). Edinburgh: Scottish Executive.

Scottish Human Rights Commission, (2017). *PANEL Principles.* Edinburgh: Scottish Human Rights Commission.

Sumner, L. (1987) *The Moral Foundations of Rights.* Oxford: Oxford University Press.

Sweeney, A., Clement, C., Filson, B. and Kennedy, A. (2016) 'Trauma-informed mental healthcare in the UK: what is it and how can we further its development?', *Mental Health Review Journal,* 21, pp. 174–92.

Szasz, T. S. (1973) 'Mental illness as a metaphor', *Nature,* 242, pp. 305–07.

The Patient Rights (Scotland) Act 2011. a.s.p 5. Available at: www.legislation.gov.uk/asp/2011/5/pdfs/asp_20110005_en.pdf (Accessed: 13 January 2018)

The Scottish Government (2012) *Charter of Patient Rights and Responsibilities.* Edinburgh: The Scottish Government.

United Nations (2008) *Convention on the Rights of Persons with Disabilities.* New York, NY: United Nations.

United Nations (1948) *Universal Declaration of Human Rights.* New York, NY: United Nations.

To Learn More

Cohen, J. and Ezer, T. (2013) 'Human rights in patient care: a theoretical and practical framework'. *Health and Human Rights,* 15, pp. 7–19.

Mental Welfare Commission for Scotland (2017) *Rights in Mind: A Pathway to Patients' Rights in Mental Health Services.* Edinburgh: Mental Welfare Commission for Scotland.

Trachsel, M., Irwin, S. A., Biller-Andorno, N., Hoff, P. and Riese, F. (2016) 'Palliative psychiatry for severe persistent mental illness as a new approach to psychiatry? Definition, scope, benefits, and risks'. *BMC Psychiatry,* 16, p. 260.

ANSWERS TO SELF-ASSESSMENT EXERCISE 8.2

Time: 15 minutes
1. b
2. c
3. c
4. a
5. d
6. a

CHAPTER 9

Symptom Management Framework

John Richard Ashcroft and Laura Henry

INTRODUCTION

It is generally accepted that the diagnosis and treatment of mental health conditions are fundamentally different to other specialties in medicine. Diagnosis of mental disorder according to the two principal diagnostic classification systems, namely the International Classification of Mental and Behavioural Disorders (ICD-10) (World Health Organisation 1992) and Diagnostic and Statistical Manual of Mental Disorders (DSM-V) (American Psychiatric Association 2013), in their tenth and fifth version respectively is based on collections of symptoms, also known as syndromes, which occur together consistently to allow for descriptive terms to be used.

Therapeutic intervention, whether by way of medication, psychology or environmental change is focused on alleviating such symptoms as opposed to directly addressing underlying pathology. Of course, if such pathology is known, efforts will be made to address cause, although all too often in mental health settings causes are at best suspected or theorised and the aims of intervention are to alleviate suffering and to achieve symptomatic relief.

COMORBIDITY AND TREATMENT RESISTANCE

Comorbidity is extremely frequent in mental health settings (Maj 2005) and refers to the presence of two or more disorders occurring in any one individual usually at the same time although sometimes the term refers to the sequential development or overlap of a second condition. An example would be the presence of an anxiety disorder in conjunction with a mood disorder such as Bipolar Disorder or Major Depressive Disorder. In contrast, a single symptom may be acknowledged as an intrinsic feature of any one of a number of mental disorders or syndromes. For example, poor attention or difficulty with concentration may be seen across a range of conditions such as Attention Deficit Hyperactivity Disorder (ADHD), Obsessive Compulsive Disorder, Schizophrenia, Bipolar Disorder or Acquired Brain Injury. Where two or more conditions exist in any one individual, how do we determine to which disorder a single symptom belongs? A treatment or intervention may result in alleviation of one symptom or set of symptoms, but result in the emergence of others (side effects). All too often an individual's response to any particular treatment is partial at best and there is often some degree of treatment resistance frequently as a result of confounding factors (Casher et al. 2012).

THE INDIVIDUAL SYMPTOMS APPROACH

Therefore, upon consideration of the above facts it becomes increasingly apparent that to address mental health problems simply by focusing on an overarching disorder and diagnostic label alone could be seen as disadvantageous and an approach for managing symptoms regardless of a diagnosis may be more appropriate in many cases. It could be argued that the syndromal approach to treatment is akin to a rather non-specific 'scatter gun' type strategy, whereby several symptoms of a disorder are addressed at once. For example, antipsychotic medications prescribed for psychotic experiences have the effect of reducing the intensity and frequency of auditory hallucinations yet also impact (positively or negatively depending on subjective reports) on aspects of mood, cognition and behaviour. There may also be physical health effects such as central nervous system and endocrine disturbance.

Once the desired outcome has been achieved (for example in the case of a prescription for antipsychotics for a reduction in psychotic symptoms) is the goal of treatment achieved? Invariably the job is only half complete as it is as important at this stage to assess for the presence of side effects and to revaluate the situation for the presence of additional features of ill-health that may not have been immediately evident.

KEY POINT 9.1

It is imperative that this phase of treatment be considered an integral part of management and that sufficient time is spent in planning, assessing and reviewing treatment.

Without a symptomatic approach this crucial stage of treatment may be overlooked and what appears to have been treatment success could be regarded as simply a swap from one set of symptoms to another. It is this feature which may explain, at least in part, the reason for non-concordance of medication and other forms of treatment, disengagement from services and a poor therapeutic alliance.

AN EFFECTIVE SYMPTOMATIC APPROACH

Such a symptomatic approach is often adopted in the treatment of people experiencing neuropsychiatric manifestations of traumatic brain injury and acquired brain injury. The clinical presentation of individuals experiencing brain injury often crosses traditional classification boundaries (Hurley & Taber 2002) whereby an individual may present with a combination of neurobehavioural, neurocognitive and emotional disturbances, which does not allow for the use of any one diagnosis. Indeed, it would be wholly inappropriate to attempt to do so as this would likely lead to unnecessary complications or unwanted side effect profiles if treatment were to follow. Rather, specific symptoms are targeted based on individual symptoms, knowledge of the location of the site of injury, and an understanding of neuronal circuitry. Interestingly in individuals experiencing brain injury, severity of a lesion sustained does not predict the degree of psychological disturbance (Hiploylee et al. 2016; Malec and Kean 2016) and it is extremely important to evaluate an individual's insight into their difficulties such as the awareness of change in personality. Although an experience may be distressing and or painful and consequently lead to a secondary reaction by virtue of the unpleasantness of the experience, an additional layer of suffering must be considered, namely the **meaning** or **significance** of the symptom.

INDIVIDUAL SYMPTOMS

For a mental health disorder to be diagnosed, particular criteria need to be met. For example, for a diagnosis of mild depression (World Health Organisation, ICD-10 F32) two of the following symptoms must be present for a period of at least two weeks
1. Depressed mood
2. Loss of interest and enjoyment
3. Increased fatigability.

However, how should an individual presenting with only a single feature be approached? Seemingly an individual experiencing persistent low mood only who is otherwise functioning extremely well would not meet the threshold criteria for depression. Similarly, individuals experiencing symptoms of both anxiety and depression, often fail to meet the threshold to achieve a formal diagnosis of either depressive disorder or anxiety disorder because of the changeable nature of their presentation and their ability to otherwise function. Such a quantitative approach seems rather arbitrary when compared to the more qualitative approach favoured by a symptom management framework.

Where an individual's symptoms do not fit smoothly into a diagnostic categorical framework it may be tempting to minimise the extent and or severity of ill-health ('the diagnostic criteria has not been met and therefore the individual is not as unwell or suffering as much as reported') or equally disconcerting, efforts may be made to fit the individual's symptoms into established diagnostic entities, by way of exaggerating associated features and minimising others.

A highly functioning individual with marked subjective anxiety and/or low mood may become angry at being told that he/she is not severely unwell as a consequence of his or her high functioning and his or her disclosed regular thoughts of suicide, deemed to be evidence of an Emotionally Unstable Personality Disorder.

Similarly, an adult with a history of sexual abuse as a child who experiences strong visual and auditory imagery (deemed to be evidence of hallucinatory phenomena) and significant anxiety (subjective and not reported) associated with persecutory ideation (as observed by suspiciousness and odd behaviour deemed more so by a lack of appreciation of subjective distress) may receive a diagnosis of schizophrenia rather than an assessment for individual symptoms of post-traumatic stress disorder (*See* Chapter 11) because 'the disorder should not generally be diagnosed unless there is evidence that it arose within 6 months of a traumatic event of exceptional severity' (World Health Organisation, ICD-10 F43.1).

Clearly, in such circumstances if one is to assume that the aim of treatment is to alleviate subjective distress and suffering, an approach which addresses symptoms separately, albeit acknowledging that there may be an association between one symptom and another, is preferable than an effort to make sense of the presentation by means of matching sets of symptoms to pre-existing diagnoses.

THE REHABILITATION SETTING

Often individuals are referred to specialist rehabilitation services after there has been a series of unsuccessful admissions to hospital and or significant treatment resistance for a particular disorder. As discussed above, to continue to make efforts to treat any individually diagnosed disorder might not always be in the best interest of the individual. We need to remain conscious of the limitations of psychiatric diagnostic classification systems. It may therefore be more appropriate to break down the individual's presentation into a series of individual problems and to address each in a systematic, controlled and considered way. Such an approach has previously been suggested by other professionals in other clinical settings such as the management of symptoms of advanced cancer in palliative care (Hill 2006, pp. 40–76). A ten-step symptom management framework is detailed below:

1. Identification of symptoms.
2. Prioritisation of symptoms.
3. Causation of symptoms.
4. Isolation of the cause and causes of most aetiological significance.
5. Exploration of the concerns and expectations of the individual.
6. Discussion of likely diagnosis/diagnoses.
7. Negotiation of an agreed treatment approach.
8. Maintenance of treatment.
9. Evaluation assessment of an individual.
10. Repetition and review of an individual's response to the agreed intervention and approach.

1. Identification: What are the symptoms?

Case Study 9.1

Jake is a 30-year-old gentleman with a diagnosis of treatment-resistant schizophrenia whose psychotic symptoms have considerably improved since the introduction of anti-psychotic medication. The frequency of intrusive and distressing voices has considerably reduced. However, Jake has put on 10kg in weight in the last two years and has developed borderline type 2 diabetes. He lacks motivation and has difficulty getting out of bed in the morning. He often feels tired in the day and lacks motivation to attend to his personal care for which he often needs to be prompted. Jake does not appear to be depressed in mood and subjectively denies feeling so. He demonstrates little interest in activities he would previously find pleasurable such as listening to music and watching films. He is smoking more.

SELF-ASSESSMENT EXERCISE 9.1

Time: 30 minutes
- Discussion points
- Has medication been effective?
- What are Jake's symptoms?
- What are Jakes signs?
- Can all signs and symptoms be attributable to a single diagnosis or disorder?
- What would Jake describe as his main problems?

The first step in the assessment process is to identify the complaints of the individual in his or her own words. Although often used interchangeably the terms symptom and sign are distinct (Kraft and Keeley 2015). The process of identification of an individual's complaints requires an understanding of the difference between subjectively experienced symptoms and objectively observed and measurable signs.

2. Prioritisation: Prioritise symptoms to be dealt with first

Case Study 9.2

Dave is a teacher with a diagnosis of bipolar disorder recently prescribed quetiapine XL as a mood stabiliser. The severity and frequency of his mood swings have reduced although he is aware of a subjective sense of reduced concentration span and inability to remained focused for the whole day. He is extremely fatigued upon returning home from work. His wife feels that their relationship has improved greatly as a result of his calmer demeanour although Dave's sex drive has reduced. Dave is happy that his mood swings have improved although is concerned about the change in his circumstances. He has discussed his concerns with his psychiatrist although he was told that he must continue to take medication as prescribed.

SELF-ASSESSMENT EXERCISE 9.2

Time: 30 minutes
- Discussion points
- What are the issues in terms of prioritisation of treatment?
- What are Dave's concerns?
- What are the concerns of his treating psychiatrist?
- What would you advise?

Ideally the individual experiencing mental ill-health should be encouraged to prioritise which symptoms need to be addressed by virtue of the fact that often individuals will wish to first alleviate those symptoms that are causing the most distress. However, the priority of the treating professional may differ from that of the individual experiencing symptoms. An understanding of the distinction between the definition of signs and symptoms may explain this discrepancy to some degree as a result of differing perspectives. For example, how much time should be spent managing 10 per cent increase in symptoms of anxiety following a 50 per cent reduction in psychotic experiences manifesting in odd behaviour? The answer of course is that it depends greatly on the distress experienced by the individual in treatment although . . .

KEY POINT 9.2

It is crucially important that the individual with any symptom determines the severity, the importance, and the significance of that symptom.

Consideration of Risk

In contrast to disorders of physical health, mental ill-health may be associated with risk, whether to the individual by way of deliberate self-harm for example or to others (*See* Chapter 19). That is not to say that mental and physical ill-health do not overlap, or that purely physical health conditions are not associated with risk (take for example the risk of suicide in people experiencing severe chronic pain) but as a rule mental ill-health by virtue of the commonly associated features of behavioural and perception disturbance are much more likely to require a detailed consideration of risk when prioritising intervention and treatment goals.

For example, an individual with a diagnosis of treatment resistant schizophrenia may have very well controlled positive symptoms of psychosis, although experiencing side effects of disturbed sleep and poor motivation. The treating professional may determine that the current medication regime is appropriate and that there is an acceptable balance between symptom control and risk. However, the individual may disagree and may deem a dose reduction to be preferable regardless of the possible re-emergence of psychotic experiences.

3. Causation: It is important to compile a list of potential causes for any symptom

Case Study 9.3

Steve has a diagnosis of schizophrenia for which he is prescribed olanzapine. He is worried about his father's health; his father was recently diagnosed with prostate cancer. Steve has informed his care coordinator that he has been hearing voices. Steve has an appointment with his psychiatrist. He has been told that his medication dose is likely to be increased. This is causing Steve to feel anxious.

SELF-ASSESSMENT EXERCISE 9.3

Time: 30 minutes

Discussion points
- What are Steve's symptoms?
- What types of 'voices' are there?
- Are all voices psychotic in nature?
- Can anxiety and ruminations present as voices?
- What treatment options are available for Steve's voices?

KEY POINT 9.3

It is imperative not to jump to conclusions as to the cause of the symptom or indeed the nature of the symptom itself.

All too often additional medication is prescribed without consideration of the possible presence of psychological factors, social and environmental disturbance such as relationship difficulties, and physical health concerns. Iatrogenic causes (the effects of treatment itself) also need to be considered. Antidepressants may cause anxiety (Sinclair et al. 2009), and antipsychotic drugs may be associated with dopamine super sensitivity and psychosis (Yin et al. 2017).

In addition, it is extremely important that the treating professionals regularly assess, and re-evaluate the nature of the presenting symptom. Failure to do so may deflect from identification of cause and associated factors of aetiological significance. In Steve's case a diagnosis of schizophrenia may lead to a presumption that the 'voices' as reported are psychotic in nature, and by virtue of this fact, that the cause is in some way related to the primary diagnosis (albeit acknowledging that such a diagnosis of schizophrenia is one of a diagnosis of exclusion). However, voices manifest in a variety of guises and intrusive worries and thoughts may present as and be described as 'voices'. The treatment approach to the latter would be very different than the treatment of true auditory hallucinations.

4. Establish the Probable Cause of the Symptom – Isolation of the Cause(s) of Most Aetiological Significance

Having compiled a list of potential causes of any individual symptom, it is imperative to gather as much information as possible to determine the likelihood of any suggested theories. It is likely that any individual entering mental health services for the first time would undergo a full history and examination and although such documentation is often detailed and accurate at the time of the assessment, it is most certainly in the best interests of all for the history to be revisited to ensure that the information is correct; a diagnosis in mental health made upon admission to hospital or secondary services should by no means go unchallenged. As stated above, given the significant comorbidity in mental health settings, we should remain mindful of the possibility of other causes for symptoms. Mental ill-health diagnoses are diagnoses of exclusion, and where possible all non-psychiatric causes should be excluded before a mental health problem is diagnosed.

There may be a complex interplay between a number of causes and associated symptoms and the identification of a singular cause may not be possible. There is often a reciprocal relationship between symptoms of depression, anxiety and physical pain, for example, by way of one symptom impacting negatively on another in terms of exacerbation and perpetuation of symptom severity. Similarly, alleviation of one symptom may have a positive effect on others. A narrative may ensue by way of the process of informed formulation.

For example, in the presence of prolonged affective symptoms following brain injury it is often difficult to differentiate between symptoms directly attributable to brain injury and those relating to the psychological reaction to neuropsychiatric sequelae. There is very likely a complex interplay between an individual's symptoms of low mood, anxiety and physical pain. Anxiety and depression are associated with somatic symptoms and chronic physical pain is associated with affective disturbance.

Equally, in the comorbid presence of anxiety disorders and chronic pain the situation is more complicated as not all somatic symptoms can or should be regarded as psychosomatic/psychogenic (by virtue of the fact that many such symptoms will be unrelated) and not all symptoms of anxiety and depression should be regarded as a psychological reaction to chronic pain (as in the case of premorbid symptoms of anxiety). However, the subjective experience of each negatively impacts the other.

5. Exploration of the Concerns, Ideas, and Expectations of the Individual

Treatment Expectations

In all cases it is extremely important to identify what the individual knows and understands about his or her diagnosis and symptoms. The individual's expectations of treatment and their individual concerns should be noted, as it has been well established that such expectations and preconceived ideas could significantly impact on treatment outcome (Bowden 1980). A simple change in expectation may itself be sufficient to alleviate a symptom or indeed set of symptoms, or allow improved acceptance to receive, or willingness and or motivation to engage in a proposed treatment or intervention.

Meta Suffering

KEY POINT 9.4

Efforts should be made to explore the significance of the perceived experience or symptom, whether physical or psychological, rather than simply aim to treat symptoms alone.

The on-going presence of physical pain and anxiety may contribute to further anxiety by virtue of associated thoughts (significance) and fear of further ill-health and possibly death. Layers of anxiety or depression may be present whereby an individual may be anxious about feeling anxious for example or depressed because they feel depressed not simply as a consequence of the experience but because of what the symptom signifies and means to them.

6. Discussion of the Likely Diagnosis/Diagnoses

For some individuals the provision of a diagnosis can be a significant moment in their treatment journey, an 'I knew something was wrong' moment and or a validation of suffering. However, diagnosis in mental health can be extremely stigmatising and it is important to discuss with the individual their views and opinion of the subject. It may be appropriate to discuss the limitations of psychiatric diagnosis with some individuals although this may not always be possible or advisable. In contrast, the absence of an identifiable diagnosis does not and should not negate or preclude the presence of suffering.

SELF-ASSESSMENT EXERCISE 9.4

Time: 30 minutes

Discussion points
Mental Health Diagnosis
- Is it useful?
- Is the previous diagnosis correct?
- Has the diagnosis changed?
- Are there more than one appropriate diagnoses?

An individual's preconceived ideas of mental ill-health may itself be significantly contributing to the on-going presence of symptoms and or treatment resistance. For example, an individual with a particularly negative view of those who experience depression and who later develop depression, may experience significant symptoms of anxiety and be of an increased susceptibility to medication side effects and treatment resistance.

7. Deciding on the Best Treatment – Negotiation of an Agreed Treatment Approach

There is considerable evidence for the importance of good therapeutic alliance in improving clinical outcomes (Chaplin et al. 2007). Individuals should be included in the treatment making process and this should be regarded as a key element for good clinical practice (Goss & Moretti 2008). All side effects of medication should be explained. Medical and non-medical options should be discussed in detail. The individual should be made aware of all treatment options available. It is imperative to involve the individual and family in all aspects of the decision-making process pertaining to treatment wherever possible. Therefore the 'best treatment' for one individual may not necessary be the same as that for another regardless of what the literature may say in regards evidence based practice. Adopting a textbook bio-psycho-socio approach to individual symptoms and to address predisposing, precipitating and maintaining factors may be best practice although approaches may simply be excluded as possibilities sometimes without explanation. It is often necessary to negotiate alternative strategies. Occasionally a decision may be made not to treat a primary symptom and an intervention may focus on aspects of motivation.

8. Setting Realistic Treatment Goals and Maintaining Hope

To maximise levels of engagement in any treatment regime, individuals should be made aware of the likelihood of treatment. Unrealistic goals and expectations should be avoided at all costs as it is extremely likely that if an individual fails to respond to suggested treatment, they will blame themselves for this and this may result in an exacerbation of existing symptoms or an emergence of others. One individual's ability or willingness to accept a particular symptom may be very different from the next. Wholesale approaches to levels of acceptable outcomes and side effect profiles should also be avoided. It may be 'realistic' to the treating clinician that a person should occasionally experience headaches as a side effect and that the benefits of a treatment greatly outweigh the risk of such a symptom. But who should decide this? It seems counterintuitive to suggest that such decisions should be determined by anybody but the individual receiving the treatment, yet in the presence of risk it is common place for individuals to be forced to take medication against their will despite such effects. At the very least options should be explored.

9. Evaluation – Assessing the Response to Treatment

Response to treatment should be evaluated through a number of sources involving a variety of objective and subjective measures to include the views of all health care professionals involved in an individual's care and the view of the individual and relatives. A set period should be determined from the outset when introducing any intervention to review the success of treatments. Clearly, in the longer term it is the view of the

Case Study 9.4

John is a 35-year-old man with a diagnosis of schizoaffective disorder for which he is prescribed depot antipsychotic medication. Following an acute exacerbation of psychotic symptoms and aggressive behaviour he was admitted to hospital for assessment and review of medication. Since the introduction of olanzapine, although John has spoken little, he is much calmer and more willing to go along with the requests of staff. He is occasionally tearful although much less aggressive than at the time of admission. The multidisciplinary team feel that John has made considerable progress since admission and his symptoms of psychosis have significantly reduced. Discharge home is expected in the next few days.

individual that truly counts although there may be observational indicators of behavioural change, which may be fed back to the individual where appropriate to maintain morale and motivation. For example, in the case of individuals experiencing depression, objective measures of sociability may be more apparent to observers than the individual themselves, who may not have experienced any change in mood state and be feeling more pessimistic than necessary about a particular intervention.

10. Review of all Above – Repetition and Review of an Individual's Response to the Agreed Intervention and Approach

KEY POINT 9.5

It is imperative that progress is reviewed on a regular basis and that any treatment approach is adjusted accordingly.

As is unfortunately often the case in people experiencing mental ill-health symptoms, treatment programmes continue regardless of response to treatment in the hope that at some point in the future things may change. This approach is extremely difficult for the person to understand and is highly unproductive. To blindly persist with any intervention simply in the hope that something will change later is nonsensical. Individuals and the close family should be involved in any decision-making process including choice and duration of treatment.

Adaptation

It is extremely important that assessing and treating clinicians adapt to the emergence of new symptom presentations in a timely and effective manner. A preoccupation with any individual's diagnosis could hinder this by a newly developed or developing symptom or presenting problem that does not fit with the previous diagnosis or theoretical paradigm. Approaching the use of diagnoses as a framework only allows for the emergence of new symptoms to come as no surprise and for such change in symptomatology not to be excluded as insignificant, unrelated or irrelevant to the current treatment plan. In effect the assessing and treating practitioner should expect all and everything.

KEY POINT 9.6

The role of formulation in the rehabilitation setting is extremely important in that there is a constant assessment, re-assessment and re-appraisal of the situation to allow for new information to be factored into the working formulation.

CONCLUSION

The aim of this chapter is to introduce a framework for addressing individual symptoms presenting in people experiencing mental health problems. Such a symptom management framework does not aim to replace the current diagnostic approach but rather to be used in conjunction with the current classification system, to enable the limitations of the current system to be addressed and compensated for.

Individuals experiencing any mental ill-health problem rarely form a homogenous group. An approach, which treats all individuals with a particular disorder in the same way, is fundamentally flawed. It could be argued that the focus on the syndromal approach is to identify individuals with the same symptoms to apply a standardised treatment approach to such collection of symptoms. In contrast to the framework of symptoms, management is focused on what makes one individual's symptoms different from the next, whether in the context of an established mental disorder or not. In this way the treatment approach will be tailored to the specific set of symptoms that are unique to the individual.

The frequency of comorbidity of disorder, the degree and diagnostic uncertainty, and the prevalence of treatment resistance requires that all too often adjustments to treatment regimes are required. A flexible approach to the ever-changing symptom presentation is required and a symptom management approach is better placed to achieve this goal than utilising an arguably rigid diagnostic classification system alone.

REFERENCES

American Psychiatric Association (2013) Diagnostic and Statistical Manual of Mental and Behavioural Disorders. 5th edition. Washington DC: American Psychiatric Association.

Bowden, C. L. (1980) 'Mental health attitudes and treatment expectations as treatment variables', Journal of Clinical Psychology, 36, pp. 653–7.

Casher, M. I., Gih, D., Bess, J. D. and Agarwala, P. (2012) Confounding factors in treatment resistant depression (part 2) Comorbidities and treatment resistance. Available at: www.psychiatrictimes.com/printpdf/159808 (Accessed 5 December 2017)

Chaplin, R., Lelliott, P., Quirk, A. and Seale, C. (2007) 'Negotiating styles adopted by consultant psychiatrists when prescribing antipsychotics', Advances in Psychiatric Treatment, 13, pp. 43–50.

Goss, C. and Moretti, F. (2008) 'Involving patients in decisions during psychiatric consultations', British Journal of Psychiatry, 193, pp. 416–21.

Hill, S. (2006) 'Symptom management: a framework', in Cooper, J. Stepping Into Palliative Care: Care and Practice. 2nd edition. Oxon, UK/New York: Radcliffe Publishing Ltd. pp. 40–76.

Hiploylee, C., Dufort, P. A., Davis, H. S., Wennberg, R. A., Tartaglia, M. C. et al. (2016) 'Longitudinal study of post concussion syndrome: not everyone recovers', Journal of Neurotrauma, 33, pp. 1–9.

Hurley, R. A. and Taber, K. H. (2002) 'Emotional disturbances following traumatic brain injury 2002', Current Treatment Options in Neurology, 4, pp. 59–75.

Kraft, N. H. and Keely, J. W. (2015) 'Sign versus symptom', *The Encyclopaedia of Clinical Psychology*. Available at: http://onlinelibrary.wiley.com/doi/10.1002/9781118625392.wbecp145/abstract;jsession id=1545A9498457FBAD7181D9DB4D67D536.f03t04 (Accessed 5 December 2017)

Maj, M. (2005) 'Psychiatric comorbidity: an artefact of current diagnostic systems?', *British Journal of Psychiatry*, 186, pp. 182–4.

Malec, J. F. and Kean, J. (2016) 'Post-inpatient brain injury rehabilitation outcomes: Report from the national outcome info database', *Journal of Neurotrauma*, 33, pp. 1371–9.

Sinclair, L. I., Christmas, D. M., Hood, S. D., Potokar, J. P., Robertson, A., Isaac, A., Srivastava, S., Nutt, D. J., and Davies, S. J. C. (2009) 'Antidepressant-induced jitteriness/anxiety syndrome: systematic review', *British Journal of Psychiatry*, 194, pp. 483–90. Available at: http://bjp.rcpsych.org/content/194/6/483 (Accessed: 5 December 2017)

World Health Organisation (1992) *International Classification of Mental and Behavioural Disorders*. 10th edition. Geneva: World Health Organisation.

Yin, J., Barr, A., M. Ramos-Migual, A. and Procyshyn, R. M. (2017) 'Antipsychotic induced dopamine super sensitivity psychosis: a comprehensive review', *Current Neuropharmacology*, 15, pp. 174–83.

To Learn More

Craddock, N. and Mynors-Wallis, L. (2014) 'Psychiatric diagnosis: impersonal, imperfect and important', *British Journal of Psychiatry*, 204, pp. 93–5.

Mayou, R. and Farmer, A. (2002) 'Functional somatic symptoms and syndromes', *British Medical Journal*, 325, pp. 265–8. www.bmj.com/content/325/73/58/265

Read, J., Mosher, L. R. and Bentall, R.P. (2004) *Models of Madness. Psychological, Social and Biological Approaches to Schizophrenia*. London and New York: Routledge.

Sacks, O. (1986) *The Man Who Mistook His Wife for a Hat*. London: Picador.

Sacks, O. (1995) *An Anthropologist on Mars*. London: Picador.

CHAPTER 10

Developing the Art of Self-Knowledge and Applying Deductive Reasoning in Clinical Practice

Subia Parveen Rasheed and Ahtisham Younas

The overarching goal of health care is to improve health outcomes of persons experiencing health problems in an efficient and effective manner. One of the much-needed skills that may help health care professionals in improving health outcomes is having sound clinical reasoning skills (Benner, Hughes & Molly 2008). In order to develop sound clinical reasoning skills, health care professionals must focus on becoming self-knowledgeable (Gardiner 2016). The terms 'self-knowledge', 'self-awareness', and 'self-knowing', are used interchangeably in the literature, but in this text, we will use the term self-knowledge. Self-awareness or self-knowledge is an 'intrapersonal process of self-discovery' (Eckroth-Bucher 2010, p. 301) that entails three types of analyses:

1. **superficial analysis** – refers to examining one's concrete personality traits such as gender, eye color, body shape, and so forth
2. **selective analysis** – refers to recognizing one's personal beliefs, biases, and attitudes
3. **deep awareness** – refers to examining and recognizing one's hidden aspects of personality.

(Eckroth-Bucher 2010)

Being self-knowledgeable means possessing the following four attributes as outlined by (Eckroth-Bucher 2010).
1. **Cerebral exercise of introspection** – cognitive examination of one's emotional states, thoughts, feelings, beliefs, biases, and pre-conceived ideas
2. **Process** – continuous examination and comparison of one's emotional states, thoughts, feelings, beliefs, biases, and pre-conceived ideas with newly developed ideas and beliefs
3. **Understanding convictions and values** – a profound examination of one's meaningful personality traits, beliefs, and experiences

4. **Guidepost** – an ability to direct one's actions consistent with personal values, beliefs, and meaningful personality traits.

Although the awareness analyses and the attributes are essential for becoming self-knowledgeable, it is important to remember that self-knowledge is contextual, should be assessed in every situation, and should involve examination of the environment (Rasheed 2015).

Similar to self-knowledge, clinical reasoning is 'a context dependent way of thinking in professional practice to guide practice actions' (Higgs 2008, p. 4). It is a process of collecting and understanding information about a person's health by reflecting and identifying cues and then developing an effective plan of care (Levett-Jones et al. 2010). Deductive reasoning refers to the logical application of general rules to specific situations (Bolton 2015). Hence, deductive clinical reasoning is the application of general rules to a specific clinical situation after a thorough contextual assessment. Thereupon, the health professional should scrutinize the assessment, and then follow through with an appropriate action plan. Self-knowledge has been positively linked to deductive clinical reasoning and both are considered contextual (Borrell-Carrió & Epstein 2004; Ashoorion, Liaghatdar & Adibi 2012; Gay, Bartlett & McKinley 2013; Sedgwick, Grigg & Dersch 2014). Moreover, it has been suggested that higher levels of self-knowledge result in enhancing one's deductive clinical reasoning skills (Sedgwick, Grigg & Dersch 2014). Within the context of mental health palliative care, a health care professional's approach to decision making and provision of care is primarily interpersonal and holistic, that is, focusing on the physical, spiritual, psychological, and emotional health and well-being of both persons and health care professionals. It could be challenging for health care professionals to connect with persons experiencing mental health problems. Therefore, the necessity of interpersonal skills (Holewa 2004). Hence, self-knowledge, being an essential interpersonal skill, plays a decisive role for success in these settings (Goswami 2013) as it allows health care providers to effectively analyze the individual information (Rasheed 2015). Such is the purpose of this text; to provide readers with a practical approach for fostering self-knowledge, enhancing deductive clinical reasoning skills, and applying self-knowledge within palliative mental health settings through the use of comprehensive reflection, deductive clinical reasoning, and ethical practice. Before further discussion, we encourage you to engage in the following reflective practice exercise 10.1.

REFLECTIVE PRACTICE EXERCISE 10.1

Time: 20 minutes
Sit at your favorite place in your home or outside, close your eyes, and without putting your hand on your chest or your wrist try to count your heart rate. Then, ask your friend or partner or anyone else to count your heart rate. Compare the readings and see if your reading is close to the reading that your friend took. The closer the reading the more self-aware you are (Davidson 2012).

This exercise directs your attention to one of the tiniest physiological changes taking place in your body and gives an idea of your personal self-knowledge. Here, it is important to note that self-knowledge is not limited to knowing your personal self, such as physiological and emotional changes and biases, but it also involves recognizing your pre-conceived biases and understanding of the environment, your previous experiences within a similar kind of environment, and the impact of those biases and intentions on your interaction with the persons involved in that situation (Gardiner 2016). Knowing about environment helps us to focus our full attention on the needs of other persons involved in the situation (Rasheed 2015). By engaging in this first exercise, we hope you have an idea of how self-knowledgeable you are. Having laid the foundation of knowing yourself and your environment . . . read the following imaginary case study 10.1 and engage in three types of self-awareness analyses at the personal as well as at the environmental level.

REFLECTIVE PRACTICE EXERCISE 10.2 – ENGAGING IN AWARENESS ANALYSES

Time: 40 minutes

Case Study 10.1

Cynthia, 32, was admitted to the mental health hospital with a history of self-neglect and two attempted suicides because of her recent break-up with her husband. On the first attempt, she ingested 20 sleeping pills and on the second attempt she tried to cut open her wrists with a sharp broken glass. She was diagnosed with severe clinical depression. The primary factors that led to her depression were: death of her mother and one child, an abusive relationship, and receiving a recent diagnosis of ovarian cysts.

As the health care professional of Cynthia, we encourage you to engage in this brief and quick self-knowledge examination and ask yourself these questions.

Superficial Analysis
- **Personal:** What is your heart rate and respiration rate as you enter Cynthia's room for the very first time? What is your body movement? Does it seem as if your body is talking to you? Are you taking short or long steps? (Analyze your body mechanics and gestures and try to recognize your physiological changes).
- **Environmental:** What is Cynthia's room like (observe windows, doors, and space in the room)? Where is she sitting? What is she doing? Is there any object of any kind in the room that *Cynthia* may use to harm herself?

Selective Analysis
If you are caring for Cynthia, we believe you have previously cared for persons with clinical depression.
- **Personal:** Do you have any pre-conceived biases about persons with depression? If so, what are your biases in this situation? Do you have a pre-developed action plan to care for Cynthia?
- **Environmental:** Do you have any pre-conceived assumptions about the room in which Cynthia is staying? Did you care for anyone else in the same room? Did you have any

good or bad memories associated with this room? If so, try to recognize those memories and their effect?

Deep Analysis

- **Personal:** What are your feelings and emotions in this situation? Do you feel anxious about caring for persons experiencing clinical depression? It is the time to quickly reflect if any one of your loved ones ever experienced stress or depression and did they share with you? How might your caring for them affect your care for Cynthia? Did the persons you cared for provide some feedback on your caring abilities?
- **Environmental:** Are Cynthia's family members or relatives or friends in the room? If yes, what are their emotions and feelings? How are they interacting with Cynthia? What are the contextual environmental factors such as workload, organizational commitments, peer pressure, and support from your management that may influence your interaction with Cynthia?

BECOMING SELF-KNOWLEDGEABLE

As previously described, becoming self-knowledgeable requires analysis at superficial, selective, and deep levels in order to gather knowledge about one's psychological, physical, ecological, and interpersonal self (Campbell 1980). Gathering knowledge about the psychological, physical, ecological, and interpersonal self falls under the three levels of awareness mentioned above.

➤ Psychological knowledge – entails one's abilities to deal with stressful situations and with negative emotions
➤ Physical knowledge – entails awareness of one's bodily sensations and personal self-image
➤ Ecological knowledge – entails the effect of different environmental factors and the interplay between different persons
➤ Interpersonal knowledge – entails superficial and deep relationships with other persons.

Within the health care context, these awareness analyses are critical for developing a therapeutic relationship experiencing persons with health problems. However, becoming self-knowledgeable is a time-consuming process (Rasheed 2015) and requires continuous use of several skills and strategies. Some of the widely suggested skills and strategies are:

➤ reflection and reflective practice
➤ practicing meditation and mindfulness
➤ seeking feedback from others.

(Rasheed 2015; Driscoll & Teh 2001)

These strategies are interrelated and should be used as a whole for developing self-knowledge because there is no one size fits all approach for developing self-knowledge.

REFLECTION AND REFLECTIVE PRACTICE

Reflection is a broad concept defined as 'a process of engaging the self in attentive, critical, exploratory and iterative interactions with one's thoughts and actions with a view to changing them and with a view on the change itself' (Nguyen et al. 2014, pp. 1182). However, reflective practice is more focused and involves the critical examination of one's practice that enables self-enquiry for empowerment and transformation of practice (Duffy 2007). It means that reflection and reflective practice allows a person to engage in an introspective examination of one's thoughts and emotions in any given situation. Reflection and reflective practice can also help health care professionals to develop self-awareness and to become more self-knowledgeable (Forrest 2008; Myers 2003; Kwiatek, McKenzie & Loads 2005) thereby enabling health professionals to become better care providers (Gallagher et al. 2017). Therefore, health care professionals should continuously foster their self-reflection and reflective practice. This can be achieved by journal writing, portfolios (Rasheed 2015), psychodramas (i.e. a critical analysis of one's action on a daily basis and identification of areas of improvement) (Oflaz et al. 2011), meditation, and seeking feedback from others (Mann, Gordon & MacLeod 2009). However, health care professionals should discern the best method to foster reflective practice by considering their preferences and circumstances (Morgan 2009).

REFLECTIVE PRACTICE EXERCISE 10.3

Time: 20 minutes
Reflect on your most memorable clinical situation and describe the following things.
- Your personal values that you operated out of in order to interact with the person in that situation
- Your obligations as health care provider that encouraged you to interact with the person
- Your most important actions or interventions that brought about any differences in the health status of the person.

PRACTICING MEDITATION AND MINDFULNESS

Meditation is a voluntary process that entails five elements, which include:

1. a deliberate choice to relax
2. use of self-induction
3. a well-defined technique
4. use of muscle relaxation strategies
5. focusing on trivial details.

(Cardoso et al. 2004)

Meditation could be done in several ways. One of the most widely used approaches to meditation in health care is mindfulness. Mindfulness is a 'transformative process where one develops an increasing ability to experience being present, with acceptance, attention and awareness' (White 2014, p. 282). It is a non-judgmental way of attending to one's perceptions without reacting to them through action or mental dialogue (Davidson 2012). Practicing mindfulness fosters self-knowledge and self-reflection (O'Rourke 2017) because it reduces activation in the amygdala and cortexes, distracts you from unnecessary thoughts, and alters your relationships with those thoughts and sensations and thereby prevents you from being hijacked by your own thoughts (Davidson 2012). Put simply, mindfulness can help health professionals to become self-knowledgeable in two ways. First, if you are less self-knowledgeable, mindfulness makes your thoughts noticeable. Second, if you are hyper-knowledgeable, it helps reduce the inner noise arising from your thoughts (Begley 2007). Emerging evidence also indicates that mindfulness practices can improve the physical and emotional well-being of persons (McCubbin et al. 2014; Abbott et al. 2014; Yang et al. 2015; Spijkerman, Pots & Bohlmeijer 2016), can improve their self-knowledge (Siegel 2007, 2009), and can help them to engage more fully in meaningful communication with persons (Beach et al. 2013) that can lead to the development of therapeutic relationships.

REFLECTIVE PRACTICE EXERCISE 10.4 – 10-MINUTE MINDFULNESS EXERCISE FOR SELF-KNOWLEDGE

Time: 10 minutes

Step I: Preparation

- At the end of your working day, sit at your favorite place, relax, grab a cup of tea/coffee or your favorite beverage and ask yourself the following questions. Please do not rationalize any of the thoughts that may arise in your mind.

Step II: What were the good things about this day?

- Who cheered me up? Who prayed for me? Who taught me something? Who said something good about me?

Step III: What were some of the bad things about this day?

- Was I rude to people? Was I anxious? Did I miss something important? Did I care for myself? Did I pass the whole day without lifting up my personal self?

Step IV: What I need to do tomorrow?

- What opportunities are available to learn something? What opportunities are available to practice kindness? How can I improve my day?

Step V: Compliment yourself that you completed all the above-mentioned steps.

SEEKING FEEDBACK FROM OTHERS

Seeking feedback from one's family and peers is a simple, yet important strategy to gain self-knowledge (Cassedy 2010). Several studies have noted the benefits of feedback for increasing self-knowledge (Miller et al. 2017; Ramani et al. 2017) as it helps learning about one's strengths, limitations, skills, unknown behaviors, and hidden talents from others' perspectives. In order to use this strategy effectively, prior to seeking feedback from others, one should engage in self-assessment of personal strengths and limitations and then compare the self-assessment findings with the feedback received from others. Comparing self-assessment and feedback from others is also important to prevent oneself from basing one's concept of oneself on inaccurate perceptions of others (Jack & Smith 2007). In order to learn more about self, critical and constructive feedback should be sought on a continuous basis and accepted in a positive manner.

APPLICATION OF SELF-KNOWLEDGE AND DEDUCTIVE CLINICAL REASONING TO CARE GIVING

In the previous sections, we discussed self-knowledge, its types, and different skills and strategies that may help in becoming more self-knowledgeable and increase awareness of clinical situations. In this section, we will discuss a process for the application of self-knowledge and deductive clinical reasoning in order to develop a care plan for persons you interact with during your practice. Figure 10.1 illustrates a schematic step-by-step process for engaging in self-knowledge and deductive clinical reasoning in order to develop a care plan for persons with whom you interact in your clinical practice.

Step I: Becoming aware of yourself and your environment

As health care professionals, we are predisposed to many pre-conceived beliefs, values, cultural norms, traditions, and perceptions of and about the persons with whom we interact on a daily basis (Jasper 2003). These pre-disposed beliefs and values are ingrained in us because of our childhood, past experiences, and social interactions that influence our thoughts and actions. We bring all our values and beliefs into our practice. Therefore, it is important to recognize those beliefs and values before interacting with persons in clinical settings so that we can better identify the needs of the persons (Borrell-Carrió & Epstein 2004). There are several frameworks that could be used to know yourself and your environment such as the Johari Window (Luft & Ingham 1961) and the three-stage Now, Transition, and Regroup Experiential Framework (Jack & Miller, 2008).
The Johari Window comprises four quadrants namely,
1. Open
2. Blind
3. Hidden
4. and unknown.

Each of these quadrants gives different information about the self. The open area indicates that we are knowledgeable about the self and so are others. The blind area means that people are aware of several of our characteristics that we are unaware of. The hidden means we know but others do not know something about us, and the unknown is something that no one, including ourselves, know. The wider the open quadrant gets, the more self-knowledgeable we become. Therefore, in order to increase the area of the open quadrant, we should talk to people about self and seek feedback from them. To decrease the area of the hidden quadrant, one needs to engage in self-disclosure. To decrease the area of the blind quadrant one needs to seek continuous feedback from others, and to decrease the area of the unknown quadrant, one needs both self-disclosure and feedback. It is worth noting that if a person wants to become self-knowledgeable, one needs to make a conscious choice because forced intervention may lead to failure. Put simply, a person's readiness and openness influence the development of self-knowledge, which in turn transforms one's behaviors and characteristics. With the received feedback, one can decrease the areas of the hidden, blind, and unknown quadrants (Luft 1982).
Based on the Johari Window, Jack & Miller (2008) developed a three-stage:
➤ Now
➤ Transition
➤ Regroup Experiential Framework

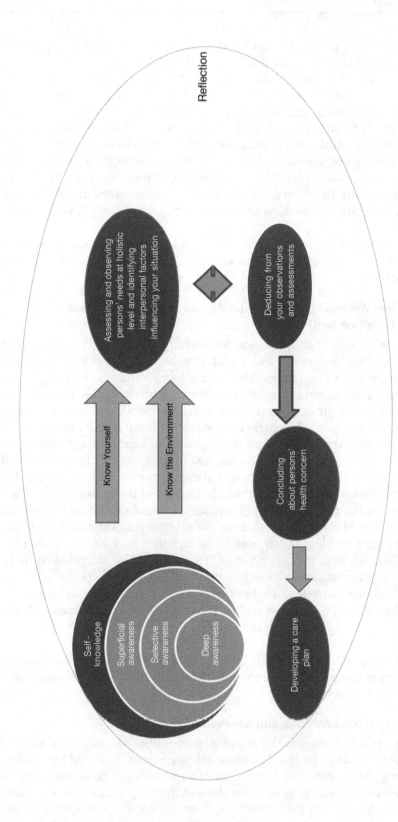

Figure 10.1 Self-knowledge and deduction

The process of self-knowledge and deduction in clinical reasoning (Key: circle represents the continuous nature of self-knowledge and deduction, double arrow headed indicates the continuous scrutinization of your assessment and deduction, arc represents the use of reflection in the process).

... that seeks answers to a different question in each stage and enables persons to recognize their way of thinking and how to change and transform it.

➤ In the 'now stage', we ask ourselves about the self, the persons with whom we are about to interact with, and our beliefs that we bring to the specific situation. Seeking answers to these questions in the 'Now Stage' provides us with more insights to reflect upon in the 'Transition Stage'. In this stage, we must ask ourselves which strengths are required to deal with the situation, which strengths we need to develop, and how we can develop our strengths. Once we identify our strengths and limitations, we need to expand on the strengths and to develop those strengths needed to overcome our limitations. Based on our understanding of ourselves, in the 'Regroup Stage', we incorporate the new learning and accept our new self (Jack & Miller 2008).

These two frameworks can be used to know ourselves and our environment prior to entering any given situation and to develop necessary skills in order to become effective health care professionals.

Step II: Observing and assessing persons' needs and identifying factors influencing your interaction with them

People observation and assessment are critical for identifying the needs of persons in a holistic manner and then developing a care plan that best fits the persons' needs as well as acknowledging the health care providers' strengths and limitations (Feely 1994). Engaging in a holistic assessment also enables health care professionals to develop a therapeutic relationship with the persons (Carniaux-Moran 2008), which in turn helps in gathering accurate information. The observation and assessment entails both objective and subjective assessments. During the objective assessment, health care professionals identify sign and symptoms, vital signs, diagnostic test findings, and different cues that may provide insights about the needs and health status of the individual. During the subjective assessment, data is gathered from the individuals and their families, and from other people involved in the given situation (Carniaux-Moran 2008; Younas 2017). An in-depth assessment should be done so that no meaningful information is left out. Therefore, it is important to identify any and all factors that may be influencing the situation. For a holistic assessment, three types of factors should be identified namely,

1. intrapersonal – within each person including personal self and others
2. interpersonal – between yourself and other persons and among other persons
3. contextual – hidden or implied factors such as the effect of the environment (Doane & Varcoe 2015).

Using these assessment approaches, health care professionals can assemble a complete understanding of their personal self, the needs of persons they care for, and deduce what course of action is best for each person.

Step III: Deducing from observations and assessments

We previously defined deductive clinical reasoning as an application of general rules to a specific clinical situation after thorough contextual assessment, followed by scrutiny of assessment. During observation and assessment of a person's needs, we used general principles of objective and subjective assessment along with interpersonal, intrapersonal, and contextual factors in order to gather relevant information. Once this information has been gathered, we break down and sort this information into useful evidence, meaningful patterns, and cues that play a substantial role in prioritizing the needs of persons and arriving at the main health concern of the person (Elstein & Schwartz 2002). The identified evidence, patterns, and cues should be examined through cause–effect relationships and discrepancies should be identified. The discrepant information should be disregarded in order to deduce accurately the central health concern of the persons (Kyriacou 2004). It is important that during deduction, health care professionals should use knowledge of themselves, of the persons, of the environments as well as their knowledge and training about mental health problems, to describe the whole situation including all the gathered information.

Step IV: Concluding about health concerns

After completing all the above-mentioned steps and scrutinizing one's deductions, one must draw conclusions about the main health concerns of the persons. The conclusions drawn should be pertinent to the gathered facts and provide an overview of the person's health situation, so that a future care plan can be developed.

Step V: Developing a care plan

Prior to developing a care plan, several important things should be done. First, validate your assessment, observations, and deductions by communicating with the person for whom the care plan is to be developed. Second, after validation, develop SMART (specific, measurable, achievable, realistic, and time bound) goals to outline a preliminary structure for the action plan. In your care plan, you should include the goals, outcome criteria, interventions, and evaluation of goals pertinent to your assessments and deductions.

We have learned the process of applying self-knowledge and deduction in clinical practice. It is time to apply these concepts to arrive at a further understanding of this process.

REFLECTIVE PRACTICE EXERCISE 10.5

> **Time: 50 minutes**
>
> **Case Study 10.2**
>
> Alex, 53, is admitted to the mental health ward with a diagnosis of severe depression. In 2015, he also received a diagnosis of end-stage Hepatocellular carcinoma. The past medical and social history shows that he drinks alcohol on a regular basis and smokes two packs of cigarettes a day. Currently, he has completed his chemotherapy and has been advised Prozac for depression. You have been assigned to care for Alex. Based on his initial assessment, the following data was gathered:
>
> Heart Rate: 93b/min, Respiratory Rate: 21b/min, Blood Pressure 140/85, Temp: 99 F
>
> As the health care professional of Alex, we encourage you to engage in a brief and quick self-knowledge examination and to integrate the process of deductive clinical reasoning to develop a care plan for Alex.

Step I: Becoming aware of yourself and your environment
- Refer to Reflective Practice Exercise 10.1 and engage in superficial, selective, deep awareness analyses
- Use the three-stage Now, Transition, and Regroup Experiential Framework
- What are your feelings? What do you know about yourself and Alex? What are your strengths and limitations for interacting with Alex? What strengths do you need to develop? How should you communicate with Alex?

Step II: Observing and assessing person's needs and identifying factors influencing your interaction with him
- Perform objective and subjective assessments
- Explore interpersonal, intrapersonal, and contextual factors that might influence your interaction. For this exploration, communicate with Alex, his family members, health care professionals, and identify cues such as social and environmental factors that may play a role in this situation.

Step III: Deducing from observations and assessments
- What are his perceived needs? Prioritize the needs.
- What is Alex's major health concern?

Step IV: Concluding about the health concerns
- What is the major health concern?
- Do you possess adequate knowledge and skills to help Alex with the management of his problem?

Step V: Developing a care plan
- Develop an action and intervention plan.

CONCLUSION

This chapter presents an overview about the importance of the arts of self-knowledge and deductive clinical reasoning, provides a theoretical understanding of these arts, outlines different types of analyses and strategies required to become self-knowledgeable, and illuminates different practical models and frameworks for the application of self-knowledge and deduction in clinical practice.

KEY POINTS 10.1

➤ The art of self-knowledge refers to a deliberate examination to discover one's personal self and is essential for improving deductive clinical reasoning
➤ Deductive clinical reasoning is the application of general rules to a specific clinical situation after a thorough contextual assessment
➤ The awareness analyses and the attributes are essential for becoming self-knowledgeable, but it is important to remember that self-knowledge is contextual,

should be assessed in every situation, and should involve examination of the environment as well

➤ Within the context of palliative mental health care, a health care professional's approach to decision making and provision of care is primarily interpersonal, and holistic focuses the physical, spiritual, psychological, and emotional health and well-being of both persons and health care providers

➤ Becoming self-knowledgeable is a time-consuming process and requires continuous use of several skills and strategies. Some of the widely suggested skills and strategies are: reflection and reflective practice, practicing meditation and mindfulness, and seeking feedback from others

➤ Seeking feedback from one's family and peers is a simple, yet important strategy to gain self-knowledge

➤ To learn more about self, critical, and constructive feedback should be sought on a continuous basis and accepted in a positive manner.

REFERENCES

Abbott, R. A., Whear, R., Rodgers, L. R., Bethel, A., Thomson Coon, J., et al. (2014) 'Effectiveness of mindfulness-based stress reduction and mindfulness based cognitive therapy in vascular disease: a systematic review and meta-analysis of randomised controlled trials', *Journal of Psychosomatic Research*, 76, pp. 341–51.

Ashoorion, V., Liaghatdar, M. J. and Adibi, P. (2012) 'What variables can influence clinical reasoning?', *Journal of Research in Medical Sciences*, 17, pp. 1170–5.

Beach, M. C., Roter, D., Korthuis, P. T., Epstein, R. M., Sharp, V. et al. (2013) 'A multicenter study of physician mindfulness and health care quality', *The Annals of Family Medicine*, 11, pp. 421–8.

Benner, P., Hughes, R. and Molly, S. (2008) 'Clinical reasoning, decision making, and action: thinking critically and clinically', in Hughes, R. (ed.). *Patient Safety and Quality: An Evidence-Based Handbook for Nurses*. Rockville (MD): Agency for Healthcare Research and Quality (US).

Begley, S. (2007) *Train Your Mind, Change Your Brain*. New York, NY: Ballantine.

Bolton, J. W. (2015) 'Varieties of clinical reasoning', *Journal of Evaluation in Clinical Practice*, 21, pp. 486–9.

Borrell-Carrió, F. and Epstein, R. M. (2004) 'Preventing errors in clinical practice: a call for self-awareness', *The Annals of Family Medicine*, 2, pp. 310–16.

Campbell, J. (1980) 'The relationship of nursing and self-awareness', *Advances in Nursing Science*, 2, pp. 15–26.

Cardoso, R., de Souza, E., Camano, L., and Leite, J. R. (2004) 'Meditation in health: an operational definition', *Brain Research Protocols*, 14, pp. 58–60.

Carniaux-Moran, C. (2008) 'The psychiatric nursing assessment', in O'Brien, P. C. and Kennedy, W. Z. (eds.). *Psychiatric Mental Health Nursing: An Introduction to Theory and Practice*. Burlington, MA: Ballard Jones and Bartlett, pp. 41–3.

Cassedy, P. (2010) *First Steps in Clinical Supervision: A Guide for Healthcare Professionals*. Berkshire, UK: McGraw-Hill Education.

Davidson, R. J. (2012) *The Emotional Life of Your Brain: How Its Unique Patterns Affect the Way You Think, Feel, and Live—and How You Can Change Them*, London, UK: Plume.

Doane, G. H. and Varcoe, C. (2015) *How to Nurse: Relational Inquiry with Individuals and Families in Changing Health and Health Care Contexts*, Wolters Kluwer Health/Lippincott Williams & Wilkins.

Driscoll, J. and Teh, B. (2001) 'The potential of reflective practice to develop individual orthopaedic nurse practitioners and their practice', *Journal of Orthopaedic Nursing*, 5, pp. 95–103.

Duffy, A. (2007) 'A concept analysis of reflective practice: determining its value to nurses', *British Journal of Nursing*, 16, pp. 1400–7.

Eckroth-Bucher, M. (2010) 'Self-awareness: a review and analysis of a basic nursing concept', *Advances in Nursing Science*, 33, pp. 297–309.

Elstein, A. S. and Schwartz, A. (2002) 'Clinical problem solving and diagnostic decision making: selective review of the cognitive literature', *British Medical Journal*, 324, pp. 729–32.

Feely, M. (1994) 'Know your patient. The importance of assessment in care delivery', *Professional Nurse*, 9, pp. 318–20.

Forrest, M. E. (2008) 'On becoming a critically reflective practitioner', *Health Information & Libraries Journal*, 25, pp. 229–32.

Gallagher, L., Lawler, D., Brady, V., O'Boyle, C., Deasy, A. and Muldoon, K. (2017) 'An evaluation of the appropriateness and effectiveness of structured reflection for midwifery students in Ireland', *Nurse Education in Practice*, 22, pp. 7–14.

Gardiner, F. W. (2016) 'The art of self-knowledge and deduction in clinical practice', *Annals of Medicine and Surgery*, 10, pp. 19–21.

Gay, S., Bartlett, M. and McKinley, R. (2013) 'Teaching clinical reasoning to medical students', *The Clinical Teacher*, 10, pp. 308–12.

Goswami, D. C. (2013) 'Understanding self-awareness in palliative care', *Journal of Pain & Palliative Care Pharmacotherapy*, 27, pp. 367–9.

Higgs, J. (2008) *Clinical Reasoning in the Health Professions* 3rd edition. Sydney, Australia: Elsevier Health Sciences.

Holewa, M. H. (2004) 'Mental health and palliative care: exploring the ideological interface', *International Journal of Psychosocial Rehabilitation*, 9, pp. 107–19.

Jack, K. and Miller, E. (2008) 'Exploring self-awareness in mental health practice', *Mental Health Practice*, 12, pp. 31–35.

Jack, K. and Smith, A. (2007) 'Promoting self-awareness in nurses to improve nursing practice', *Nursing Standard*, 21, pp. 47–52.

Jasper, M. (2003) *Beginning Reflective Practice*. Delta Place, UK: Nelson Thomas.

Kwiatek, E., McKenzie, K. and Loads, D. (2005) 'Self-awareness and reflection: exploring the "therapeutic use of self"', *Learning Disability Practice*, 8, pp. 27–31.

Kyriacou, D. N. (2004) 'Evidence-based medical decision making: deductive versus inductive logical thinking', *Academic Emergency Medicine*, 11, pp. 670–1.

Levett-Jones, T., Hoffman, K., Dempsey, J., Jeong, S. Y., Noble, D. et al. (2010) 'The 'five rights' of clinical reasoning: an educational model to enhance nursing students' ability to identify and manage clinically 'at risk' patients', *Nurse Education Today*, 30, pp. 515–20.

Luft, J. (1982) 'The Johari window: a graphic model of awareness in interpersonal relations' in Porter, L. C. and Mohr, B. (eds). *Reading Book for Human Relations Training*, NTL Institute, pp. 34–5.

Luft, J. and Ingham, H. (1961) 'The Johari window', *Human Relations Training News*, 5, pp. 6–7.

Mann, K., Gordon, J. and MacLeod, A. (2009) 'Reflection and reflective practice in health professions education: A systematic review', *Advances in Health Sciences Education*, 14, pp. 595–621.

McCubbin, T., Dimidjian, S., Kempe, K., Glassey, M. S., Ross, C. and Beck, A. (2014) 'Mindfulness-based stress reduction in an integrated care delivery system: one-year impacts on patient-centered outcomes and health care utilization', *The Permanente Journal*, 18, pp. 4–9.

Morgan, G. (2009) 'Reflective practice and self-awareness', *Perspectives in Public Health*, 129, pp. 161–2.

Miller, M. K., Mandryk, R. L., Birk, M. V., Depping, A. E. and Patel, T. (2017) 'Through the looking glass: the effects of feedback on self-awareness and conversational behaviour during video chat', in *Proceedings of the 2017 CHI Conference on Human Factors in Computing Systems*, pp. 5271–83. ACM. DOI: Available at: http://dx.doi.org/10.1145/3025453.3025548 (Accessed: 21 January 2018)

Myers, S. (2003) 'Reflections on reflecting: how self-awareness promotes personal growth', *Person-Centered Journal*, 10, pp. 3–22.

Nguyen, Q. D., Fernandez, N., Karsenti, T. and Charlin, B. (2014) 'What is reflection? A conceptual analysis of major definitions and a proposal of a five-component model', *Medical Education*, 48, pp. 1176–89.

O' Rourke, M. (2017) *Mindfulness and Reflective Practice: Enriching Personal and Professional Growth.* Available at: www.virtualhospice.ca/en_US/Main+Site+Navigation/Home/For+Professionals/For+Professionals/The+Exchange/Current/Mindfulness+and+Reflective+Practice_+Enriching+personal+and+professional+growth.aspx (Accessed 21 January 2018)

Oflaz, F., Meric, M., Yuksel, C. and Ozcan, C. T. (2011) 'Psychodrama: an innovative way of improving self-awareness of nurses', *Journal of Psychiatric and Mental Health Nursing*, 18, pp. 569–75.

Ramani, S., Könings, K., Mann, K. V. and van der Vleuten, C. (2017) 'Uncovering the unknown: a grounded theory study exploring the impact of self-awareness on the culture of feedback in residency education', *Medical Teacher*, 39, pp. 1065–73.

Rasheed, S. P. (2015) 'Self-awareness as a therapeutic tool for nurse/client relationship', *International Journal of Caring Sciences*, 8, pp. 211–16.

Sedgwick, M. G., Grigg, L. and Dersch, S. (2014) 'Deepening the quality of clinical reasoning and decision-making in rural hospital nursing practice', *Rural and Remote Health*, 14, pp. 1–12.

Siegel, D. J. (2007) 'Mindfulness training and neural integration: differentiation of distinct streams of awareness and the cultivation of well-being', *Social Cognitive and Affective Neuroscience*, 2, pp. 259–63.

Siegel, D. J. (2009) 'Mindful awareness, mindsight, and neural integration', *The Humanistic Psychologist*, 37, pp. 137–58.

Spijkerman, M. P. J., Pots, W. T. M. and Bohlmeijer, E. T. (2016) 'Effectiveness of online mindfulness-based interventions in improving mental health: a review and meta-analysis of randomised controlled trials', *Clinical Psychology Review*, 45, pp. 102–14.

White, L. (2014) 'Mindfulness in nursing: an evolutionary concept analysis', *Journal of Advanced Nursing*, 70, pp. 282–94.

Yang, Y., Liu, Y. H., Zhang, H. F. and Liu, J. Y. (2015) 'Effectiveness of mindfulness-based stress reduction and mindfulness-based cognitive therapies on people living with HIV: a systematic review and meta-analysis'. *International Journal of Nursing Sciences*, 2, pp. 283–94.

Younas, A. (2017) 'The nursing process and patient teaching', *Nursing Made Incredibly Easy*, 15, pp. 13–16.

To Learn More

Davidson, R. J. (2012) *The Emotional Life of Your Brain: How its Unique Patterns Affect the Way You Think, Feel, and Live—and How You Can Change Them*, London, UK: Plume.

Begley, S. (2007) *Train Your Mind, Change Your Brain.* New York, NY: Ballantine.

Jasper, M. (2003) *Beginning Reflective Practice.* Delta Place, UK: Nelson Thorne.

CHAPTER 11

Trauma and Post-Traumatic Stress Disorder

Nicole Newman and Lisa M. Brown

OVERVIEW

Palliative care is often provided in an emotionally challenging environment to the people who are the recipient of services, their family and friends, and the professionals who are providing care. As detailed in previous chapters, thoughtfulness and consideration should be taken when working in this setting with providing comfort and end-of-life care. In addition to the issues previously discussed, professionals providing palliative care should be mindful of actions that could be triggering for someone with a history of trauma. A trigger could be something, such as a touch or smell that elicits a symptomatic response in a person with a history of trauma that could be expressed as a flashback or a panic attack.

Settings that offer palliative care (e.g., intensive care, end-of-life care units) are often extremely stressful. The environment and medical personnel can unintentionally stress the individual in ways that have the potential to trigger previous unresolved traumas. Professionals must strive to work ethically (*See* Chapters 2 and 3) and carefully in these settings in order to best serve the people who are receiving care. The presentation, treatment, and prognosis of physical ailments may be complicated by the presence of an existing, emerging, or reemerging trauma. Such interaction calls for professionals to be cognizant of and attentive to symptoms and risks of trauma – including their own. There is substantial scientific literature pertaining to compassion fatigue, burnout, and secondary traumatic distress experienced by palliative care professionals. This chapter focuses on how to identify and address the manifestations of trauma in people who are receiving palliative care.

WHAT IS TRAUMA?

Before we delve into the ethical implications of providing care to persons experiencing a trauma history, it is important to define trauma. The trauma discussed in this chapter is psychological trauma not physical trauma, although both can occur simultaneously. It should be noted that physical types of trauma may make an individual more susceptible to psychological trauma, and therefore should not be overlooked. A universally accepted definition of trauma does not formally exist. However, psychological trauma is largely understood to be the mental or emotional distress that results from an event, or sequence of events, in which an individual experiences overwhelming stress or threats to their well-being. Trauma events or stressors can be difficult to specifically define as it depends chiefly on the perspective of the individual experiencing the event. In modern dialogues of trauma, professionals often discuss three components:

1. exposure
2. experience
3. effect(s).

Exposure, commonly referred to as the traumatic event or stressor, is the event that precipitates the distress. Said exposure can be a one-time incident, often referred to as an index event, (e.g. car accident, disaster) or as a set of repeated circumstances, often called complex trauma (e.g. child neglect, combat with multiple deployments). The individual experiencing the event ascertains the exposure's traumatic valence, thus complicating the process by which we define and treat trauma. For example, two people in a car accident may experience the event very differently. One may perceive it as a minor stressor while the other person is severely traumatized and becomes fearful about driving in a car. Experience is the internal manifestation of the event. The experience incorporates many individual factors that impact how one interfaces with the incident (Yehuda & LeDoux 2007; Sherin & Nemeroff 2011; Norris 1992). The experience of an individual is an intricate web of one's biological temperament and dispositions, past experiences, learned behaviors, and culture.

Stress and Physical Health

We cannot have a conversation about trauma without discussing the role of stress. Stress has come to be understood in primarily three ways: physiological, environmental, or transactional (Aldwin & Levenson 2013). Physiologically, stress is a biological process in which the hypothalamus activates the release of hormones, including adrenaline and cortisol. The release of these hormones increases heart rate, glucose production, respiratory processes, and blood flow to muscles. These processes occur with the intention of protecting one's body (e.g. tensing of muscles and spikes in energy). This construct of stress affects the state of an organism – the biological experience, often referred to as the strain. An environmental understanding of stress is much like the concept of exposure. When there is an external change or threat to an organism, that construct is popularly called stress or a stressor. A transactional approach emphasizes the interaction between the exposure (stressor) and the individual (strain). Usually this interaction involves the capital that a stressor requires, and the individual's available resources to cope with those requirements.

Stress typically has a bad reputation. We often associate being stressed with lower immune system functioning and cardiac diseases (Segerstrom & Miller 2004). However, stress is important to our day-to-day wellbeing. Stress motivates us to initiate and complete various activities and tasks. Like most things in life, stress is good in moderation. Without stress, we would be immobile and unmotivated. But what happens when you are too stressed? When environmental changes or exposure to a stressor exceeds our ability to cope or manage physiological arousal, the individual becomes stressed. According to the Stress and Coping Model of Trauma, over and under arousal (strain) creates distress (Aldwin 1994).

Over- or prolonged-stimulation of stress responses can have deleterious health consequences. Chronic stress is associated with several health complications including heart disease, cancer, liver disease, and pulmonary disease (Anda et al. 2006; Felitti & Anda 2010). The biological processes that keep our body safe for immediate exposure create a toxic environment for our bodies long term. Chronic stress weakens the immune system, making individuals susceptible to illnesses and complicating recovery from ill-health (Segerstrom & Miller 2004).

This finding suggests that an already 'ill' person may have further difficulty with treatment and recovery if they are stressed or have been chronically stressed. With that, it is important to consider the person receiving care as well as the environment. Palliative care provided in a stressful environment (e.g. announcements over loudspeakers, lights on in the middle of the night, interrupted sleep) and the implications of the care setting could further put the individual, professionals, and their social support network at greater risk for adverse outcomes. People experiencing a formal diagnosis of a trauma-related disorder or those experiencing an unaddressed history of trauma or exposure to significant chronic stressors may be particularly vulnerable to developing post-traumatic stress disorder (PTSD), depression, or anxiety. Those living and working in such a setting are susceptible to the deleterious effects of stress. Even an individual with no trauma history may be compromised by the daily stress of the palliative care environment.

Post-traumatic Stress Disorder and Trauma-Related Disorders

Trauma has been defined as the overwhelming stress response that occurs in response to a potentially traumatic event. So, how does stress manifest in its most extreme cases? Arguably, the most common psychiatric trauma-related diagnosis is Post-Traumatic Stress Disorder (PTSD). Trauma, or at least its exposure, is a universal phenomenon with approximately 80 percent of people experiencing a potential traumatic event during their lifetime (Benjet et al. 2016; Roberts et al. 2011). Yet, even with such a high percentage of exposure, less than 10 percent of the general population develops and is formally diagnosed with PTSD (American Psychiatric Association, 2013). Keep in mind that PTSD and its corresponding diagnosis, falls on the more severe end of the trauma response spectrum. The markedly limiting criteria of the diagnosis may contribute to its low diagnostic epidemiology. For instance, the American Psychiatric Association (APA) describes trauma as any event that confronts an individual with death, threatened death, actual or threatened serious injury, or actual or threatened sexual violence (2013). Terminal or chronic ill-health may not qualify people for a formal PTSD diagnosis; however, the diagnosis, treatment, or care of a medical ill-health can be extremely traumatizing for some individuals and their caregivers. In some cases, terminal or life-limiting physical ailments can serve as the primary traumatic exposure (Kangas, Henry & Bryant 2005). In other cases, the ill-health can reactivate past trauma or memories (Roth & Massie 2009). For example, the U.S. Army Medical Department (AMEDD) and the Veterans Health Administration (VHA) reported that PTSD is difficult to treat and that symptoms can be evident years after combat exposure (Berg et al. 2007). Although their military service ended decades ago, the estimated prevalence rate of PTSD among Vietnam veterans is 11 percent and Gulf War veterans is 12 percent (National Center for PTSD 2017). Regardless, the medical conditions that are common in palliative care can place individuals at increased risk for PTSD. Symptoms of PTSD can also further complicate treatment and care.

Post-traumatic stress disorder (PTSD), is an episodic syndrome that develops in response to a stressor event that is outside the realm of normal experience. Criteria for PTSD diagnosis listed in the APA's Diagnostic and Statistical Manual of Mental Disorders (DSM-5) include symptoms related to involuntary re-experiencing, avoidance of cues and memories, negative thoughts or feelings, and hyperarousal (2013). Some of these symptoms are archetypal characteristics of PTSD such as flashbacks, nightmares, and hypervigilance. However, many of the other symptoms tend to be subtler in nature and are also markers for an array of other mental health ill-health, such as irritability, difficulty concentrating, depression, and isolation. Given the heterogeneous nature of the disorder, it is possible for two persons to experience the debilitating effects of PTSD, but to have very different diagnostic pictures. Moreover, because of the overlap in symptomology across mental disorders, individuals experiencing PTSD can be misdiagnosed or go unnoticed.

Acute Stress Disorder (ASD) is another trauma-related, psychiatric diagnosis. In this case, symptoms appear within one month of the exposure, but do not last longer than four weeks. Because of its brief nature, ASD can go undiagnosed and undetected. If it goes untreated, individuals with ASD are at greater risk of developing PTSD (Harvey & Bryant 1998; Staab et al. 1996). Post-traumatic stress disorder can also have a delayed onset, meaning that symptoms do not appear until at least six months after the exposure (APA 2013). As such, persons receiving palliative care with a history of trauma exposure may be at an increased risk of developing delayed onset or re-activating suppressed PTSD symptoms. All in all, professionals should familiarize themselves with trauma symptomology, so that they may be able to better identify when there is a trauma-related concern. Trauma indicators can include:

➤ Irritability or hostility
➤ Treatment resistance or hesitation (avoidance)
➤ Nightmares or other sleep disturbances
➤ Isolation, withdrawal, or unresponsive behavior
➤ Heightened reactions to common medical treatments
➤ Emotionally fueled disagreements
➤ Aversion to conflict and inability to talk through issue
➤ Lack of interest in activities.

Likewise, traumatization or a positive PTSD diagnosis can further complicate and or exacerbate physical ill-health and symptoms. The case below illustrates how trauma can muddle the symptoms of a physical ill-health.

It is not uncommon for individuals suffering from diabetes to experience chronic pain. In some cases, chronic pain in diabetes can signal a complication in the disease and its treatment. However, due to Jane's history of trauma and potentially traumatic bereavement, it is unclear if her chronic pain is a result of her physical ill-health or psychological distress. Research suggests that physical distress, specifically perceived pain, and psychological distress co-occur and are closely associated (Otis, Keane, & Kerns 2003). Moreover, a growing body of research indicates that elevated resting heart rate, even while sleeping, is an indicator of a previous trauma (Bertram et al. 2014; Woodward et al. 2009). Elevated heart rate increases risk for cardiovascular disease (Diaz et al. 2005; Jouven et al. 2005; Perret-Guillaume, Joly, & Benetos 2009).

> **Case Study 11.1**
>
> Jane is an 87-year-old woman who emigrated from Japan with her family as a young girl. She met her to-be-husband while their families were forcefully living in a Civilian Assembly Center in California. While pregnant with her son, she was diagnosed with gestational diabetes, and has since developed Type 1 diabetes. Her diabetes was well-managed until two years ago when her husband died suddenly of a heart attack. Since then, she has experienced chronic pain in her feet. Jane reports that she cannot get out of bed because of the pain. Since her son has a demanding job and she cannot take care of herself, he pays for in-home palliative care.

Cultural Considerations of Trauma

Trauma's idiosyncratic nature can make it difficult to identify its presence. As are each individual's experiences, the trauma experience, and the subsequent expression of symptoms culturally bound. Language and cultural norms affect the way in which a person internalizes, externally manifests, and verbally expresses a traumatic event (*See* Chapter 6). For instance, an individual who speaks a language with only four words or phrases to express their emotional distress may have more difficulty verbally describing their experience than an individual who speaks a language that has 30 descriptors for distress. Individuals who do not have a wide, expressive trauma vernacular may find it challenging to describe their experience. Likewise, when a language discrepancy exists between individuals and professionals, language-specific idioms may go misunderstood or undetected. In such cases, symptoms or explanations of trauma can go unnoticed. Cultural humility is thus a core component of treating people who are receiving palliative care. Joshua Hook et al. (2013), a clinical psychologist who specializes in multicultural issues, describes cultural humility as 'the ability to maintain an interpersonal stance that is other-oriented (or open to the other) in relation to aspects of cultural identity that are most important to the [individual]' (p. 2).

An approach that includes cultural understanding is especially salient when trying to identify trauma in individuals who do not share the lingual or ethnic background(s) of the clinician. Because Western cultures and mental health medicine comparatively take a reductionist approach to psychological distress, researchers continue to strive to create culturally diverse and accurate measurements of trauma (Aderibigbe & Pandurangi 1995; Purnell 2008). Many cultures do not share the same, or in some cases any, nosology regarding trauma that Western cultures use in clinical settings. When applying a cultural perspective, the clinician would appropriately tailor treatment for an individual from Vietnam differently than for an individual from the United Kingdom.

When inquiring about an individual's trauma history, it is important for professionals to account for multiple-identities. In a progressively globalized and interconnected world, identity intersectionality is increasing, further individualizing the trauma experience. When appraising the emotion most commonly associated with PTSD, fear is usually the first to come to mind. However, in many cultures, it is socially inappropriate and discouraged for some cis-gender men to candidly express fear. Consequently, a man may have more emotional access to irritability and anger as a form of trauma expression, than fear or anxiety. Social norms and cultural roles blur diagnostic and symptomatic lines. When professionals adapt a culturally humble perspective, they are more open to diverse ideas and manifestations of trauma.

MINORITY STRESS

Being culturally humble comes with the acknowledgment that some people are exposed to more stress, both in quantity and variety, than others. Those who identify with stigmatized groups and minority identities often encounter more stress (Link & Phelan 2001; Meyer 2003). This phenomenon is referred to as minority stress. As a result of prejudice, discrimination, and stereotyping, minority identities fall victim to more stressors than their White, heteronormative counterparts. Keeping in mind how overwhelming amounts of stress can lead to a traumatic experience as well as how stress affects the immune system, minority status or identity does not necessarily make a person more susceptible to PTSD. Nonetheless, where there is more stress, there are more opportunities to become overwhelmed. A stance of cultural humility also compels professionals to consider age and life development as a risk factor. The case study 11.2 below is an example.

Abe's story is a reminder that an individual can develop traumatic symptoms at any point in their life and is heavily dependent on their context. An individual, who can cope with potential traumatic experiences in earlier years, may struggle in later life because resources that were once readily available are not so easily accessible in older age. With that, it is important to note that (older) age is a risk for trauma exposure (Pietrzak et al. 2012). An increase in trauma exposure is associated with a greater risk for developing trauma-related disturbances. This is especially true when an individual is receiving care in a stressful environment. Notably, older adults tend to make up most of the palliative and hospice care populations. People who have been independent and healthy for most of their lives may find the transition to an institutional environment particularly strenuous, and even traumatic.

Case Study 11.2

Abe is a 72-year-old, Black cis-gender male who served in the Vietnam War when he was 22 years old. During the war, he was badly injured and saw many of his friends die. Upon his return home and during treatment for his injuries, family members and friends took turns caring for Abe. Even though he considered his experiences in Vietnam to be disturbing, he rarely talked about them. Abe remarks that he never got 'shell shock' while serving. Through help from his sister, he was able to get a job at a local cheese shop. He met his wife while working and they married shortly thereafter. They had three children. The family described themselves as being very close and supportive of one another. Four years ago, Abe's wife died suddenly of a heart attack. His children moved home to be with Abe, but characterized him as always having been well adjusted and balanced. Abe was admitted into palliative care treatment six months ago after being diagnosed with an advanced stage cancer. Since his admission, he has been markedly irritable. The nurses and staff describe his behavior as 'rude' and 'difficult'. His night nurse reports that he has trouble sleeping and refuses sleep medication.

ASSESSMENT AND TREATMENT

An exact prevalence of PTSD and trauma-related symptoms in palliative and hospice care settings is unknown and likely due to psychological treatment not being a priority in facilities providing palliative and end-of-life care. In a sample taken from a Veterans Affairs (VA) facility in 2010, roughly 17 percent of patients demonstrated PTSD symptomology in the last month of life (Alici et al. 2010). Most of this sample did not enter care with a PTSD or related diagnosis, which suggests that their symptoms had been undetected or not reported during their lifetime or that they developed PTSD-related symptoms after admission into end-of-life care. Other research implies that being critically ill can be traumatic, further spiking prevalence rates up to 60 percent (Schelling et al. 2001; Jackson et al. 2007). There are a growing number of evidence-based treatments that target trauma-related diagnoses. Some of the most commonly used treatments for PTSD include Prolonged Exposure Therapy, Cognitive Processing Therapy, Eye Movement Desensitization and Reprocessing, and Present-Centered Therapy (Bradley et al. 2005; American Psychological Assessment (APA) Division 12 2016). Yet, without a clear-cut history or a formal diagnosis, how should non-mental health professionals assess for trauma when they suspect it might be contributing to current problems?

Screeners

Individuals may not display traumata-related symptoms at the time of their admission or previous to receiving palliative care, which can make assessment for and treatment of trauma challenging. One way to circumvent this issue is to include PTSD and trauma-related screeners into admission paperwork. Screeners are assessment instruments often used by psychologists and medical professionals to indicate risk of a condition or need for further evaluation. Unlike an assessment, screeners are brief, sometimes truncated versions of longer instruments, and indeterminate in nature. Currently, there is not one comprehensive screener that delineates risk and or exposure for trauma-related experiences and symptoms. However, many government organizations are creating and utilizing screeners. One of these organizations is the Veteran Affairs (VA), which has established a program to screen for PTSD (Spoont et al. 2013).

As noted previously, trauma is a unique experience and exposure does not necessarily maintain that someone will have trauma-related distress. Professionals looking to utilize screeners should keep this in mind when deliberating which to choose. Screeners that aim to measure or identify exposure to potentially traumatic events are less helpful in assessing one's propensity for trauma-related symptoms (Wang et al. 2005; Galea et al. 2012). Perhaps the most popular and validated screener is the PTSD Checklist (PCL). In accordance with the DSM 5, the most recent version of the screener is the PCL-5. The screener is a brief, taking approximately ten minutes, self-report measure (Weathers et al. 2013), making it an ideal addition to admission paperwork and evaluation in palliative care. Using screeners allows for professionals to account for possible trauma experiences without significant inconvenience or treatment distraction. Screeners are not only helpful for determining risk for PTSD, but also help catalyze conversations about mental health (Gaynes et al. 2010). When an individual presents with and/or is being cared for a debilitating or chronic physical health issue, mental health can fall low on treatment priority. Using a screener can open up avenues for people to speak with their care professionals about all aspects of their health.

However, even when using a screener people may be unwilling or unable to recognize or report their symptoms due to such factors as amnesia, avoidance, ill-health, or cognitive impairment. For people who are gravely ill, the burden to recognize distress and encourage treatment increasingly falls on family and friends. Given that this responsibility is placed on others, it is useful to know which symptoms are amenable to detection by informants. One study found that the ability of female spouses of Vietnam veterans to report on various indicators of PTSD using the Mississippi Scale for Combat-Related PTSD varied across item content and that items themselves were not diagnostic at the same level for detecting presence of PTSD. Overall, veterans showed greater sensitivity to their own symptoms and were able to provide more information than their spouses. However, some items on the measure provided greater information when endorsed by the spouse instead of the veteran. In general, items were endorsed by the spouse only when the PTSD symptoms had become severe (Niles et al. 1993; Taft et al. 1999).

Although reexperiencing symptoms may be intra-personally disturbing, these symptoms are usually not disturbing to others because they are primarily an internal experience (Evans et al. 2010). In contrast, avoidance and hyperarousal symptoms have both affective and behavioral external expressions that are often distressing to family and friends (Solomon, Dekel, & Zerach 2008). Hyperarousal is often expressed as heightened physiological reactivity, anger, and irritability. Avoidance manifests as detachment from others and diminished interest in previously enjoyed activities (Taylor et al. 1998). The effectiveness of informant reports to detect PTSD vary based on the degree to which the symptoms are overt (i.e. behaviors or actions) or covert (i.e. thoughts or feelings) (Gallagher et al. 1998). It is well recognized that multiple assessment of different domains and informants may improve diagnostic accuracy (Wilson & Keane 2004).

Considerations for Evidence-Based Treatment

Once the presence of trauma symptoms has been detected or the potential for future traumatization is anticipated, appropriate services and treatment should be offered. Given the growing research of trauma's impact on physical health, it may be in the best interest of the person receiving palliative care to address their PTSD and trauma-related symptoms. However, just because a person would benefit from treatment does not mean that they are appropriate candidates for all evidence-based interventions.

Keep in mind that much of the work done in settings such as palliative and hospice care involves comfort and quality of life improvement (Rome et al. 2011). Yet, the goals of palliative care may be directly contradicted in trauma-related treatment. Arguably the most significant detail concerning the treatments offered in this chapter is that they are efficacious for physically healthy individuals (Cukor et al. 2010). Treatment for PTSD, and other stress and trauma-related disorders, can be demanding. Often, persons receiving care, experience and confront painful memories and feelings, which can be adverse for persons in fragile physical states. Physically healthy people undergoing treatment usually report symptoms worsening or intensifying before subsiding (Hembree et al. 2003; Nishith et al. 2002). In addition to cognitive-behavioral therapy, below is a brief description of three trauma-focused evidence-based therapies that are commonly used by psychologists treating traumatized people.

1. Prolonged Exposure

Prolonged Exposure (PE) is a trauma-focused psychotherapy where people repeatedly talk about the details of their traumatic event using a technique called imaginal exposure. Prolonged Exposure (PE) is intended to address avoidance issues and the fear associated with certain activities, people, and places. With repeated exposure to the details of the trauma, PTSD symptoms decrease and the ability to confront safe situations that have been previously avoided increase. The PE protocol requires that substantial time be allocated to preparation of the individual to engage in imaginal exposure. Psycho-education, homework, breath work, developing a list of avoided places use of the Subjective Unites of Distress Scale, and in vivo exposure assignments are typically carried out over the course of 12 weeks. Prolonged Exposure may not be suitable for people receiving palliative care as many healthy people report that this type of treatment can be difficult and stressful. It takes considerable motivation and regular practice to achieve a positive outcome. People who are receiving palliative care may not be optimal candidates for starting a rigorous, intense, evidence-based therapy.

2. Cognitive Processing Therapy

Cognitive Processing Therapy (CPT) is a 12-session therapy that teaches people to evaluate and change their upsetting thoughts about their trauma. The premise of CPT is that traumatic events negatively change the way that people view themselves and the world. To counter these negative thoughts, individuals are taught how to decide whether there might be more accurate and helpful ways to think about their trauma. The information generated by examining whether the facts support their thoughts provides new information that can be used to determine if it makes sense to have a different perspective. If negative thoughts are changed, feelings will change as well. However, the cognitive demands of CPT may make it a challenging therapy to learn and master required skills when receiving palliative care. Appreciating that this type of therapy also requires effort and energy, it may be too much to undertake simultaneously when dealing with serious physical health problems.

3. Eye Movement Desensitization and Reprocessing (EMDR)

Eye Movement Desensitization and Reprocessing (EMDR) is a therapy that helps people process their trauma-related thoughts, memories, and feelings. A variety of different EMDR protocols exist and there is no consensus about the right approach. Some recommend that the individual focuses their attention on a back-and-forth movement made by the therapist's fingers or a light bar. Another approach suggests use of a sound that beeps in one ear at a time. Both require that the individual recalls the traumatic event until the way the memory is recalled shifts and becomes less distressing. Most people report that they benefit from the experience and that the effort and discomfort is minimal. For select individuals, this might be a good approach because it requires minimal times (i.e. no homework or practice between sessions) and only involves thinking and not speaking about the trauma. Although the demands are less than other types of therapy, it still requires weekly visits for one to three months.

This begs the question, "How does one know when and how to address trauma"? Professionals should consider whether the end, in this case PTSD symptom relief, justifies the means (i.e. time commitment, adversity of treatment, expended effort).

When determining if a person is suitable for treatment, professionals should primarily consider three ethical principles:
1. Nonmaleficience
2. Justice
3. Respect for autonomy.

1. Nonmaleficence – the first ethical principle, necessitates that care providers inflict the least harm, distress, or disturbance to ensure a beneficial outcome. When attempting to maximize palliation, professionals should consider the ways in which relief will be achieved. A person at the end-of-life with active PTSD should not be considered for strenuous or long-term psychological treatment. This principle works as a preventative value on palliative care and treatment. Nonmaleficence posits that the individual under care's safety and well-being be the top priority of treatment.
2. Justice – the ethical principle of justice asks professionals to conduct a cost-benefit analysis regarding treatment. Individuals living in palliative care settings are particularly vulnerable, often at the mercy of their care providers. When considering any kind of treatment for these individuals, whether it be pharmaceutical or psychological, the individual should be the center of the decision. Especially when considering PTSD treatment for people at the end-of-life, professionals should consider whether the distress caused by treatment justifies the relief the individual will, hopefully, experience. Individuals should not be encouraged to enter treatment that they do not have the capacity to participate in or that may perpetuate discomfort and distress. With this in mind, before beginning treatment, professionals should account for an individual's capacity, life expectancy, and potential prognosis.
3. Respect of Autonomy – the ethical principle asks that providers allow for the Respect for Autonomy of the individuals under care. It can be difficult to prioritize an individual's autonomy and agency in their care when professionals must follow a strict treatment plan to maintain their quality of life, comfort, or physical safety. Simon Woods provided the following definition of Respect for Autonomy: 'Giving moral weight to a person's interests [and a means of] shaping and directing his or her own life' (2005 p. 109)

Giving individuals a voice in their care can make a significant difference in their receptiveness to treatment. Validating individuals' feelings towards their treatment and incorporating their personal goals into treatment can enhance care effectiveness. An example of an individual reluctant to receive treatment can be found here.

For individuals such as Christopher, who feel that they lack independence and control over their situation, it may be even more salient to afford them autonomy in their care when possible. Christopher's care team should consider involving him in the planning of his treatment, such as scheduling and care trajectory. When possible, care providers should incorporate the individual and their preferences into their care. Respecting an individual's right and capacity to make decisions in their care promotes empowerment. Consider the person who is resistant to taking their medication, whether it is oral or by injection. Merely having them administer their own medication or choose the method by which they receive, when appropriate, can enhance feelings of control and agency in their care. Equally, when considering psychological treatment, having an open conversation with the individual in which they make the determination for treatment

Case Study 11.3

Christopher is a 17-year-old male of Salvadoran American descent. Two years ago, he was in a motor vehicle accident that left him paralyzed from the waist down. His parents report that Christopher often gets down on himself and feels hopeless about treatment and rehabilitation. He states that the accident has robbed him of any resemblance of independence and his care often gets in the way of him being a regular teenager. Christopher says his parents bring him to his medical appointments and rehabilitative therapy against his wishes, and his team of physical and occupational therapists report that he is unwilling to try the exercises.

can facilitate a smoother treatment trajectory. Similarly, this principle requires that professionals reflect on the reasons why autonomy is limited or constrained (Woods 2005). Individuals should be respected as independents who have agency in their own life and care, especially in places where that independence is often limited.

TRAUMA INFORMED APPROACH TO CARE

With the high demand on professionals in palliative care settings, it can seem daunting, and even unrealistic to some, to suggest that they incorporate mental health diagnosis or treatment into their care responsibilities. Considering the high-stress environment of palliative care and the propensity for traumatization with severe physical ill-health and end-of-life care, it would be unethical to not address said risk. Recently, there has been a push within residential and in-patient care settings to adopt a more systematic approach in which trauma is a consideration of health care. Formally, this organizational trend has been referred to as 'trauma informed care' (TIC). As an approach to care, TIC values patient safety, empowerment, and agency (Huckshorn & LeBel 2013). Perhaps the most attractive component of TIC is that it is not a treatment, but instead a way to organize care systems and treatment to compensate for possible trauma. The Substance Abuse and Mental Health Services Administration (SAMHSA) endorses the use of treatment informed approaches in care-giving settings, especially in residential settings (2015). Substance Abuse and Mental Health Services Administration developed the following definition of trauma-informed approach: 'A program, organization, or system that is trauma-informed realizes the widespread impact of trauma and understands potential paths for healing, recognizes the signs and symptoms of trauma in staff, clients, and others involved with the system; and responds by fully integrating knowledge about trauma into policies, procedures, practices, and settings'. (2015 www.samhsa.gov/nctic/trauma-interventions).

Incorporating a trauma-informed approach to palliative care may require reorganization of administration and systems of treatment. Trauma-informed environments can act as a precursor to formal modes of psychological therapy. Growth and healing are the forefront objectives of TIC. There have been several proposed structures to TIC, each incorporating three similar principles:

1. safety
2. connection
3. emotion management (Bath 2008).

These principles are commonly referred to as the pillars of TIC. When working with those who have been exposed to or suffer from trauma, it is imperative that they feel safe, both physically and emotionally. An often-defining feature of PTSD or trauma-related experiences is feeling unsafe or the inability to ensure one's consistent safety. This can lead to the exacerbation of PTSD symptoms such as irritability and avoidance, and create distrust in care providers. Building a safe environment for individuals under care requires providers to be consistent, reliable, and transparent. Informing and explaining an individual's treatment plan in a way that is comprehensible, minimizes uncertainty among individuals about their care. Making care predictable for individuals, such as providing medication at the same time by the same provider, can increase feelings of safety and trust.

Safety may largely depend on the second pillar, individuals' connection with their care providers. Social support, actual and perceived, can impact mental and physical prognosis. Encouraging professionals to be compassionate and genuine with individuals receiving care creates pathways for connection. Positive relationships aid in healing; specifically, positive professional–individual relationship is associated with better treatment outcomes and quality of life (Rambiharilal Shrivastava, Saurabh Shrivastava, & Ramasamy 2014). The third pillar is an effect of the first two – without safety and connection, it is difficult for individuals and their care providers to manage emotion. Affect dysregulation is a key feature of mental health disturbances, and trauma is not an exception. When individuals under care cannot appropriately or effectively regulate emotions, care providers can help by being supportive and managing the affect activation that is occurring. Managing emotions can make treatment more palatable and be a protective factor against developing or maintaining PTSD. Awareness that care providers may trigger individuals when attempting to be helpful can reduce providers from becoming defensive and increase ability to meet individuals with understanding during their activation.

It is often difficult for providers to effectively prepare treatment or accommodate for an individual's trauma exposure when they are unaware of the precipitating event or experience (Ganzel 2016). As mentioned previously, using a screener can help inform care providers of possible trauma-related experiences or symptoms. Adopting a trauma-informed approach encourages the use of appropriate screens, but does not require that administration do so. Trauma informed care (TIC) creates a system in which potential traumatic experiences are considered and accounted for.

CONCLUSION

Much of the focus of this chapter has been dedicated to how health care professionals' treat people who are receiving palliative care and may have a trauma history or be prone to traumatization in the medical setting. Care providers in palliation make up a diverse community with multifaceted roles. These include physicians and medical treatment professionals, nurses, volunteers, family, and friends alike. The need to be cared for, loved and valued is an integral part of being human. Therefore, it is no surprise that social support is important in the prognoses of both physical and mental health. Throughout the chapter, we have discussed several risk factors to stress and trauma. However, social support and life satisfaction work as a protective influence against life stress (Uchino 2006; Cobb 1976). Perceived support is not only vital to maintaining healthy biochemical mechanisms, but also strongly influences our behaviors. For example, treatment and medication adherence is vital in all medical treatment settings, especially palliation. Individuals with more cohesive support networks or who are living with another caring person were found to adhere more to their required medical treatments (DiMatteo 2004). With regard to trauma, those who were more satisfied with the social support they received tended to report less PTSD symptoms or severity (Andrews, Brewin, and Rose 2003) or recall the second pillar of TIC, connection. Perceived closeness, or strength of a social connection, can determine the impact of the relationship's consequences (Abbey, Abramis, & Caplan 1985). Thus, it is in the person's best interests for care providers to invest in and build genuine and stable connections.

Unfortunately, there are tradeoffs to our need for social support and connection. Negative social support and conflict can lend to worse prognosis (DiMatteo 2004; Andrews, Brewin, and Rose 2003). This finding emphasizes the importance of an expansive social network. An extensive social system in palliative care minimizes the impact of taxed care providers or systems on the individual. Likewise, extensive support networks amplify the opportunities for individuals to be cared for in a way that is aligned with their choices and values, especially when the network is compiled of several close relationships.

KEY POINTS 11.1

➤ Trauma is a unique, internal experience that will differ from person to person
➤ Treatment may exacerbate or worsen symptoms before they do or don't improve
➤ Cultural humility is a stance professionals can take to better identify and address symptoms of trauma
➤ When developing a treatment plan, psychologists should consider principles of justice, non-maleficence, and respect for person's autonomy
➤ Professionals' and caregivers' personal care should not be overlooked
➤ Professionals and caregivers in palliative care are susceptible to second hand trauma.

SELF-ASSESSMENT EXERCISE 11.1 – SEE P. 152 FOR ANSWERS

Time: 30 minutes

1. Which of the following is an indicator of trauma?
   a) reduced interest in activities
   b) irritability
   c) treatment resistance
   d) all of the above

2. True or False? If a person does not meet criteria to diagnose PTSD, the psychologist should not treat the trauma.

3. Which of the following is not an ethical principal of trauma-related palliative care?
   a) Justice
   b) Trauma Informed Care
   c) Respect for Autonomy
   d) Nonmaleficence

4. Why should palliative care professionals make trauma a consideration in their work?
   a) Untreated trauma can complicate the diagnosis and treatment of physical health conditions
   b) Health care providers are ethically obligated to treat trauma-related symptoms and PTSD
   c) Trauma should not be a consideration for medical professionals

5. When receiving palliative care, who is at risk for developing trauma-related distress?
   a) Individuals receiving treatment
   b) Family and friends of the individual
   c) Health care professionals
   d) All of the above

REFERENCES

Abbey, A., Abramis, D. J. and Caplan, R. D. (1985) 'Effects of different sources of social support and social conflict on emotional well-being'. *Basic and Applied Social Psychology*, 6, pp. 111–29.

Aderibigbe, Y. A. and Pandurangi, A. K. (1995) 'The neglect of culture in psychiatric nosology: the case of culture bound syndromes'. *International Journal of Social Psychiatry*, 41, pp. 235–41.

Aldwin, C. M. (1994) *Stress, Coping and Development: An Integrative Perspective*. New York: Guilford Press.

Aldwin, C. M. and Levenson, M. R. (2013) 'Stress', in *Encyclopedia of Sciences and Religions* (pp. 2216–26). Netherlands: Springer.

Alici, Y., Smith, D., Lu, H. L., Bailey, A., Shreve, S., et al. (2010) 'Families' perceptions of veterans' distress due to post-traumatic stress disorder-related symptoms at the end of life'. *Journal of Pain and Symptom Management*, 39, pp. 507–14.

American Psychiatric Association 2013. *Diagnostic and Statistical Manual of Mental Disorders (DSM-5(r))*. Arlington, VA: American Psychiatric Pub.

American Psychological Association Division 12. (2016) 'Psychological Treatments. Division 12 of The American Psychological Association'. *Society of Clinical Psychology*. Available at: www.div12.org/psychological-treatments/treatments/ (Accessed 29 November 2017).

Anda, R. F., Felitti, V. J., Bremner, J. D., Walker, J. D., Whitfield, C. H., et al. (2006) 'The enduring effects of abuse and related adverse experiences in childhood'. *European Archives of Psychiatry and Clinical Neuroscience*, 256, pp. 174–86.

Andrews, B., Brewin, C. R. and Rose, S. (2003) 'Gender, social support, and PTSD in victims of violent crime'. *Journal of Traumatic Stress*, 16, pp. 421–7.

Bath, H. (2008) 'The three pillars of trauma-informed care'. *Reclaiming Children and Youth*, 17, pp. 17–21.

Benjet, C., Bromet, E., Karam, E. G., Kessler, R. C., McLaughlin, K. A., et al. (2016) 'The epidemiology of traumatic event exposure worldwide: results from the World Mental Health Survey Consortium'. *Psychological Medicine*, 46, pp. 327–43.

Berg, A. O., Breslau, N., Goodman, S. N., Lezak, M., Matchar, D., et al. (2007) *Treatment of PTSD: An Assessment of The Evidence*. Washington, DC: National Academies Press.

Bertram, F., Jamison, A. L., Slightam, C., Kim, S., Roth, H. L. and Roth, W. T. (2014) 'Autonomic arousal during actigraphically estimated waking and sleep in male veterans with PTSD'. *Journal of Traumatic Stress*, 27, pp. 610–17.

Bradley, R., Greene, J., Russ, E., Dutra, L. and Westen, D. (2005) 'A multidimensional meta-analysis of psychotherapy for PTSD'. *American Journal of Psychiatry*, 162, pp. 214–27.

Cobb, S. (1976) 'Social support as a moderator of life stress'. *Psychosomatic Medicine*, 38, pp. 300–14.

Cukor, J., Olden, M., Lee, F. and Difede, J. (2010) 'Evidence-based treatments for PTSD, new directions, and special challenges'. *Annals of the New York Academy of Sciences*, 1208, pp. 82–9.

Diaz, A., Bourassa, M. G., Guertin, M. C. and Tardif, J. C. (2005) 'Long-term prognostic value of resting heart rate in patients with suspected or proven coronary artery disease'. *European Heart Journal*, 26, pp. 967–74.

DiMatteo, M. R. (2004) 'Social support and patient adherence to medical treatment: a meta-analysis'. *Health Psychology*, 23, pp. 207–18.

Evans, L., Cowlishaw, S., Forbes, D., Parslow, R. and Lewis, V. (2010) 'Longitudinal analyses of family functioning in veterans and their partners across treatment'. *Journal of Consulting and Clinical Psychology*, 78, pp. 611–22.

Felitti, V. J. and Anda, R. F. (2010) 'The relationship of adverse childhood experiences to adult medical disease, psychiatric disorders and sexual behavior: implications for healthcare', in Lanius, R. A. and Vermetten, E. (eds). *The Impact of Early Life Trauma an Health and Disease: The Hidden Epidemic*, 1st edition. New York: Cambridge University Press, pp. 77–87.

Galea, S., Basham, K., Culpepper, L., Davidson, J., Foa, E., et al. (2012) *Treatment for Posttraumatic Stress Disorder in Military and Veteran Populations: Initial Assessment*. Washington, DC: The National Academies.

Gallagher, J., Riggs, D., Byrne, C. and Weathers, F. (1998) 'Female partners' estimations of male veterans' combat-related PTSD severity'. *Journal of Traumatic Stress*, 11, pp. 367–74.

Ganzel, B. L. (2016) 'Trauma-informed hospice and palliative care'. *The Gerontologist*, pii, pp. gnw146.

Gaynes, B. N., DeVeaugh-Geiss, J., Weir, S., Gu, H., MacPherson, C., et al. (2010) 'Feasibility and diagnostic validity of the M-3 checklist: a brief, self-rated screen for depressive, bipolar, anxiety, and post-traumatic stress disorders in primary care'. *The Annals of Family Medicine*, 8, pp. 160–9.

Gradus, J. L. National Center for Post-Traumatic Stress Disorder. (2017) *Epidemiology of PTSD*. Available at: www.ptsd.va.gov/professional/ptsd-overview/epidemiological-facts-ptsd.asp (Accessed: 29 November 2017)

Harvey, A. G. and Bryant, R. A. (1998) 'The relationship between acute stress disorder and posttraumatic stress disorder: a prospective evaluation of motor vehicle accident survivors'. *Journal of Consulting and Clinical Psychology*, 66, p. 507.

Hembree, E. A., Foa, E. B., Dorfan, N. M., Street, G. P., Kowalski, J. and Tu, X. (2003) 'Do patients drop out prematurely from exposure therapy for PTSD'? *Journal of Traumatic Stress*, 16, pp. 555–62.

Hook, J. N., Davis, D. E., Owen, J., Worthington, E. L. and Utsey, S. O. (2013) 'Cultural humility: measuring openness to culturally diverse clients'. *Journal of Counseling Psychology*, 60, pp. 353–66.

Huckshorn, K. and LeBel, J. L. (2013) 'Trauma-informed care', in: Yeager, K., Cutler, D., Svendesn, D. and Sills, G. (eds). *Modern Community Mental Health Work: An Interdisciplinary Approach*, 1st edition. New York: Oxford University Press pp. 62–83.

Jackson, J. C., Hart, R. P., Gordon, S. M., Hopkins, R. O., Girard, T. D. and Ely, E. (2007) 'Post-traumatic stress disorder and post-traumatic stress symptoms following critical illness in medical intensive care unit patients: assessing the magnitude of the problem'. *Critical Care*, 11, pp. R27.

Jouven, X., Empana, J. P., Schwartz, P. J., Desnos, M. Courbon, D. and Ducimetière, P. (2005) 'Heart-rate profile during exercise as a predictor of sudden death'. *New England Journal of Medicine*, 352, pp. 1951–8.

Kangas, M., Henry, J. L. and Bryant, R. A. (2005) 'Predictors of posttraumatic stress disorder following cancer'. *Health Psychology*, 24, p. 579.

Link, B. and Phelan, J. (2001) 'Conceptualizing stigma'. *Annual Review of Sociology*, 27, pp. 363–85.

Meyer, I. H. (2003) 'Prejudice, social stress, and mental health in lesbian, gay, and bisexual populations: conceptual issues and research evidence'. *Psychological Bulletin*, 129, p. 674.

National Center for Post-Traumatic Stress Disorder. (2017) US Department of Veteran Affairs. Available at: www.ptsd.va.gov/ (Accessed: 12 December 2017).

Nishith, P., Resick, P. A. and Griffin, M. G. (2002) 'Pattern of change in prolonged exposure and cognitive-processing therapy for female rape victims with posttraumatic stress disorder'. *Journal of Consulting and Clinical Psychology*, 70, p. 880.

Niles, B. L., Herman, D. S., Segura-Schultz, S., Joaquim, S. J. and Litz, B. T. (1993) *The Spouse/Partner Mississippi Scale: How Does It Compare?* Paper presented at the 32-annual meeting of the International Society for Traumatic Stress Studies, San Antonio, Texas.

Norris, F. H. (1992) 'Epidemiology of trauma: frequency and impact of different potentially traumatic events on different demographic groups'. *Journal of Consulting and Clinical Psychology*, 60, pp. 409–18.

Otis, J. D., Keane, T. M. and Kerns, R. D. (2003) 'An examination of the relationship between chronic pain and post-traumatic stress disorder'. *Journal of Rehabilitation Research and Development*, 40, p. 397.

Perret-Guillaume, C., Joly, L. and Benetos, A. (2009) 'Heart rate as a risk factor for cardiovascular disease'. *Progress in Cardiovascular Diseases*, 52, pp. 6–10.

Pietrzak, R. H., Goldstein, R. B., Southwick, S. M. and Grant, B. F. (2012) 'Psychiatric comorbidity of full and partial posttraumatic stress disorder among older adults in the United States: results from wave 2 of the National Epidemiologic Survey on Alcohol and Related Conditions'. *The American Journal of Geriatric Psychiatry*, 20, pp. 380–90.

Purnell, L. D. (2008) 'Traditional Vietnamese health and healing'. *Urologic Nursing*, 28, p. 63.

Rambiharilal Shrivastava, S., Saurabh Shrivastava, P. and Ramasamy, J. (2014) 'Exploring the dimensions of doctor-patient relationship in clinical practice in hospital settings', *International Journal of Health Policy*, 2, pp. 159–60.

Roberts, A. L., Gilman, S. E., Breslau, J., Breslau, N. and Koenen, K. C. (2011) 'Race/ethnic differences in exposure to traumatic events, development of post-traumatic stress disorder, and treatment-seeking for post-traumatic stress disorder in the United States', *Psychological Medicine*, 41, pp. 71–83.

Rome, R. B., Luminais, H. H., Bourgeois, D. A. and Blais, C. M. (2011) 'The role of palliative care at the end of life'. *The Ochsner Journal*, 11, pp. 348–52.

Roth, J. R. and Massie, M. J. (2009) 'Anxiety in palliative care', in Chochinov, H. M. and Breitbart, W. (eds). *Handbook of Psychiatry in Palliative Medicine*, 2nd edition. New York: Oxford University Press, pp. 69–74.

Schelling, G., Briegel, J., Roozendaal, B., Stoll, C., Rothenhäusler, H. B. et al. (2001) 'The effect of stress doses of hydrocortisone during septic shock on posttraumatic stress disorder in survivors'. *Biological Psychiatry*, 50, pp. 978–85.

Segerstrom, S. C. and Miller, G. E. (2004) 'Psychological stress and the human immune system: a meta-analytic study of 30 years of inquiry'. *Psychological Bulletin*, 130, p. 601.

Sherin, J. E. and Nemeroff, C. B. (2011) 'Post-traumatic stress disorder: the neurobiological impact of psychological trauma'. *Dialogues in Clinical Neuroscience*, 13, p. 263.

Solomon, Z., Dekel, R. and Zerach, G. (2008) 'The relationships between posttraumatic stress symptom clusters and marital intimacy among war veterans'. *Journal of Family Psychology*, 22, 659–66.

Spoont, M., Arbisi, P., Fu, S., Greer, N., Kehle-Forbes, S., et al. (2013) 'Screening for post-traumatic stress disorder (PTSD) in primary care: A systematic review'. Available at: www.ncbi.nlm.nih.gov/books/NBK126691/ (Accessed: 29 November 2017)

Staab, J. P., Grieger, T. A., Fullerton, C. S. and Ursano, R. J. (1996) 'Acute stress disorder, subsequent posttraumatic stress disorder and depression after a series of typhoons'. *Anxiety*, 2, pp. 219–25.

Substance Abuse and Mental Health Services Administration. (2015) 'Mental Health Services Administration. Trauma-Informed Approach and Trauma Specific Interventions'. *National Center for Trauma-Informed Care (NCTIC)*. Accessed 2 December 2017, <www.samhsa.gov/nctic/trauma-interventions>

Taft, C., King, L., King, D., Leskin, G. and Riggs, D. (1999) 'Partners' ratings of combat veterans' PTSD symptomatology'. *Journal of Traumatic Stress*, 12, pp. 327–34.

Taylor, S., Kuch, K., Koch, W., Crockett, D. and Passey, G. (1998) 'The structure of posttraumatic stress symptoms'. *Journal of Abnormal Psychology*, 107, pp. 154–60.

Uchino, B. N. (2006) 'Social support and health: a review of physiological processes potentially underlying links to disease outcomes'. *Journal of Behavioral Medicine*, 29, pp. 377–87.

Wang, P. S., Berglund, P., Olfson, M., Pincus, H. A., Wells, K. B. and Kessler, R. C. (2005) 'Failure and delay in initial treatment contact after first onset of mental disorders in the National Comorbidity Survey Replication'. *Archives of General Psychiatry*, 62, pp. 603–13.

Weathers, F. W., Litz, B. T., Keane, T. M., Palmieri, P. A., Marx, B. P. and Schnurr, P. P. (2013) 'The PTSD Checklist for *DSM-5* (PCL-5). Scale available from the National Center for PTSD'. Available at: www.ptsd.va.gov/professional/assessment/adult-sr/ptsd-checklist.asp (Accessed: 29 November 2017)

Wilson, J. P. and Keane, T. M. (2004) *Assessing Psychological Trauma and PTSD*. New York: Guilford Press.

Woods, S. (2005) 'Respect for persons, autonomy and palliative care'. *Medicine, Health Care and Philosophy*, 8, pp. 243–53.

Woodward, S. H., Arsenault, N. J., Voelker, K., Nguyen, T., Lynch, J., et al. (2009) 'Autonomic activation during sleep in posttraumatic stress disorder and panic: a mattress actigraphic study'. *Biological Psychiatry*, 66, pp. 41–6.

Yehuda, R. and LeDoux, J. (2007) 'Response variation following trauma: a translational neuroscience approach to understanding PTSD'. *Neuron*, 56, pp. 19–32.

To Learn More

National Center for Trauma-Informed Care (SAMHSA). www.samhsa.gov/nctic

National Center for PTSD (U.S. Department of Veterans Affairs); www.ptsd.va.gov

Rothschild, R. (2000) *The Body Remembers: The Psychophysiology of Trauma and Trauma Treatment*. New York: Norton Professional Books.

van der Kolk, B. A. (2014) *The Body Keeps the Score: Brain, Mind, and Body in the Healing of Trauma*. New York: Penguin Books.

ANSWERS TO SELF-ASSESSMENT EXERCISE 11.1 – *SEE* P. 148 FOR QUESTIONS

1. D. All of the above. Trauma and its related symptoms are idiosyncratic and unique to each individual, which means that it can present in a multitude of ways.

2. False. Subthreshold presentations of PTSD still indicate distress and should not go untreated. The type of treatment selected will be determined by the desires and values of the individual and the appropriateness of the therapy given the person's current health status.

3. B. Trauma Informed Care. Trauma Informed Care is a value or approach that is adopted by all who are working in a medical environment. Trauma informed care (TIC) can enhance the treatment of trauma, quality of life, and satisfaction with treatment but is not an ethical principle.

4. A. It can complicate the diagnosis and treatment of physical health conditions. There is a physiological response and consequence to trauma and chronic stress, which can impact or exacerbate medical ailments.

5. D. All of the above. Social support is an important mediator of trauma distress and symptoms. Lack of social connectedness can make any of the listed persons above more susceptible to trauma stressors.

CHAPTER 12

Specific Needs of the Child, Adolescent, and Young Adult

Geraldine S. Pearson

INTRODUCTION

Children and adolescents present particular challenges to individuals providing mental health care. These challenges include their legal, social, and economic dependence on their caregivers, their status as individuals who are NOT mini-adults, and the transitional nature of their developmental status and functioning. While these issues may vary slightly by culture and geography the inherent dependence of pediatric populations on caregivers makes them vulnerable to ethical breaches (*See* Chapter 6). Consideration of the individual's rights, combined with caregiver rights, and responsibility of mental health providers has the potential to result in ethically driven care that preserves and protects the pediatric population (*See* Chapter 8). Already vulnerable because of difficulties with mental health, that vulnerability needs to be recognized and dealt with early in assessment and into treatment.

This chapter will explore the ethical issues that might confront professionals providing mental health treatment to a pediatric population, recognizing that the needs of a 4-year-old child might vary greatly from that of a young adult at the end of adolescence at age 19 or 20. The intellectual capacities and value structures of the individual develop in childhood and change as the individual moves into adolescence and young adulthood. Autonomy and competence ideally grow and develop with maturation (Matthews 2016). For the child or adolescent experiencing mental health issues, this development of autonomy and competence is potentially threatened or derailed. This complicates ethical care and forces reliance on the caregiver or parent as the primary manager of the child or adolescent. The particular issues influencing these differing age ranges will be discussed.

DEVELOPMENTAL STAGES

This chapter aims to discuss ethical issues in treatment for populations from infancy into early 20s. While the definitions of infancy and toddlerhood (birth to three), preschool years (three to six years), and school age (seven to 11 years) have remained generally unchanged, the age boundaries of adolescence (beginning at age 12–13) have shifted. Adolescence is now thought to extend into the early 20s with the social and developmental characteristics shifting depending on geography and culture. Many individuals in their early 20s continue to be dependent on caregivers or parents for financial and emotional support. This has coincided with later marriage and child-bearing occurring in the late 20s. The predominant goal of adolescence has consistently been a striving for autonomy (Cuffe 2010).

The legal ages of consent, which vary by culture and location, and the ability to handle increasing autonomy, a common goal of adolescence regardless of global location, influence ethical decision making. Most individuals over the age of 18 are seen as legally capable of making their own decisions about their mental health care. Certainly, impairment and ill-health might influence this but they can sign consents for treatment, release of information, and medication management.

RIGHTS OF CHILDREN AND ADOLESCENTS

Historically children were not seen as having rights in Ancient Greece, during the Middle Ages, through the Renaissance and into the Industrial Revolution. By the twentieth century, in the contemporary world, childhood was increasingly viewed as a time when individuals needed to have rights irrespective of age, color, or creed (Sousa & Araujo 2011). In 1959 the 'Declaration of the Rights of the Child' was adopted by UNICEF (United Nations International Children's Emergency Fund – UNICEF 2008) and outlined children's rights to freedom of speech, though, choice, and ownership of one's body. This led to the 'United Nations Convention on the Rights of the Child' in 1989 and 'Barcelona Declaration' from the III World Congress on Children and Adolescents Rights (UNICEF 2008). These documents specified that children and adolescents have a right to live a life outside of poverty, should not be abused or experience discrimination, and should have adequate health care, education, and social participation in the world.

Despite these international declarations children are still seen, in many parts of contemporary society, as small adults with fewer rights and entitlements. Children of many cultures and ethnicities still live in poverty, with few rights, and with limited access to health care, education, and safety. The difficulty with declarations around children's rights comes with the extreme diversity of children's lives across the world. If culture is defined as the common values, beliefs, and social behaviors of individuals with a shared heritage, this culture will likely influence access to mental health services, the role of stigma in mental health problems, and the overall population's view of mental health (Stewart, Simmons, & Habibpour 2012).

> [While] heterogeneity is assumed within a named cultural or racial group, the terms Hispanic, Asian, and African-American incorporate subgroups . . . different in linguistic, historical, and geographical ancestry.
>
> (Stewart, Simmons, & Habibpour 2012, p. 72)

Stewart and colleagues (2012) make the point that even among populations with historical ties, values, beliefs, and social behaviors, there can be wide variation in the culture and identification with the mainstream culture. This is further influenced by social class, which in turn, can influence access to mental health treatment. Disparities in accessing services are multi-determined and can involve economics, the individual, and provider variables.

KEY POINT 12.1

Rights of the individual child, adolescent, or young adult will vary according to geography, and culture and may vary between countries.

ETHICAL ISSUES INFLUENCING TREATMENT

The general principles about treating children and adolescents with respect, dignity, kindness, and caring are applicable to any professional working with this population. The concept of caring involves a natural and fundamental part of human existence. This caring also translates into ethical management of the mental health care of children and adolescents. Ethical care involves understanding and working effectively with children, adolescents, and families. These principles of ethical management involve the following concepts, as outlined by the American Academy of Child and Adolescent Psychiatry (AACAP 2014). Paraphrased for use more broadly by psychiatric professionals they include:

Principle I, Developmental Perspective

The professionals working alongside children and adolescents are obligated to understand the developmental context of individuals in their care. This means including children in treatment decisions according to their developmental level, their ability to understand, and influence of their social and emotional difficulties. It involves knowing and understanding the knowledge and ability of caregivers and using this knowledge in involving the child in decision making.

This principle involves professionals who know and understand the differences between adults and children and recognize that children's development is on a changing trajectory. The developmental challenges presented by a five-year-old, beginning school will be vastly different from someone in their late teens or early 20s, launching into the work force or finishing secondary school. Similarly, the ethical issues facing these populations will be at least partially dependent on age and developmental level. Five-year-olds are very dependent on their families and caregivers for all basic needs while individuals in later adolescence are developing increasing autonomy and independence from caregivers.

Principle II, Promoting the Welfare of Children and Adolescents (Beneficence)

This principle focuses on the professional's obligation to promote optimal functioning in children and adolescents. The professional's needs take a secondary role to those of the individual in care. The welfare and needs of the child should be paramount (AACAP 2014). Clinical decisions should be based on reasoning that examines what best promotes a child's welfare. American Academy of Child and Adolescent Psychiatry (AACAP) notes that a child's social, economic, and cultural environment contributes to the complexities of the principle of beneficence. Professionals are urged to understand all the influences on a child or adolescent's behavior and presentation considering these cultural issues.

All developmental issues are understood in the context of culture, spiritual beliefs (*See* Chapter 23), and ethnicity. Cultural competence (*See* Chapter 6) is essential for any professional providing treatment to diverse populations (Pumariega, Rothe,

& Rogers 2009). This competence involves an awareness of common presentations and an understanding of shared values and beliefs of a specific population within a community. Recognition of the differences within groups might make application of specific cultural information difficult (Stewart, Simmons, & Habibpour 2012). Fields (2010) recommends that professionals be aware of their own assumptions and consistently challenge and test these as they treat populations from cultures different from theirs.

Principle III, Minimizing Harmful Effects (Non-maleficence)

This principle embodies the concept of "do no harm" and avoiding any actions detrimental to the optimal functioning and development of children and adolescents. This also involves attempting to minimize harm at multiple levels including individual, family, community, and societal levels. It cautions against exploitation and avoiding adverse impacts on patient care. Keeping boundaries between professionals and children and adolescents in care is essential (*See* Box 12.1).

BOX 12.1 Steps for Mental Health Professionals and Students to Identify, Avoid or Correct Ethical Difficulties

- Students are taught about ethics, vulnerabilities, and corrective actions through curriculum, practicum training, supervision, and consultation
- Understand the emotions and situational factors that influence professional behavior
- Faculty and supervisors emphasize going beyond minimum standards of care and model ethical excellence and increased self-awareness
- Balance self-care issues with the emotional demands of providing care to individuals with mental health problems
- Identify personal values self-assessment and understand how they influence ethical decision making
- Utilize corrective action through interventions such as supervision, consultation, or personal psychotherapy when ethical dilemmas are identified, and the dilemma has been compounded by the professional's personal issues.

Adapted from Tjeltveit and Gottlieb (2010)

Principle IV, Assent and Consent (Autonomy)

This principle involves the ability of children and adolescents to make their own decisions about their care. Individuals under the age of 18 are generally seen as needing parent or guardian consent for treatment decisions. Consent and assent guidelines will vary greatly by country or local state regulations. In some areas individuals over the age of 7 must assent to treatment, meaning they must agree to the care. This is complicated by competence, degree of impairment, capability, developmental status, and the ability to understand risks, benefits, and side effects of treatment. Like other principles, this one is influenced by cultural and community normative factors, family structure, health status, and setting of care.

> Informed consent has been defined as having three elements: information sharing, decision-making capacity and voluntariness.

> (AACAP 2014)

Case Study 12.1

A nine-year-old male is brought to the mental health clinic for evaluation of symptoms of Attention Deficit Disorder. The professional has done a thorough evaluation with family history, history of current difficulties in school, and adequacy of parenting skills. The professional recommends a trial of stimulant medication at the same time the family receives treatment for conflicts between the individual and his siblings. When this treatment plan is discussed the nine-year-old adamantly refuses to consider taking any pill. He is adamant about this despite his parents' attempts to obtain compliance with the plan. Later his mother calls the professional and suggests that they crush the medication and put it in his morning yogurt. The professional explains that while parents have the right to provide legal consent for the treatment, the nine-year-old must assent to this and agree to the intervention. It is unethical to crush his medicine without his knowledge and put it in his food. Treatment efforts were focused on the professional understanding better the reasons behind the boy's refusal for medication management. He later revealed, as part of play therapy that "only crazy people take pills and I'm not crazy". Alternative treatment models were used with the individual and the family. He never gave assent for the medication.

Information needs to be tailored to the individual's developmental level, the preferred language, and literacy. Can the individual communicate a preference for care, understand the presented information, and be able to view the larger effect on their life? It is not acceptable to deceive or withhold information from an individual under age 18. Appreciation of ability to understand and attempts to communicate at the individual's development level are imperative.

Principle V, Confidentiality (Autonomy/Fidelity)

Individuals have the right to have their information kept private and confidential. It is essential that professionals inform children and adolescents about the principles of confidentiality and the limits of this if there is any chance of the individual being a danger to self or others. All releases of information must have the individual's assent and the guardian's consent. The balance involves protecting the individual's privacy while keeping parents and guardians informed about care.

For older adolescents these confidentiality issues are somewhat different in that they do not require parental permission for care if over age 18 in most countries. However, the tenets about professional confidentiality in the face of threat to self or others are the same. The goal of the care is to keep the individual safe regardless of their age and confidentiality rules are suspended.

Professionals need to share the risk of providing care for any individual who presents as a danger to self or others. Peer consultation and supervision are excellent ways of sharing the risk of managing these individuals.

Principle VI, Third Party Influence (Fidelity)

This principle involves focusing on influences to care from outside entities. Professionals need to put the welfare of individuals above all other interests. These conflicts of interest might include responsibilities to other agencies providing care, child custody disputes, or research activities. Commercial entities involving products or pharmaceuticals can create a conflict of interest for professionals. Many agencies have limited or banned the professional in their employ from receiving any products from commercial entities as a strategy to limit conflicts of interest.

Principle VII, Research Activities

This principle involves minimizing risk of research to the individual child or adolescent. It recommends never forcing people, regardless of age, to participate in research against their will. Research must follow the ethical standards of the culture and the priority must be protection of the child or adolescent. It is usually recommended that research involving individuals be separated from clinical care. The activities and associated ethical issues, while similar, have different goals and objectives.

Principle VIII, Advocacy, and Equity (Justice)

Competent mental health care should be available to all children, adolescents, and families. Professionals must support the improved access to care while minimizing exposure to injustice. This principle involves maintaining an awareness of vulnerable populations and avoiding exploitation of them in treatment or research situations.

Some research has pointed to there being a higher stigma against mental ill-health in minority groups. These stigmas can be subtle and adverse to facilitating care (Stewart, Simmons, & Habibpour 2012).

Principle IX, Professional Rewards

This Principle has applicability to all professionals working with children and families. It asks that professionals be aware of the possible influence of rewards on their judgments and actions. Examples might be products that advertise a particular medication, free samples of medication to dispense to individuals, and in the past, dinners and trips for individual providers who used or recommended a particular product. Avoiding compromises to integrity helps the public trust the individuals providing care to their children and adolescents. This involves not taking gifts from commercial entities. Many institutions have banned salespeople from directly marketing a product to individuals who could recommend this as part of treatment.

KEY POINT 12.2

The American Academy of Child and Adolescent Psychiatry (www.aacap.org) offers free resources to mental health practitioners including this 'Code of Ethics'.

SPECIFIC ETHICAL DILEMMAS WITH AN ADOLESCENT POPULATION: ACCESSING CONFIDENTIAL CARE

According to the World Health Organization (2013), 1.3 million adolescents worldwide died from preventable or treatable causes. These included motor vehicle accidents, accidental injuries, interpersonal violence, suicide, chronic ill-health, and human immunodeficiency virus (HIV). High-risk behaviors such as unprotected sex and substance use (*See* Chapter 17) also maximized risk to this age group. At the same time, maximizing adolescent health involves access to care. This has to address the boundaries of confidentiality and the adolescent's expectations of this as they seek care (Alderman 2017).

Assuring confidentiality for an adolescent seeking health care supports the ethical principle of respect for the adolescent's developing autonomy. Beneficence is also supported by confidentiality (Alderman 2017). Confidentiality cannot always be assured. State and local laws, the individual's age, developmental level and relationship with caregiver must also be considered. Many states in the U.S. have laws that protect confidential care for adolescents based on the type of care, i.e. sexual health, outpatient mental health, and substance use. Other non-diagnostic influences on confidentiality can include billing issues or specific conditions that require parental consent (such as HIV treatment in some countries).

Professionals providing mental health treatment to an adolescent population should know and understand the legal boundaries and limits of the geographic area of their practice. It is imperative that this be communicated to the adolescent and caregivers before care commences.

SPECIAL ETHICAL DILEMMAS: THE INDIVIDUAL WITH A DEVELOPMENTAL DISORDER

Delivering mental health services to an individual experiencing developmental disabilities can be ethically complex, presenting concerns for professionals. Ramisch and Franklin (2008) note that care issues have shifted as there is more emphasis on community management. They note that it is imperative that professionals examine and recognize 'their own biases, stereotypes, and attributional errors' (Ramisch & Franklin 2008, p. 313) when working with individuals with developmental disorders and their families. What are their attitudes about individuals with disabilities and how does this translate consciously or unconsciously into care.

Professionals need to understand that individuals experiencing developmental disorders might also have a dual diagnosis that involves a psychiatric disorder. This situation is particularly challenging to professionals since the symptoms often overlap. Treatment addresses both issues and considers that family involvement might be more prominent if the individual is dependent on family members because of their disability.

Treatment must also address associated ethical issues. These can include balancing the rights and needs of the individual with the caregiving rights of the individual providing care. There are three predominant ethical concerns when treating an individual with developmental issues. These include obtaining a voluntary consent for treatment, developing treatment goals where the individual has input, and maintaining confidentiality (Lynch 2004). The clarity of a consent process will set the frame for beginning treatment. This must be balanced with the ability of the individual to understand the consent and their legal rights. Can they legally offer consent if under the care of a guardian or does legal consent for care rest with the guardian? Regardless of the answer to this, individuals experiencing developmental disorders can give assent, or agreement to the mental health treatment. Assessment and intervention has to be tailored to the level of functioning of the individual. Professionals are challenged to hold a high ethical standard when offering treatment to an individual with a developmental disability (Ramisch & Franklin 2008).

Similarity, the issue of confidentiality with this population might be difficult to discuss or define, particularly in situations where the individual is enmeshed with family caregivers. Professionals are urged to define confidentiality to the individual and family, detailing the situations when confidentiality would not apply, i.e. danger to self or others, but also noting the need for mutual agreement between the individual and professional about information shared with caregivers (Sori & Hecker 2006). In all situations treatment goals have to be based on the assumption that individuals have the right to choose whether or not to engage in treatment regardless of differing caregiver goals (Ramisch & Franklin 2008). Professionals must apply ethical standards to treatment of this population despite their disability.

KEY PONT 12.3

Despite having a developmental disability, the individual child, adolescent, or young adult has rights within the context of their mental health treatment. Families may need to be educated regarding these rights. Professionals must tailor their explanations to the functioning level of the individual.

CONSIDERING STIGMA IN ETHICAL PSYCHIATRIC CARE OF CHILDREN, ADOLESCENTS, AND YOUNG ADULTS

Stigma has far-reaching influences in terms of access to care, use, or underuse of mental health services, and increasing caregiver burden (Mukolo, Heflinger, & Wallston 2010). From an ethical perspective it has implications for public perceptions of individuals experiencing mental health disorders and for the professionals who provide their care.

REFLECTIVE PRACTICE EXERCISE 12.1

Time: 15 minutes
What are my personal biases or stigma around populations or disorders?

Mukolo and colleagues (2010) found that there were three dimensions of stigma involving childhood mental disorders. These involved negative stereotypes, devaluation, and discrimination. Additionally, they identified in their literature review that self and general public comprised the two contexts of stigma; the targets of stigma were self/individual, and family. They identified the lack of literature describing stigmatizing contexts related to children's emotional and behavioral problems.

Stigma has pertinence to this chapter in that recognition of the dimensions, context, and targets of stigma is essential for ethical practice with children, adolescents, and young adults. The core of this is understanding self-attitudes and biases while maintaining an awareness of the biases inherent in organizational policies and procedures that might adversely affect the mental health treatment received by these individuals and their families.

Family members are targets of stigma simply by their association with an individual who is experiencing mental health issues. The shame of being a 'bad parent' or somehow 'causing' the mental health problems in a child or adolescent cannot be underestimated and crosses cultural and socioeconomic boundaries throughout the world.

Understanding stigma requires that professionals understand 'the socioculturally defined idiosyncrasies of mental disorders' [and the] 'potential interactions between mental illness and other socially devalued statuses' (Mukolo, Heflinger, & Wallston 2010, p. 100).

These could include idiosyncrasies further defined by ethnicity, race, or socioeconomic group. Professionals need to first identify their own potential stigmatizing attitudes, those of the agency where they provide care, and the perceived stigma of individuals and their families in the community. Stigma exists and for many professionals and families it is so pervasive that it becomes an expected part of involvement with a child, adolescent, or young adult experiencing mental health problems. Complacency should be avoided and pursuit of systematic understanding of an individual or population will assist in addressing it in provision of mental health care. Advocacy efforts must be ongoing so that confronting stigma becomes as commonplace as recognizing it.

KEY POINT 12.4

Stigma is a powerful and pervasive influence on individuals who struggle with mental health issues. Professionals must maintain constant awareness of this and the influence it has on treatment.

SELF-ASSESSMENT OF ETHICAL VALUES

Mental health professionals working alongside children, adolescents, and young adults should embody health care values fundamental to the practice of compassionate, ethical, and safe relationship-centered care (Rider et al. 2014). The International Charter for Human Values in Healthcare details these core values and supports their adoption by health professionals. They identified five fundamental categories of human values for every health care interaction and have applicability to professionals working with young populations. They are compassion, respect for persons, commitment to integrity and ethical practice, commitment to excellence, and justice in health care.

It is recommended that these values inform every health care interaction and be embedded in educational and clinical training programs. The goal is fostering a movement that 'restores the primacy of human values, to place them at the center, and to make values, and the communication skills necessary to demonstrate them, the foundation of every effort in healthcare' (Rider et al. 2014, p. 279).

Such a movement has to begin with individual professionals examining their practice and defining their personal ethical standards in tandem with the ethical standards of their work environment. Tjeltveit and Gottlieb (2010, p. 98) identify four general dimensions of evaluation that have applicability to those professionals working alongside children and adolescents. They are:
1. the desire to facilitate positive (good) outcomes
2. the powerful opportunities given to professionals to effect change
3. personal values
4. education (p. 98).

Addressing these dimensions reduces vulnerability to ethical violations, intentional or unintentional, while enhancing the professional's resilience, and generally improving quality of work (*See* Box 12.2).

BOX 12.2 First Steps to Providing an Ethical Framework

1. Know and identify the ethical practice values of clinical practice
   a. Do they reflect the values of the community?
   b. Are they articulated?
   c. What are the supports if professionals face an ethical dilemma while providing care?

2. What are the local laws around consent of children and adolescents, confidentiality, and caregiver involvement in treatment?
   a. How stringently are the laws enforced?
   b. What are the documentation requirements around consent and confidentiality?
   c. How do the requirements of caregiver involvement differ between a 9-year-old and a 19-year-old?

3. What are the ethical supports available to mental health professionals in the community?
   a. Is there regular clinical supervision for those treating children, adolescents, and young adults?
   b. Is there institutional stigma for those professionals who are seeking their own mental health treatment?
   c. Do professionals in the agency trust their supervisors?

Multiple factors influence the ethical responses of individual professionals: "... the awareness that ethical issues are present, social and cultural influences, habits, emotions, intuitions, identity, virtues and character, multiple or competing motivations, prior decisions, and the executive and organizational skills needed to implement decisions" (Tjeltveit & Gottlieb 2010, p. 99).

Research suggests that emotions, social, and cultural factors influence moral judgments and behaviors more than moral reasoning (Haidt 2007). Mental health professionals must constantly examine their behavior for these influencing factors.

SELF-ASSESSMENT EXERCISE 12.1

Time: 20 minutes
What steps can a professional working with children, adolescents, and young adults take to ensure that their practice with a vulnerable population is of the highest ethical standard?

The roots of ethical practice begin with recognizing that professionals have childhood, upbringing, family values, and adult personal and professional experiences that all influence their ethical values and behaviors. Regularly examining this either through self-reflection, supervision, or personal psychotherapy will assist in making conscious the values that could influence ethical behaviors in practice.

[Tjeltveit & Gottlieb (2010, pp. 99–100) note] '. . . because personal feelings, motivations, and values so powerfully shape the ethical lives of professionals, we must be cognizant of them. Vulnerability to ethical infractions increases when one's understanding of these basic processes is inadequate or deteriorates' (pp. 99–100).

All humans have biases and prejudices. For professionals working alongside children, adolescents, and young adults these biases are likely complicated by the vulnerability presented by a young population. This can be influenced by the developmental stage of the professional and the influence this stage has on personal issues, whether new in practice, young, parenting, or near retirement. The key to ethical practice is examining this, acknowledging the influences, but maintaining an ethical standard of care that is applied to all individuals.

SELF-ASSESSMENT EXERCISE 12.2

Time: 120–240 minutes
- Access your local or regional laws around confidentiality with adolescents and children, consent and assent for treatment.
- Review the policies and procedures in your agency of practice around consent, confidentiality, and dealing with psychiatric emergencies in a pediatric population.

CONCLUSION

Children, adolescents, and young adults present unique ethical challenges to the mental health professionals who provide their treatment regardless of geography and culture. While the goal of treatment is nearly always maintenance of or improvement of functioning, this needs to be provided within a professional ethical framework identified by the professional, supported by the care environment, and clear to the individual.

While ethical issues will always present themselves to professionals, the key is recognizing them and taking corrective action to ensure that there are no adverse events for individuals in care. This is especially important with individuals experiencing chronic mental health issues that potentially compromise development and make them more vulnerable. Maintaining an ethical practice requires lifelong diligence and attention to the process.

REFERENCES

Alderman, E. M. (2017) 'Confidentiality in pediatric and adolescent gynecology: when we can, when we can't, and when we're challenged'. *Pediatric Adolescent Gynecology*, 30, pp. 176–83.

American Academy of Child and Adolescent Psychiatry. (2014) 'Code of ethics'. Available at: www.aacap.org/App_Themes/AACAP/docs/about_us/transparency_portal/aacap_code_of_ethics_2012.pdf (Accessed: 17 October 2017).

Cuffe, S. P. (2010) 'Assessing adolescents', in *Dulcan's Textbook of Child and Adolescent Psychiatry*. Washington, DC: American Psychiatric Publishing, Inc.

Fields, A. J. (2010) 'Multicultural research and practice: theoretical issues and maximizing cultural exchange'. *Professional Psychological Research and Practice*, 41, pp. 196–201.

Haidt, J. (2007) 'The new synthesis in moral psychology'. *Science*, 216, pp. 998–1002.

Lynch, C. (2004) 'Psychotherapy for persons with mental retardation'. *Mental Retardation*, 22, pp. 170–5.

Matthews, E. (2016) 'Respect for personhood in medical and psychiatric ethics', *Ethics, Medicine and Public Health*, 2, pp. 490–8.

Mukolo, A., Heflinger, C. A. and Wallston, K. A. (2010) 'The stigma of childhood mental disorders: a conceptual framework'. *Journal of the American Academy of Child and Adolescent Psychiatry*, 49, pp. 92–103.

Pumariega, A. J., Rothe, E. and Rogers, K. (2009) 'Cultural competence in child psychiatric practice'. *Journal of the American Academy of Child & Adolescent Psychiatry*, 48, pp. 362–6.

Ramisch, J. L. and Franklin, D. (2008) 'Families with a member with mental retardation and the ethical implications of therapeutic treatment by marriage and family therapists'. *The American Journal of Family Therapy*, 36, pp. 312–22.

Rider, E. A., Kurtz, S., Slade, D., Esterbrook Longmaid, H., Ho, M-J., et al. (2014) 'The international charter for human values in healthcare: an interprofessional global collaboration to enhance values and communication in healthcare'. *Patient Education and Counseling*, 96, pp. 273–80.

Sousa, C. and Araujo, C. (2011) 'The ethical rights of children: yesterday and today'. *Pediatric Nursing*, 37, pp. 141–4.

Sori, C. F. and Hecker, L. L. (2006) 'Ethical and legal considerations when counseling children and families', in Sori, C. F. *Engaging Children in Family Therapy*. New York: Routledge, pp. 159–74.

Stewart, S. M., Simmons, A. and Habibpour, E. (2012) 'Treatment of culturally diverse children and adolescents with depression'. *Journal of Child and Adolescent Psychopharmacology*, 22, pp. 72–9.

Tjeltveit, A. C. and Gottlieb, M. C. (2010) 'Avoiding the road to ethical disaster: overcoming vulnerabilities and developing resilience'. *American Psychological Association*, 47, pp. 98–110.

United Nations International Children's Emergency Fund (UNICEF). (2008) *Third World Congress on Avoiding the Exploitation of Children and Adolescents*. Available at: www.unicef.org/protection/brazil_46520.html. (Accessed: 17 October 2017).

World Health Organization. (2013) *Women's and Children's Health: Evidence of Impact of Human Rights*. Available at: www.who.int/maternal_child_adolescent/documents/women_children_human_rights/en/ (Accessed: 17 October 2017)

To Learn More

Pelto-Piri, V., Lindvall, C. and Engstrom, I. (2016) 'Justifications for coercive care in child and adolescent psychiatry, a content analysis of medical documentation in Sweden'. *BMC Health Services Research*, 16, pp. 1–8.

Sandman, L., Granger, B. B., Ekman, I. and Munthe, C. (2011) 'Adherence, shared decision-making, and patient autonomy'. *Medical Health Care and Philosophy*, 15, pp. 115–27.

Smith, M. C., Turkel, M. C. and Wolf, Z. R. (2013) *Caring in Nursing Classics: An Essential Resource*. New York: Springer Publishing Company.

CHAPTER 13

Specific Needs of the Female Adult

Siân Bensa

INTRODUCTION

It might be asked "what has palliative care got to do with mental health difficulties"? Palliative care is a term usually associated with the physical health care of the terminally ill and dying. However, the principles of palliative care may translate well into the area of mental health, where people may be experiencing long term, subjectively disabling difficulties, which may or may not worsen over time, and that prevent people from living the lives they might ordinarily have hoped for.

In Western societies, there is an underlying expectation that health care services and health care professionals exist to 'cure' individuals of their 'ill-health'. As with many difficulties, people do not always make a full recovery, and often need to experience their difficulties as best they can. For those who do not make a full recovery, public and health care professionals may begin to feel frustrated and let down. This may lead to the overtreatment of people in an effort to get them better, and health care professionals may attempt various and multiple interventions whether these may or may not be wanted and or suitable. Medical models, particularly in physical health, have traditionally taken a paternalistic position, which may at times be helpful, but also asserts a position of authority, taking the 'expert' position and assuming they know what is right for people, weighing up the cost–benefits themselves. This could even lead to potentially harmful and punitive interventions when people are seen not to be responding adequately: people may be blamed for not recovering as they 'should', or labelled as being 'treatment resistant'. There is a case for a move away from focusing on cure to supporting people to live with the difficulties they experience.

The essential components of palliative care have been quoted as the 'effective control of symptoms and effective communication with patients, their families, and others involved in their care'. Rehabilitation, with the aim of maximising independence, is essential to providing good support.

> As a disease progresses, continuity of care becomes increasingly important—coordination between services is required, and information must be transferred promptly and efficiently between professionals in the community, in hospitals, and in hospices.
>
> (O'Neill & Fallon 1997, p. 801)

Although we might not wish to call mental health difficulties 'diseases', the principles of palliation may generalise when considering how to support people experiencing long-term mental health challenges. Palliative care ideas become very relevant and applicable when there is no cure as such, and instead offer 'symptom' management (*See* Chapter 9). In addition, a palliative care analogy may be helpful and more aligned with medically orientated thinking and contexts when considering how to support individuals with long-term difficulties.

The person-centred philosophy of palliative care is fundamentally based on compassion with the focus being on helping people and their families/supporters with difficulties as well as attempting to determine and meet the needs of the whole person (Cooper & Cooper 2014, p. 4). In some respects, palliative care parallels and overlaps many of the 'Recovery' principles in mental health (Repper & Perkins 2003) where the emphasis and focus of support has been directed more to the 'living with' instead of the 'eradication of' disabling and distressing mental health experiences. What follows is a discussion about gender differences in relation to mental health, gender and society and the role of trauma and trauma informed practice, to provide a case illustration of how such ideas might meet some of the specific needs of women. To exemplify how such principles might be operationalized within services, a brief psychological formulation of a woman experiencing emotional regulation difficulties is presented, and an outline of how services might intervene to support her to live with her difficulties derived from this formulation.

GENDER DIFFERENCES IN MENTAL HEALTH

Women make up just over half of the population in the UK, provide most of the care for others, and significantly contribute to the workforce. Hence, the effects of mental health difficulties on women are systemically important as they go beyond the impact on individuals, having wide reaching implications for the wellbeing of others (e.g. dependents and their attachments) and society as a whole. In order to develop mental health services that are responsive and effective to the needs of women, an understanding in relation to the specific nature and causes of mental health difficulties for women needs to be ascertained so that these can be used as a basis to inform holistic supportive care. Moreover, it is necessary to consider individuals' possible triggers and factors that may maintain difficulties in order to provide good and individualised care.

There are obvious and not so obvious sex and gender differences between men and women: sex can be thought of as relating to biological factors and differences such as reproduction systems and physical differences; gender can be thought of in terms of how people see themselves and how society views them in terms of social role and functioning, the latter being influenced by 'rules' and expectations derived from particular cultures and social norms (*See* Chapter 7). Research has demonstrated that because of sex and gender differences, both men and women may experience 'the same diseases at different rates or with different symptoms, or they may experience different kinds of illness altogether' (Brittle & Bird 2007, p. 2).

For example, anxiety, depression, and somatic complaints are more commonly diagnosed for women than men; substance use and anti-social personality disorder are more commonly diagnosed from men (World Health Organization – WHO 2017). However, substance use (See Chapter 17 – alcohol and other drugs) amongst women should not be ruled out as problems can occur pre-mental health problem, during mental health problem, as a consequence of a mental health problem and or post-mental health problem. For schizophrenia, men (*See* Chapter 14) have an earlier onset of symptoms than women and poorer premorbid psychosocial development and functioning (Piccinelli & Homen 1997). Some studies report that women experience a higher frequency of hallucinations or more positive psychotic symptoms than men (Lindamer et al. 1999). For bipolar disorder, women are more likely to develop the rapid cycling, exhibit more comorbidity (Leibenluft1997) and have a greater likelihood of being hospitalised during the manic phase of the disorder (Hendrick et al. 2000).

Surprisingly, the development and implementation of mental health services in the UK does not usually consider gender differences in relation to both probable causes and interventions, grouping evidence together to provide a service for people as a whole. However, biomedical models might propose that there are biological differences in relation to neurotransmitters, neuroanatomy and/or physiology (Ruigrok et al. 2014). Due to biological sex differences, there are some difficulties that only occur for women, which may be associated with social factors, for example, postpartum depression and psychosis. Why these develop is not clear, perhaps a mixture of biological and social factors: having a baby is physically stressful, involves hormonal changes, can lead to sleep deprivation and incorporates many positive and/or negative experiences. Seguin et al. (1995) reported that new mothers of low socioeconomic power had higher rates of postpartum depressive symptoms at two months postpartum compared with– women of high socioeconomic power, stating that this difference may be accounted for – to some degree – the limited social networks providing emotional support for low-income women.

Another issue affecting men and women differently is the possible side effects associated with taking pharmacological treatments for mental health difficulties. It has been reported that in general, women tend to have more side effects with psychotropic medication than men (Jacobson 2014). Women's monthly variations in sex hormones may alter the metabolism, distribution and elimination of drugs, which will affect response to treatment. In addition, women become pregnant, breastfeed, go through menopause, and may take hormone replacement therapy, which may all impact on the psychotropic medication used, dosage required and response. There is literature regarding teratology and perinatal mental health in regard to the use of taking psychotropic medication (McAllister-Williams et al. 2017). Hence, women need to be able to access specialist advice and consultation if they are thinking of having children or are pregnant.

Side effects from taking psychotropic medication can also have a profound negative effect on women's self-image. Seeman (2011, p. 142) for example, reported findings from a 'Pubmed' search that the use of antipsychotics amongst women can 'increase weight ... lead to dry mouth and bad breath, cataracts, hirsutism, acne, and voice changes; they may disturb symmetry of gait and heighten the risk for tics and spasms and incontinence, potentially undermining a person's attractiveness' (p. 142), which will potentially and significantly adversely affect women's self-esteem and social functioning. Women have also reported sexual dysfunction secondary to psychotropic medication (Michelson et al. 2000). Lethargy secondary to antidepressant use may mean that women struggle to maintain caring roles for others including their children, and this may even result in them having children removed. The psychological sequelae of these effects may add further to mental health difficulties. Thus, it is important for the professionals to understand how physiology varies over a woman's lifetime and how this may affect her response to psychotropic treatment, as well as the possible impact of side effects. An open discussion about the pros and cons, and the choice to change her mind, is required. Shared decision making is advocated. This is an approach through which providers and individuals of health care services are informed and collaborate openly and explicitly to determine the best course of treatment and support. Not only may this approach increase individuals' knowledge and awareness of the interventions they are in receipt of, this may also increase their sense of power and choice within the system (Substance Abuse and Mental Health Services Administration – SAMHSA 2017). This might even mean that they are more likely to undergo and continue treatments, especially if they perceive they have been informed and been given a choice in it (e.g. adequately provided informed consent (*See* Chapter 8) as opposed to not being informed sufficiently or even coerced, potentially evoking control and powerless feelings.

GENDER AND SOCIETY

Gender is consistently reported as a critical factor of mental health difficulties and determines the differential power and control men and women have, their social position, status and treatment within society. A key to developing female specific services is therefore to gain an understanding and acknowledgement of the effects that living as a female in a male-based society might have.

Feminist psychological theories propose a difference in the development of relationships between genders. Miller (1992), discusses how a woman is concerned with developing connections with others and her 'sense of self becomes organized around being able to make affiliations and relationships' (p. 83).

It is proposed that threats to disruptions of connections are seen as losses of relationships but also as something intrinsic, such as a loss of herself. Services that emphasize women's needs for high-quality relationships and being connected, rather than seeing this as a weakness that may benefit women's well-being. Feminist psychology also suggests that traditional theories that emphasize the primacy of separation and independence from others as indicators of health and maturity, downplay the positive aspects of mutuality and sensitivity to others, and the ability for women to experience, comprehend and respond to the inner state of another person, which is highly complex and an ego strength (Walker, Kaplan & Surrey 1984). In relation to this, the 'buffer hypothesis' (Cohen & Wills 1985), which theorises that social support or supportive social networks may mediate mental health by buffering the negative effect of stress on a person's mental well-being, may demonstrate the significance of maintaining social relationships, especially for women. It has been suggested that mental health outcomes for developing countries are at least as good and probably better compared to the West (Bentall 2003; WHO 1979), whereby social networks may be more robust. Hence, the development, maintenance and reciprocity of social relationships with others and social support are perhaps critical for women to sustain healthy psychological well-being, something that should perhaps be considered when thinking about female specific needs.

Similarly, the Relational–Cultural Theory (Jordan et al. 1991) proposes that a primary motivation for women throughout life is the desire for a strong sense of connection with others: females develop a sense of self and self-worth when their actions develop from and feed into connections with others. Hence, connectedness and disconnections determine the degree of mental health well-being experienced. For women, changes in social relationships and support therefore, may significantly impact on mental health.

Social-constructionist ideas suggest that an individual's understanding of themselves and the world is influenced by personal experiences, which people have encountered during their life, affected by social, cultural, economic, biological and genetic factors.

Studies suggest that the number of people experiencing mental health difficulties at a certain point in time does not differ between women and men, however gender leads to a difference in susceptibility to mental health difficulties as well as mental health outcomes. Anxiety, depression, emotionally unstable personality disorder and eating disorders are all more commonly diagnosed or reported for women, whereas substance use and anti-social personality disorders are more commonly diagnosed or seen amongst men (Kessler et al. 1994; Kessler 2003). Socioeconomic position, associated with poverty and low income, has been consistently demonstrated to be related to the risk of anxiety and depressive disorders among women (Mazure, Keita & Blehar 2002).

GENDER, TRAUMA AND MENTAL HEALTH

A major difference between genders is the extent to which men and women experience adversities, which lead to distress and mental health difficulties. Research has consistently demonstrated that traumatic events are more frequently experienced by people in low socioeconomic groups and from minority ethnic communities (Hatch & Dohrenwend 2007). Moreover, it has been reported that between 13 per cent and 25 per cent of women in general have been found to have experienced sexual assault sometime in their lives compared to 0.6–7.2 per cent of men (Kilpatrick, Edmunds, & Seymour 1992).

Trauma refers to events or circumstances that are experienced as harmful or life-threatening and that have lasting impacts on mental, physical, emotional and/or social well-being (SAMHSA 2017) and can include sexual abuse, physical abuse, severe neglect, loss, threat, domestic violence, and/or the witnessing of violence, terrorism or disasters. It could be conceptualised that any mental health difficulty or 'symptom' is a person's coping response to distress of some kind. With this in mind, the approach to support individuals experiencing difficulties should be aimed at supporting people to help them cope better.

The Adverse Childhood Experiences (ACE) longitudinal study investigated the association between childhood trauma and adult health in over 17,000 people. Results revealed that the more adverse life events people experience prior to the age of 18, the greater the impact on health and well-being over the lifespan, including poor mental health (Anda et al. 2010). Evidence is increasingly growing and supporting the notion that trauma may predispose individuals to the development of mental health difficulties (Bentall et al. 2014; Varese, Smeets & Drakker 2012); borderline and antisocial personality disorder, eating, affective and sexual disorders, and substance misuse difficulties (van der Kolk 2005). The Mental Health Foundation Report (2016) states that women with mental health difficulties are more likely to have been exposed to domestic violence and poverty (McManus, Scott, & Sosenko 2016) as well as sexual abuse (Roberts et al. 2014). Dillon, Johnstone & Longden (2012), reported evidence for a dose-dependent relationship between the severity, frequency and range of adverse traumatic experiences and the future impact on mental health. Abuse in childhood is also more likely to affect the degree of difficulties individuals experience. For example, people who have experienced sexual or physical abuse in childhood who use mental health services typically have longer and more frequent admissions to hospital, are prescribed more medication, are more likely to self-harm, and are more likely to attempt to kill themselves than people without experiences of childhood abuse (Read et al. 2005).

Although it still remains unclear as to exactly why this might be, contemporary neuroscience theories propose that trauma may predispose individuals to mental health difficulties as it may impact on the structure and function of the developing brain (Perry 2000). This has led to the development of a trauma-genic neurodevelopmental model to possibly explain and account for the link between childhood adversity and adult psychosis (Read et al. 2001). Disruptions in neural connectivity and integration development (Nelson 2011) and the neurological damage caused by distress and trauma suggests that people who have experienced trauma could even be 'primed' to respond to current situations that replicate the experience of loss of power, choice, control and safety in ways that may appear extreme, or even abnormal. This may be demonstrated by behaviours people experiencing emotional dysregulation difficulties perform, for example, self-injury in people diagnosed with emotionally unstable personality disorder, something which is much more commonly diagnosed in women than men. If trauma may account for some of the mental health problems experienced by females, then a trauma informed approach might be helpful when working with women.

Female-specific services need to recognise the significance of the social context and possible psychological neglect and abuse women have encountered. Without this recognition, mental health services will struggle to adequately meet the needs of women. The report 'Women and Girls at risk: evidence across the life course (McNeish & Scott 2014) summarises the vast range of abuse faced by many women over their lifetimes and how women entering services are often viewed through a lens of what is wrong with them rather than through the lens of what has happened to them (Dillon, Johnstone & Longden 2012). For mental health services, this requires services to promote safety, respect and take the complexity of women's lives seriously, and to be provided in a

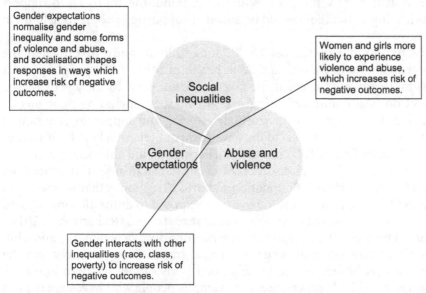

Figure 13.1 Social context, which increases risk to women and girls

Source: McNneish & Scott 2014

holistic, integrated and seamless manner. However, this may be difficult to achieve due to the multiple agencies often involved and the many systems operating, each with different priorities and cultures. Figure 13.1 below demonstrates how services to support the mental health needs of women need to be coordinated and interconnected, with consideration of the social context in which difficulties arise.

TRAUMA INFORMED APPROACHES

Trauma informed approaches in the delivery of mental health services are rapidly growing, evidence-based frameworks, based on understanding, recognising and responding to the effects of all types of events and trauma that people within services may have experienced (Harris & Fallot 2001). The rationale for this approach is the issue around the huge number of upsetting events, trauma and/or abuse that people with significant difficulties have undergone. An article by Sweeney et al. (2016) provides a detailed overview of how services might become more trauma informed. It emphasises the physical, psychological and emotional safety for both providers and individuals with the aim of rebuilding a sense of control and empowerment for the individual (Hopper, Bassuk & Olivet 2010). A trauma-informed service requires an understanding of trauma and an awareness of the impact it can have across settings, services and populations, attempting to adopt a broader view of people and their environments, including an understanding of the role and impact of neurological damage, thus adhering to the principles of using a holistic, whole system approach to support individuals (Paterson et al. 2013). It involves attending to, anticipating and avoiding institutional processes and individual practices that may be likely to re-traumatise individuals who already have experienced trauma. It advocates the importance of person-centred participation in the development, delivery and evaluation of services, for example collaboration and shared decision making. In 2014, SAMHSA convened a group of 'experts' who identified three key elements to providing a trauma-informed approach:

1. realizing the prevalence of trauma
2. recognizing how trauma affects all individuals involved with the program, organization, or system, including its own workforce
3. responding by putting this knowledge into practice.

(Center for Substance Abuse Treatment 2014)

It is suggested that mental health professionals should come from the position that people using services have probably experienced some kind of distress and trauma in their lives. This would encourage staff to consider that individuals may find it difficult to develop trusting relationships and feel safe within services and with professionals hence, the service needs to provide and organise support and interventions that promote relational and emotional safety. National Institute for Mental Health (NIMHE – 2008), recommends asking all individuals about abuse routinely. Read, Hammersley, and Rudegeair (2007) propose that all are asked at the initial assessment (or if in crisis, as soon as person is settled), in the context of a general psychosocial history, prefaced with brief normalising statements, use of specific questions and with clear examples of what you are asking about (p. 105). Despite clinical guidance on the role of mental health professionals to enquire and identify abuse and responding appropriately, poor identification continues and can lead individuals to have poor engagement with services and poor response to treatment. There needs to be a shift in thinking: instead of the professional asking individuals, "what is wrong with you", this approach needs to change so people can be asked "what has happened to you". Dillon, Johnstone and Longden (2012) and others such as the Hearing Voices Network (2017) in the UK advocate this perspective and approach to working alongside people experiencing mental health difficulties to develop a Power Threat Meaning Framework (Johnstone 2016) to help understand how power and threat may be impacting on the individual.

Relational and emotional safety is vitally important in providing mental health services for women as services may inadvertently re-traumatise individuals who they are supposed to be supporting. Re-traumatisation occurs when a person experiences something in the present that is reminiscent of a past traumatic event. The current event may evoke a similar emotional and physiological response associated with the original event. Mental health systems inadvertently can re-traumatise individuals within services through operating principles of coercion and control (Bloom & Farragher 2010). For example, acts such as restraining a person who has been sexually abused as a child, pressuring people to take medications or withholding leave, may mimic previous experiences of feeling powerlessness and controlled. Freuh et al. (2005) reported that such practices may be widespread within inpatient settings. The National Institute for Mental Health (NIMHE 2008) outlines how services might incidentally re-exert power and control over women in acute inpatient services (p. 17). For example, services might tolerate low level sexual harassment; hand out sanitary wear items rather than making them available; not seek permission before entering a woman's bedroom, sitting on the edge of her bed; conduct one to one observations by male members of staff; not appreciating individual differences in maintaining interpersonal physical and psychological boundaries; and use language to 'put women down' happens in services as well as the wider society. Collaboratively undertaking safety plans and relapse plans may help to identify specific triggers that often relate to prior upsetting experiences, and providing debriefs with individuals after they have been restrained or secluded to explore what happened and what could be done by the individual and professional to prevent a re-occurrence has been shown to be useful (LeBel, Huckshorn & Caldwell 2010). Re-traumatising may have consequences for effectiveness of support: research into treatment effectiveness has consistently shown that it is the quality of relationships between people who use services and health professionals, which is the main predictor of outcomes (Berry, Barrowclough & Wearden 2011; Hovarth & Bedi 2002; Meier, Barrowclough & Donmall 2005). If services do not take the impact of trauma into account, they may re-traumatise and possibly worsen an individual's mental health, and cause people harm as a consequence. Ultimately this will lead to increased expenditure.

Power struggles and issues of blame can start when a service identifies a woman as engaging in 'difficult' or socially unacceptable behaviour (e.g. impulsivity, promiscuity, excessive food intake and self-injury). People can be said to be "attention seeking, manipulative and time wasters" (personal experience). However, the function of such challenging behaviours needs to be understood. These behaviours might be because of needs not being met, poor attachment, poor boundaries, unhelpful ways of communicating and/or coping with distress etc. Attempts from health care professionals to prevent women from using their own coping strategies, be they maladaptive or not, might result in power struggles that may contribute to individuals' distress and psychological pain. A trauma-informed care approach advocates for people to undergo a trauma assessment involving a collaborative development of crisis/safety plans, increased understanding of the importance of environmental changes toward 'reducing triggers', and assisting people to manage emotions in less harmful and risky ways.

Service provision might be best founded upon relational aspects, considering the role of attachment, abuse and trauma. Parry-Crooke and Stafford (2009) outline key characteristics of an ideal women's service (see Box 13.1 below), drawing on women's needs to connect to others.

BOX 13.1 Key Characteristics of an ideal women's service (Parry-Crooke & Stafford 2009)

- Relational security: therapeutic relationship with staff
- Trust and positive expectations of self and others
- Empowerment and reduction in social isolation
- Meaningful days and daily staff support
- Holistic approach: person-centred
- Offering a range of interventions to meet emotional needs

So how might we operationalise palliative care approaches for women with ongoing mental health difficulties founded on the discussions above? Below is an example of how psychological formulation may be used as a basis upon which concepts outlined above might be drawn together to provide services for a woman in inpatient services experiencing emotion regulation difficulties.

A FORMULATION APPROACH

In line with principles of palliative care, mental health services could adopt formulation driven support plans to inform interventions for individuals, incorporating a bio-psychosocial approach and increasing the awareness of people's experiences and possible trauma, to facilitate a compassionate understanding for planning possible interventions for people to help them cope with their distress. Formulation can be done with individuals but also with professional teams (Bensa & Aitchison 2015).

Formulation with individuals is the process of making sense of someone's difficulties in the context of their relationships, social circumstances, life events. It is a personal narrative or account of how they make sense of their difficulties. Information and perspectives from health care professionals, family members (*See* Chapter 16), and friends can also help in the development of a person's formulation and a person's formulation can be re-formulated as 'new information' arises. Team formulation is described as 'the process of facilitating a group or team of professionals to construct a shared understanding of a service user's difficulties' (Johnstone 2014, p. 216) and a number of national policies have recommended the use of team formulation (e.g. Clinical Psychology Leadership Framework, Skinner & Toogood 2010; Health and Care Professions Council's Standards of Proficiency for Practitioner Psychologists 2010). Even when people's difficulties can seem complex and even perplexing at times, as Butler (1998) states, 'at some level it all makes sense (p. 2).

In a sample of professionals working in mental health rehabilitation, Berry, Barrowclough and Wearden (2009), reported many benefits to generating formulations within teams, which could enhance empathy and compassion for individuals within the service. They reported an increase in the degree of effort they felt individuals were making in coping, reductions in blame, more optimism about treatment and more positive feelings. If health professionals are more aware of the personal histories, difficulties, triggers and possible maintenance factors, then they may be able to offer individually focused support and interventions, be more compassionate and empathetic and hopefully reduce the chances of the service potentially and inadvertently re-traumatising people they are supposed to be supporting.

Additionally, a formulation approach may work particularly well for women due to the emphasis on meaning of experiences, as there has been a suggestion that there are gender differences in men and women's recovery processes. A qualitative study by Schön (2010), reported that female gender norms seemed to have an advantage over men's in regard to how they regain a positive sense of themselves and develop new meanings compared to males; women were focused more on meaning making, while men focused

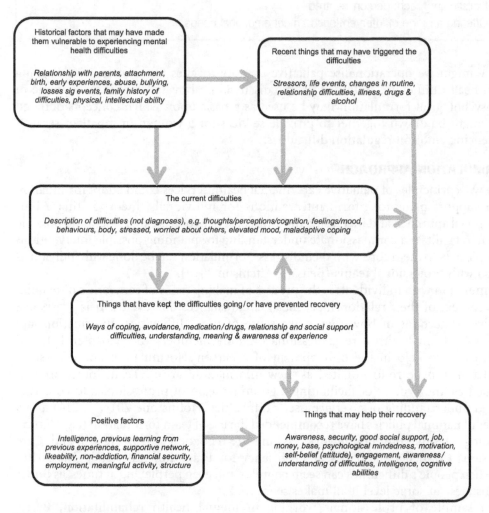

Figure 13.2 5Ps Formulation

Source: Modified from Dudley & Kuyken 2014

more on control over their experiences and the reinforcements of traditional gender roles such as occupation and independence, despite structural or societal inequalities.

There are many ways of developing formulations based on various psychological models. A cognitive behavioural approach may base the development of understanding someone's difficulties using a '5Ps model' (Dudley & Kuyken 2014; *See* Figure 13.2). Formulation involves exploring people's histories (including attachments and trauma backgrounds) to help them and staff understand the context of difficulties and this might help keep the trauma experience at the forefront of the professionals' mind when working alongside the individual. It may help the health professional understand behaviours and presentations when they happen. In this way, when a person gets verbally aggressive or harms him or herself, the behaviour does not become the focus, but the possible reasons that underlie the behaviour. Thus, services and individuals can consider together what might be going on for the person and attempt strategies that might help, thereby facilitating people to live and function more safely and hopefully experience less disruption in their and other people's lives.

Case Study 13.1

To demonstrate how formulation may help support palliative care approaches, a brief case study (13.1) is outlined below. The case study is fictitious, but may reflect fairly accurately a woman in receipt of support from secondary care mental health services in the UK.

Susan is 25 years old. She was admitted to an adult inpatient female acute mental health unit six months ago following an attempt to take her life in the community by ligaturing. She had been experiencing extreme mood swings, and was finding the "frustration" intolerable. She had felt these things this since she was about 14 and had become very hopeless that she could recover, and was low in mood. She has had three previous inpatient admissions, the longest lasting four months. When distressed she hears the voice of a man telling her to "kill your- [her-] self" and criticising her. Her suicide attempt was in response to wanting the "frustration" to end. The psychiatric diagnosis is likely to be 'emotionally unstable personality disorder' with 'psychosis', which could be considered to mean she is experiencing long-term mental health difficulties. An individual formulation with Susan could look something like this:

> You had an unhappy childhood and that your father physically abused you and your younger brother. You think, although are not certain, that your father sexually abused you from around the age of three until you were about eight years old. You were very close to your brother and used to "take the beatings" for him, but sometimes you could not protect him, and he would get hit anyway. As a child, you also witnessed physical violence towards your mother. Your father left the home suddenly when you were eight and you have not seen him since. You attended school, had one close friend and worked hard, achieving good grades. When you were about 14 you were really unhappy and tried to end your life. Following this you told your mother about the abuse, but she did not believe you and threatened you not to tell anyone. Your mother re-married

continued . . .

and when your stepfather started to abuse you, you did not feel able to confide in anyone or risk the breakup of the marriage. You left home as soon as you could age 16, and got a job in a business and the boss let you a room. However, you found it increasingly hard to deal with your boss, who was controlling and bullying in ways that reminded you of father and step-father. However, you had nowhere to go. One day you started to hear a male voice telling you to kill yourself and that you were no good to anyone. This seemed to relate to how the abuse made you feel, and it also reminded you of things that your father and stepfather said to you. You found day-to-day life increasingly difficult, as past events caught up with you and many feelings came to the surface, such as the overwhelming sense of frustration and low mood, accompanied by the male voice. At times you found it difficult to recall days and have been aggressive towards others when you have felt threatened. Despite this, you have many strengths, including intelligence, determination and self-awareness, care for others, and you have a desire to live although this can diminish when feeling overwhelmed and low in mood. You have been on the ward, which you find controlling, noisy and sometimes frightening. At times you have tried to end your life by ligaturing and at other times you are keen to keep yourself safe and look to the future. You have plans to be a nursery worker. Your mother visits once a month and you have a friend that you text regularly. She wants you to go on holiday with her next year.

FORMULATION DRIVEN INTERVENTIONS

The following is an example of possible evidence-based interventions, which may be helpful to support Susan in line with palliative care principles, based on the formulation. This list is not exhaustive.

Develop Meaning

➤ The formulation should identify her current difficulties, specific triggers and personal background, which may indicate predispositions associated with her life experiences and highlight strengths and resources, and possible maintenance factors (e.g. a 5Ps formulation *See* Figure 13.2)
➤ The assessment needs to include asking about her trauma, as shame factors that may inhibit conversation
➤ The formulation should be shared with the team(s) supporting Susan
➤ Undertake collaborative development of a working biopsychosocial formulation to develop shared understanding of difficulties to inform agreed support plans and re-formulate with 'new' information.

Ward Culture

➤ Consider relational safety and team working to provide an environment that adopts trauma informed care principles
➤ Instil trauma informed approaches into the culture of ward and individual needs

➤ Provide reflective groups when team are struggling with behaviours which are stressful and anxiety provoking (e.g. ligaturing, aggression), maintaining least restrictive approaches and keep in mind the longer-term view

➤ Ensure professionals have good awareness of possible triggers, such as shouting, aggression on the ward

➤ Hold formulation meetings with the team to develop shared knowledge, under-standing, awareness of issues.

Support from Staff

➤ Provide consistent and reliable support to health professionals, and adopt a validating stance. If something is agreed, try and ensure it happens

➤ Avoid letting Susan down, which might evoke invalidation

➤ Develop therapeutic relationship that is trusting and non-rejecting

➤ Undertake twice weekly one-to-one session

➤ Provide psychoeducation around emotion regulation, consider chain analysis of self-injury behaviours, problem-solving strategies

➤ Validate distress but be mindful not to over soothe or be too restrictive (Hamilton 2010)

➤ Avoid employing boundaries that might be seen as punitive

➤ Clear collaborative care plan development and updates.

Risks to Susan of Suicide

➤ Collaborative and explicit risk management arrangements with Susan, to validate the distress she experiences and concerns for welfare, discuss with her that the team does not want her to die

➤ Consider ways she may attempt to end her life (e.g. ligature); understand times when risky behaviours occur (e.g. associated with times of the day, night time when abuse happened, when staff are busy)

➤ Appropriate level of observation, observation by female staff where possible, least restrictive and least invasive to minimise possible feelings of control, maintain personal dignity (e.g. when attending to hygiene needs).

Safety Plans

➤ Develop safety plans collaboratively with Susan to encourage shared understanding of possible triggers, internal (mood state shift, hormonal cycle, voice experience) and external (changes on the ward, interpersonal relationships); what she can do to help; what the health professional can do to support

➤ Share details of safety plan with team

➤ Give responsibility and power to Susan, to help keep herself safe (e.g. minimise power and control perceptions), consider appropriate removal of items at specific times, positive risk taking so Susan may learn that she is able to keep herself safe (e.g. cords from clothing, shoelaces)

Mood

➤ Assessment and monitoring using formal rating scale to allow clinical discussion of risk (e.g. Columbia Severity Rating Scale; Posner et al. 2011) and informal measures, such as observation

➤ Support Susan to achieve her basic care needs, sleep, dietary factors, hygiene, structure and routine

➤ Offer and support Susan with medications for low mood

➤ Support behavioural activation on the ward, and strategies to enhance mood

➤ Chart progress to demonstrate changes and consider reasons for change with Susan. Specialist psychological assessment for personality disorder (International Personality Disorder Examination – IDE; Loranger et al. 1994) and dissociation (Structured Clinical Interview for DSM-IV Dissociative Disorders – SCID-D; First et al. 1997) to identify specific needs, and inform decisions about most appropriate post discharge support (e.g. Structured Clinical Management *See* www.annafreud.org/media/3020/scm-brochure.pdf).

Psychologically Informed Interventions

➤ Develop collaborative formulation, psychoeducation about emotional dysregulation, ABC chain analysis (Linehan 2015)

➤ Voice diaries to develop awareness of any possible relationship between mood, voice and activity, which might enhance understanding and a sense of control

➤ Therapeutic interventions, such as distress tolerance, anxiety management, compassion focused interventions, mindfulness

➤ Relapse prevention work.

Social Needs, Family and Support

➤ Include family (mother and brother) in support, so Susan does not feel alone and abandoned (as she wishes)

➤ Develop opportunities for social interaction and relationship building

➤ Develop collaborative and explicit plans for safe leave from ward (escorted/unescorted)

➤ Develop plans for the future based on Susan's interests and strengths (e.g. vocational, educational)

➤ Consider potential side effects of psychotropic medication on social functioning and self-esteem, monitor and discuss with Susan

➤ Use goal setting (based on SMART – specific, measurable, attainable, relevant, timed – principles – *See* www.projectsmart.co.uk/smart-goals.php)

➤ Engage with third sector organisations to support vocational and education needs to achieve goals

➤ Ensure strengths and personal resources highlighted.

Social role and function

➤ Promote independence and self-management of difficulties

➤ Support goals identified that might lead to employment

➤ Support to find suitable accommodation

➤ Support goals that allow enjoyment and closeness and proximity to others.

CONCLUSIONS

Palliative care approaches for people experiencing mental health difficulties advocate for a compassionate, individualised and whole systems approach to supporting people with long-standing and complex experiences. There are differences between men and women's mental health in regard to type of problems: women are more likely to be diagnosed with anxiety, depression, somatic complaints and emotional dysregulation difficulties than men. The possible causes of mental health difficulties may differ also: women are more likely to be socially disadvantaged and have experienced some kind of abuse and neglect compared to men. The cause of their problems should ideally influence and inform the type of support services should provide, taking account of specific gender issues and medication, individual stories and making meaning of their difficulties. Formulation driven interventions are advocated in order to promote more individualised, holistic and biopsychosocial interventions, which might enhance empathy and understanding amongst health professionals, making services more compassionate and hopefully effective, in order to meet the specific needs of women.

REFERENCES

Anda, R. F., Butchart, A., Felitti, V. J. and Brown, D. W. (2010) 'Building a framework for global surveillance of the public health: implications of adverse childhood experiences'. *Preventive Medicine*, 39, pp. 93–8.

Bensa, S. and Aitchison, R. (2015) 'An evaluation of inpatient staff perceptions of psychological formulation meetings'. *Clinical Psychology Forum*, 287, pp. 33–8.

Bentall, R. P. (2003) *Madness Explained: Psychosis and Human Nature.* London: Penguin Books Ltd.

Bentall, R., de Sousa, P., Varese, F., Wickham, S., Sitko, K., et al. (2014) 'From adversity to psychosis: pathways and mechanisms from specific adversities to specific symptoms', *Social Psychiatry and Psychiatric Epidemiology*, 49, pp. 1011–22.

Berry, K., Barrowclough, C. and Wearden, A. (2009) 'A pilot study investigating the use of psychological formulations to modify psychiatric staff perceptions of service users with psychosis'. *Behavioural and Cognitive Psychotherapy*, 37, p. 39.

Bloom, S. and Farragher, B. (2010) *Destroying Sanctuary: The Crisis in Human Service Delivery Systems.* Oxford University Press, New York: NY.

Brittle, C. and Bird, C. E. (2007) *Literature review on effective sex- and gender-based systems/models of care.* Rockville, MD: Office on Women's Health, U.S. Department of Health and Human Services: LLC. Available at: https://permanent.access.gpo.gov/lps100484/www.4woman.gov/owh/multidisci plinary/reports/GenderBasedMedicine/FinalOWHReport.pdf (Accessed: 23 October 2017)

Butler, G. (1998) 'Clinical formulation', in Bellack, A. S. and Hersen, M. (eds), *Comprehensive Clinical Psychology.* Oxford: Pergamon.

Center for Substance Abuse Treatment (US) (2014) 'Trauma-Informed Care: A Sociocultural Perspective', in Trauma-Informed Care in Behavioral Health Services. Rockville (MD): Substance Abuse and Mental Health Services Administration (US). Available from: www.ncbi.nlm.nih.gov/ books/NBK207195/ (Accessed: 24 October 2017)

Cohen, S. and Wills, T. A. (1985) 'Stress, social support, and the buffering hypothesis', *Psychological Bulletin*, 98, pp. 310–57.

Cooper, D. and Cooper, J. (2014). 'Palliative care within mental health: the need', in Cooper, D. and Cooper, J. (eds) *Palliative Care Within Mental Health: Care and Practice*, London: CRC Press.

Dillon, J., Johnstone, L. and Longden, E. (2012) 'Trauma, dissociation, attachment & neuroscience: a new paradigm for understanding severe mental distress'. *Journal of Critical Psychology, Counselling and Psychotherapy*, 12, pp. 145–55.

Dudley, R. and Kuyken, W. (2014) 'Case formulation in cognitive behavioural therapy', in Johnstone, L. and Dallos, R. (eds) *Formulation in Psychology and Psychotherapy; Making Sense of People's Problems.* (2nd edition.) Hove: Routledge, pp. 18–44.

First, M. B., Spitzer, R. L., Gibbon, M. and Williams, J. B. W. (1997) *Structured Clinical Interview for DSM-IV Personality Disorders, (SCID-II).* Washington, DC: American Psychiatric Press, Inc.

Freuh, C., Knapp, R., Cusack, K., Grubaugh, A., Sauvageot, J., et al. (2005) 'Patients' reports of traumatic or harmful experiences within the psychiatric setting'. *Psychiatric Services*, 56, pp. 1123–33.

Hamilton, L. (2010) 'Boundary seesaw model: good fences make for good neighbours', in Tennant, A. and Howells, K. (eds) *Using Time, Not Doing Time: Practitioner Perspectives on Personality Disorder & Risk*. Chichester: Wiley-Blackwell, pp. 181–94.

Harris, M. and Fallot, R. (2001) *Using Trauma Theory to Design Service Systems. New Directions for Mental Health Services*. San Francisco, CA: Jossey-Bass.

Hatch, S. and Dohrenwend, B. (2007) 'Distribution of traumatic and other stressful life events by race/ethnicity, gender, SES and age: a review of the research'. *American Journal of Community Psychology*, 40, pp. 313–32.

Health and care professions Council. (2010) *Standards of proficiency: practitioner psychologist*. Available at: www.hcpc-uk.co.uk/assets/documents/10002963SOP_Practitioner_psychologists.pdf (Accessed: 29 October 2017)

Hearing Voices Network. (2017) *The Hearing Voices Movement: Beyond Critiquing the Status Quo*. Available at: www.hearing-voices.org/news/the-hearing-voices-movement/ (Accessed: 23 October 2017).

PubMed www.ncbi.nlm.nih.gov/pubmed/

Google Scholar https://scholar.google.co.uk

Hendrick, V., Altshuler, L. L., Gitlin, M. J., Delrahim, S. and Hammen, C. (2000) 'Gender and bipolar illness'. *Journal of Clinical Psychiatry*, 61, pp. 393–6.

Hopper, E. K., Bassuk, E. and Olivet, J. (2010) 'Shelter from the storm: trauma-informed care in homelessness services setting'. *The Open Health Services and Policy Journal*, 2, pp. 131–51.

Horvath, A. O. and Bedi, R. P. (2002) 'The alliance', in Norcross, J. C. (ed.) *Psychotherapy Relationships That Work: Therapist Contributions and Responsiveness to Patients*. New York: Oxford University Press, pp. 37–70.

Jacobson, R. (2014) 'Psychotropic drugs affect men and women differently: prescription painkillers, antidepressants and other brain drugs have gender-specific effects'. *Scientific American Mind*. Available at: www.scientificamerican.com/article/psychotropic-drugs-affect-men-and-women-differently (Accessed: 21 October 2017)

Johnstone, L. (2014) 'Using formulation in teams', in Johnstone, L. and Dallos, R. (eds.) *Formulation in Psychology and Psychotherapy; Making Sense of People's Problems* (2nd edition). Hove: Routledge, pp. 216–42.

Johnstone, L. (2016) *Formulation Across Cultures – Can There Be Such A Thing? 'Minorities Group'*. Available at: www.bps.org.uk/system/files/user-files/Division%20of%Clinical%20psychology/public/Minorities%20conference%20July%202016%Lucy.pdf (Accessed: 23 October 2017)

Jordan, J. V., Kaplan, A. G., Miller, J. B., Stiver, I. P. and Surrey, J. L. (1991) *Women's Growth in Connection: Writings from the Stone Center*. New York: Guilford Press.

Kessler, R. (2003) 'Epidemiology of women and depression'. *Journal of Affective Disorders*, 74, pp. 5–13.

Kessler, R. C., McGonagle, K. A., Zhao, S., Nelson, C. B., Hughes, M., et al. (1994) 'Lifetime and 12-month prevalence of DSM-111-R psychiatric disorders in the United States'. *Archives of General Psychiatry*, 51, pp. 8–19.

Kilpatrick, D. G., Edmunds, C. and Seymour, A. (1992) *Rape in America: A Report to the Nation*. Washington, DC: National Victim Center.

LeBel, J., Huckshorn, K. A. and Caldwell, B. (2010) 'Restraint use in residential programs: Why are best practices ignored'. *Child Welfare*, 89, pp. 169–87.

Leibenluft, E. (1997) 'Women with bipolar illness: clinical and research issues', *American Journal of Psychiatry*, 153, pp. 163–73.

Lindamer, L. A., Lohr, J. B., Harris, M. J. and Jeste, D. V. (1999) 'Gender-related clinical differences in older patients with schizophrenia'. *Journal of Clinical Psychiatry*, 60, pp. 61–7.

Linehan, M. M. (2015) *DBT Skills Training: Manual*. (2nd edition). Guilford Press: New York.

Loranger, A. W., Sartorius, N. A., Andreoli, A., Berger, P., Buchheim, P., et al. (1994) 'The International Personality Disorder Examination (IPDE): The World Health Organisation/alcohol, drug abuse, and mental health administration international pilot study of personality disorders'. *Archives of General Psychiatry*, 51, pp. 215–24.

Mazure, C., Keita, G. and Blehar, M. (2002) *Summit on Women and Depression: Proceedings and Recommendations*. Washington, DC: American Psychological Association.

McAllister-Williams, R. H., Baldwin, D. S., Cantwell, R., Easter, A., Gilvarry, E., et al. (2017) 'British Association for Psychopharmacology consensus guidance on the use of psychotropic medication preconception, in pregnancy and postpartum', *Journal of Psychopharmacology*, pp. 1–34. Available at: www.bap.org.uk/pdfs/BAP_Guidelines-Perinatal.pdf. (Accessed: 21 October 2017)

McManus, S., Scott, S. and Sosenko, F. (2016) *Joining the dots: The combined burden of violence, abuse and poverty in the lives of women*. Agenda. Available at: https://weareagenda.org/policy-research/agendas-reports (Accessed: 21 October 2017)

McNeish, D. and Scott, S. (2014) *Women and Girls at Risk: Evidence Across the Life Course*, Lankelly Chase. Available at http://lankellychase.org.uk/wp-content/uploads/2015/12/Women-Girls-at-Risk-Evidence-Review-040814.pdf (Accessed: 23 October 2017)

Mental Health Foundation (2016) *Fundamental Facts about Mental Health*. www.mentalhealth.org.uk/publications/fundamental-facts-about-mental-health-2016 (Accessed: 21 October 2017)

Meier, P. S., Barrowclough, C. and Donmall, M. C. (2005) 'The role of the therapeutic alliance in the treatment of substance misuse: A critical review of the literature'. *Addiction*, 100, pp. 304–16.

Michelson, J., Bancroft, S., Targum, S., Yongman, K. and Tepner, R. (2000) 'Female sexual dysfunction associated with antidepressant administration: a randomized, placebo-controlled study of pharmacologic intervention'. *American Journal of Psychiatry*, 157, pp. 239–43.

Miller, J. B. (1992) *Toward a New Psychology of Women*. 2nd edition. Boston: Beacon Press.

Nelson, C. (2011) 'Neural development and lifelong plasticity', in Keating, D. (ed.) *Nature and Nurture in Early Child Development*. New York, Cambridge: Cambridge University Press, pp. 45–69.

National Institute for Mental Health. (2008) *Informed Gender Practice Mental Health Acute Care that Works for Women*. Available at: http://webarchive.nationalarchives.gov.uk/20110512085546/www.nmhdu.org.uk/silo/files/informedgenderpractice.pdf (Accessed: 21 October 2017).

O'Neill, B. and Fallon, M. (1997) 'ABC of palliative care: principles of palliative care and pain control', *British Medical Journal*, 315, pp. 801–4.

Parry-Crooke, G. and Stafford, P. (2009) '*My Life: In Safe Hands? Summary Report of an Evaluation of Women's Medium Secure Services*', London Metropolitan University. Available at: http://archive.londonmet.ac.uk/dass-research/metranet.londonmet.ac.uk/londonmet/fms/MRSite/acad/dass/CSER/Summary%20report%20of%20an%20evaluation%20of%20women%27s%20medium%20secure%20services%202009.pdf (Accessed: 21 October 2017)

Paterson, B., McIntosh, I., Wilkinson, D., McComish, S. and Smith, I. (2013) 'Corrupted cultures in mental health inpatient settings. Is restraint reduction the answer?'. *Journal of Psychiatric Mental Health Nursing*, 20, pp. 228–35.

Perry, B. D. (2000) *Maltreated Children: Experience, Brain Development, and the Next Generation*. New York: W.W. Norton.

Piccinelli, M. and Homen, F. G. (1997) *Gender Differences in the Epidemiology of Affective Disorders and Schizophrenia*. Geneva: World Health Organization.

Posner, K., Brown, G. K., Stanley, B., Brent, D. A., Yershova, K. V., et al. (2011) 'The Columbia–suicide severity rating scale: initial validity and internal consistency findings from three multisite studies with adolescents and adults'. *American Journal Psychiatry*, 168, pp. 1266–77.

Read, J., van Os, J., Morrison, A. P. and Ross, C. A. (2005) 'Childhood trauma, psychosis and schizophrenia: A literature review with theoretical and clinical implications'. *Acta Psychiatrica Scandinavica*, 112, pp. 330–50.

Read, J., Hammersley, P. and Rudegeair, T. (2007) 'Why, when and how to ask about childhood abuse', *Advances in Psychiatric Treatment*, 13, pp. 101–10. Available at: [Online] DOI: 10.1192/apt.bp.106.002840 (Accessed: 23 October 2017).

Read, J., Perry, B., Moskowitz, A. and Connolly, J. (2001) 'The contribution of early traumatic events to schizophrenia in some patients: A traumagenic neurodevelopmental model'. *Psychiatry: Interpersonal and Biological Processes*, 64, pp. 319–45.

Repper, J. and Perkins, R. (2003) *Social Inclusion and Recovery: A Model for Mental Health Practice*. London: Bailliere Tindall.

Roberts, R., O'Connor, T., Dunn, J. and Golding, J. (2014) 'The effects of child sexual abuse in later family life: Mental health, parenting and adjustment of offspring'. *Child Abuse and Neglect*, 28, pp. 525–45.

Ruigrok, A. V. M., Salami-Khorshidi, L., Meng Chuan, S., Baron-Cohen, M. V., Lombardo, R. J. et al. (2014) 'A meta-analysis of sex differences in human brain structure'. *Neuroscience & Behavioural Reviews*, 39, pp. 34–50.

Substance Abuse and Mental Health Services Administration (SAMHSA). (2011) *Shared Decision-Making in Mental Health Care: Practice, Research, and Future Directions*. Available at: https://store.samhsa.gov/shin/content/SMA09-4371/SMA09-4371.pdf (Accessed: 21 October 2017)

Substance Abuse and Mental Health Services Administration (SAMHSA). (2017) *Trauma and Violence*. Available at: https://www.samhsa.gov/trauma-violence (Accessed: 23 October 2017)

Schön, U. K. (2010) 'Recovery from severe mental illness, a gender perspective'. *Scandinavian Journal Caring Sciences*, 24, pp. 557–64.

Seeman, M. (2011) 'Antipsychotics and physical attractiveness'. *Clinical Schizophrenia & Related Psychoses*, 5, pp. 142–6.

Seguin, L., Potvin, L., St-Denis, M. and Loiselle, J. (1995) 'Chronic stressors, social support, and depression during pregnancy'. *Obstetrics Gynaecologist*, 85, pp. 563–89.

Skinner, P. and Toogood, R. (2010) *Clinical Psychology Leadership Development Framework*. Leicester: British Psychological Society.

Sweeney, A., Clement, S., Filson, B. and Kennedy, A. (2016) 'Trauma-informed mental healthcare in the UK: what is it and how can we further its development?' *Mental Health Journal Review*, 21, pp. 174–92.

Van der Kolk, B. A. (2005) 'Developmental trauma disorder: towards a rational diagnosis for chronically traumatized children'. *Psychiatric Annals*, 35, pp. 401–8.

Varese, F., Smeets, F. and Drukker, M. (2012) 'Childhood trauma increases the risk of psychosis: a meta-analysis of patient-control, prospective and cross-sectional cohort studies. *Schizophrenia Bulletin*, 38(4), 661–71. Available at: http://schizophreniabulletin.oxfordjournals.org/content/early/2012/03/28/schbul.sbs050.full.pdf+htm (Accessed: 23 October 2017).

Walker, L. E., Kaplan, A. G. and Surrey, J. L. (1984) 'The relational self in women. Developmental theory and public policy', in Walker, L. E. (ed.) *Women and Mental Health Policy*. Beverley Hills: Sage Publications, pp. 59–94.

World Health Organization. (1979) *Schizophrenia: An International Follow-up Study Chichester, UK*. Chichester, UK: John Wiley & Sons.

World Health Organization. (2017) *The core components of a gender sensitive service for women experiencing multiple disadvantage: A review of the literature*. Available at: www.barrowcadbury.org.uk/wp-content/uploads/2017/02/Mapping-the-Maze-The-core-components-of-a-gender-sensitive-service-for-women-experiencin-multiple-disadvantage-January-2017.pdf (Accessed: 21 October 2017).

To Learn More

Agenda: Alliance for Women and Girls at Risk (2017) https://weareagenda.org/

Advancing Quality Alliance (2017) *REsTRAIN Yourself Toolkit*. www.aquanw.nhs.uk/resources/restrain-yourself-toolkit/20917

Bentall, R. P. (2010) *Doctoring the Mind: Why Psychiatric Treatments Fail*. London: Penguin Books.

National Institute of Clinical Excellence (2009) Borderline personality disorder: recognition and management clinical guideline [CG78] www.nice.org.uk/guidance/cg78

CHAPTER 14

Specific Needs of the Male Adult

W.J. Wayne Skinner, Marilyn White-Campbell and Carl A. Kent

MEN'S MENTAL HEALTH IN AN AGE OF DIVERSITY

We live in an age of diversity. Most of the cultural fabric out of which modern society is woven draws on traditions, values and practices that are strongly gendered, with deep roots in patriarchy (*See* Chapter 6). Given that patriarchy confers advantages on men over women, it would be easy to presume that it would have measurable advantages for men when it comes to health and well-being. Yet even with longevity increasing around the world, men on average live less long than women, with the difference being about 4.5 years (World Health Organisation (WHO) 2015).

Murder and collective violence around the world accounts for over 10 per cent of injury-related deaths. Four-fifths (80%) of murder victims are men, with 60 per cent of victims being males between the ages of 15 and 44. Nine of 10 people killed during war are men. Yet, for all of that, at least as many people die from suicide (*See* Chapter 19) than from murder and warfare combined (Wilkinson & Marmot 2003; WHO 2015). In the developed world, three-quarters (75%) of suicides are men. In the developing world, two out of every three suicides are men (WHO 2015). For every death by suicide, murder or warfare, there are many events that leave people suffering physical and psychological injuries. The combined impact of these events directly on victims and indirectly on families and communities, if difficult to quantify, is not hard to imagine (Värnik 2012).

These points set the scene for a discussion of men's mental health. Certainly, the high rate of suicide among men points to underlying issues related to depression, trauma and emotional distress. Some might suggest that men suffer higher rates of morbidity and mortality because men are aggressive risk-takers by nature. Most murders are committed by men, and most soldiers are male. While it is an easy reflex to invoke stereotypic notions that essentially blame men for their misfortunes, we see such convenient reductions as a problematic evasion of a real consideration of men's mental health. We view suffering as endemic to human life and human communities. The challenge – and the opportunity – this chapter offers, is to open an active and reflective dialogue about the nature of mental suffering in adult men: causes, consequences and how to address it effectively and compassionately.

Vulnerability to stress is inversely related to social location (Wilkinson & Marmot 2003). While those with higher location (even the top 1%) undoubtedly experience stress, vulnerability to stress increases the lower down the social hierarchy you go. Those in the lowest quintile are the ones most disadvantaged by the effects of stress in their lives. This is manifest in lowered quality of life, increased morbidity and a shorter life span (Wilkinson & Pickett 2011). A consideration of men's mental health requires that we go beyond just biological and psychological dimensions, and include social factors. The social dimension includes not only the proximal relationships we experience in family and community life, but also the larger socio-structural factors as well. In our view, the traditional bio–psycho–social model (Engel 1977) needs to be further elaborated to include the social system, culture and spirituality, seeing all five dimensions as interdependent and requiring a comprehensive approach we call BioPsychoSocial Plus (BPS+) (Skinner & Herie 2014).

Not so long ago, the bias was towards what we have in common, not the ways in which we are different: we are all human beings, with equal rights, joined by a shared humanity. What this meant was something we presumed to understand. As necessary as these foundational values are, we have come to see how insufficient they are if we want to study health and ill-health and their determinants. We now see that social inequality is measurably related to such factors as class, race and gender, not because they reveal innate differences among human beings, but due to the way these are socially constructed. This gestalt of shared humanity and our vast differences shapes the context that opens when individuals, families, community members and health care providers face the reality of mental suffering and how to address it effectively.

Our invitation is to reflect on what that means for you. For us, it is important to acknowledge that most societies, including our own, are informed and governed by models of patriarchy that are both explicit and implicit. In its most direct form, this construct 'patriarchy' points to the persistence of gender-based power dynamics that give men power over women. However, it also constructs a social order where most men are subordinate to others, most likely men, in a world that is profoundly hierarchical and inequitable. The limited scope of the chapter does not allow us to explicate these starting points as fully as some may require. We encourage the reader to take a critically reflective look at the approach we develop here. We also refer the reader to the other chapters of this book, where many of the foundational and more extensive considerations of an ethics of palliative care in mental health are considered in more detail.

A point of departure for our exploration of an ethics of palliative care in mental health services for male adults is that most men have never been not well served by patriarchy, the dominant socio-structural worldview constructed over centuries. Patriarchy continues to be actively re-shaped even today, hiding the actual lived lives of men behind an essentialised frame of patriarchal masculinity. Importantly, patriarchy continues to be contested, particularly by humanistic approaches to well-being and human flourishing that are starting to reveal the shapes and forms of suffering and distress that inequality and hierarchy create for men.

THE BURDEN OF MASCULINITY

Patriarchy does not produce systemic and structural disadvantages just for women but for anyone falling outside the implicit hierarchies that patriarchy creates. Many males, who are the presumed beneficiaries of patriarchal social and economic hierarchies, are subjected to burdens that affect the quality of their lives, restrict the horizons of their possibilities, and consign them to identities that narrow their human potential (Niero & Bretan 2011).

Pathologies (understood as forms of mental suffering), in which men are over-represented include suicide (*See* Chapter 19). Men are significantly more at risk for substance use and other addictive disorders (*See* Chapter 17), where the male to female ratio is about 3 to 1. Males have a 40 per cent higher risk of schizophrenia, and a much higher likelihood of being diagnosed with anti-social personality disorder (Golomb et al. 1995; Picchioni & Murray 2007; Ochoa et al. 2012; Moffit et al. 2001).

Post-traumatic Stress Disorder

Post-Traumatic Disorder (PTSD – *See* Chapter 11) as a psychiatric diagnosis was very much the result of a study of soldiers and veterans who experienced what in World War I was called 'shellshock' on the battlefield. Subsequent armed conflicts, particularly the Vietnam War, led to the discovery that more people with wartime service experienced psychological injuries than were physically wounded. These psychological injuries would affect their mental health, ability to function in civilian life, and interpersonal relation-ships. It remains a challenge to come to grips with the extent of these problems because of the reluctance of men in seeking help for mental suffering and distress, especially in the context of a masculinist military and civilian culture that challenges men to suffer stoically and 'take it like a man'.

If military service is a particularly taxing occupation, there are many other 'male dominated' jobs that are hazardous in terms of mortality, morbidity and chronic mental ill-health. The growth of people experiencing chronic pain from workplace injuries, now understood as a complex problem with biopsychosocial dimensions, is causing increased rates of opioid dependence, and other problems related to loss of income and social status associated with unemployment.

Homelessness

Homelessness is another social reality in which males, particularly single men, are overrepresented (Fichtner 2010). In Canada about three-quarters of those using shelters are men, while among the homeless who do not use shelters, the percentage is higher again (Segaert 2012). These data are similar to those from other countries, including the UK and USA (Folsom et al. 2005).

There is a quip that people in the field make about the two places where it is easiest to find people suffering from serious mental health and substance use problems: in the criminal justice system and among the homeless. Canadian data indicate that over 70 per cent of offenders in federal institutions have either a mental ill-health, a substance use problem or, in many cases, both (Standing Committee Report 2010). Men represent about 95 per cent of the prison population worldwide (ChartsBin 2010).

Among those experiencing schizophrenia, men make up the larger number, with earlier onset, more relapses and poorer treatment outcomes than women. These men have higher rates of death by unnatural causes related to suicide, homicide and accidents. The male to female ratio is 1.4 to 1 (Ochoa et al. 2012; McGrath 2006).

The point of these data is not to compare in a competitive way who suffers most from mental health issues, males or females, rich or poor. Even when one gender is less diagnosed, such as depression in men, from a population basis, because of the high prevalence rates, this still means that vast numbers may have this problem. The evidence shows that, while rates will vary, all populations experience mental health problems. It is important to advocate for mental health services from an inclusive perspective that seeks to understand and respond effectively to the ways that mental health problems occur in particular populations. This ideally starts with prevention, a pragmatic understanding of the social determinants of health, and practical and structural responses that advance mental health in all communities and populations.

Recently, Mayock and Bretherton (2016), reported on women's homelessness in Europe, indicating with alarm that the percentage of homeless people who are women ranged from a low of 24 per cent in Denmark and Poland to a high of 42 per cent in Ireland.

REFLECTIVE PRACTICE EXERCISE 14.1

Time: 50 minutes

- What are your first reactions to this information?
- What concerns does this raise for you about the vulnerabilities this creates for women?
- If this report had presented the information keying on the data that most of those who are homelessness in Europe are men, with the percent ranging between 58 per cent to 76 per cent, what would your reaction be?
- In what ways might homeless women be more vulnerable than homeless men? In what ways might homeless men be more vulnerable?
- Given that homeless, marginalized people have higher rates of mental ill-health, how does this affect your view of people who are homeless?
- In what way might the differences among men and women be at least as important as the differences between men and women?
- How do stereotype and social convention shape the discourse on men's health and women's health?
- What are the advantages and disadvantages of approaches that focus on these essentially gendered issues?
- What are the barriers to going beyond a logic of comparison to an ethic of compassion that includes men as readily as women and children?

THE PARADOX OF MEN'S TREATMENT – TREATMENT AS USUAL VERSUS HOLISTIC CARE

Another challenge in framing a palliative approach to mental health in adult males is that in many ways, as treatments have advanced to become more holistic for 'special populations', a designation that implicitly excludes adult males, the interventive options that are available for men too often are drawn from the rather stagnant pool of 'treatments-as-usual'. All too often men's mental health issues have been constructed using a reductive medical paradigm of mental disorders and subjected to bio-pharmacological interventions, with the other elements of an integrated approach to care being at best subordinated and at times simply missing. One example of this is the recognition that women in recovery need social support. This has led to the development of supportive housing services for women as an essential component in a comprehensive approach to recovery. Yet while marginalised men outnumber women significantly, investment in such supportive resources for men is lacking.

THE LESSONS OF PROGRESSIVE PROGRAMMING FOR SPECIAL POPULATIONS

There is much to be learned from the more person-centred, comprehensive, integrated approaches to mental health treatment and recovery that have emerged to support women and other 'special populations', including diversity populations such as racialised (*See* Chapter 6) and marginalised groups. A key element in these more progressive approaches is a philosophical and practical shift towards seeing the person, their family and social supports, and the community as collaborating partners in planning and providing care. In doing so, approaches to care are de-centred away from a person whose ill-health makes them a less-than-adequate partner in the business of treatment and recovery, moving instead towards models that reconstruct care at the intersectional points where person, family, community and professional expertise meet and interact.

PALLIATIVE PERSPECTIVES

These considerations create the context for an ethics of palliative care for men's mental health. This requires that we move from an interventive regimen that is stuck in the provision of ad-hoc episodes of care usually governed by urgency, to approaches that intentionally work to intersect care pathways that effectively join and partner with people experiencing mental health issues. This leads to care-based healing journeys that are authored collaboratively on the basis of respect, candor, dialogue and mutual negotiation.

The principles of palliative care that we particularly want to work with are those defined by Cooper and Cooper (2012):

➤ Person-centred practice
➤ Relationship-based connectedness
➤ A belief in compassionate care
➤ Respect for autonomy and choice
➤ Quality of life issues
➤ Family as the unit of care
➤ Democratic and interdisciplinary team work.

The importance of including the family (*See* Chapter 16) (understood as the significant others who are actively involved in the person's life, as the person sees it) has radical implications that take care beyond the traditional narrow view of the person (O'Grady & Skinner, 2012).

KEY POINT 14.1

One key aspect of an ethics of palliative care is to not subject the person to unnecessary suffering. It can happen that the unrelenting search for a cure subjects the person to needless and futile investigations and interventions that allow the cure-driven health care practitioner to conclude they are doing everything that is within their power interventively, when what might really matter to the person is that the care team does everything they can to work collaboratively with the person to optimise in every way possible the person's quality of life. In a palliative approach, the person's needs and goals are what guides care delivery.

These principles resonate with the values that shape a public health approach to mental ill-health. They are strongly aligned with approaches that focus on the pragmatics of care, such as those based on harm reduction and risk mitigation. Moreover, they take what could be called a 'long' view of health, ill-health, recovery, change and wellbeing. Looking first to population-based approaches that start with universal health promotion, targeted prevention, it then proceeds stepwise along the care continuum from primary and secondary care to tertiary and specialised interventions focused on specific populations and individuals and their unique health care needs. That can be contrasted with a 'short view', which looks at acuity, without looking at anything beyond an episode of care, usually brief in nature.

We have chosen to use the word 'recovery' as a validating and organising idea that is important in a palliative care ethic in mental health. The word might seem to promise too much, but the connotation that people will get their health back is not the point here. Instead, a palliative approach allows us to recognise a deeper project of recovery in mental health care, which is helping people make the best of their circumstances, by working with the person and their family to make decisions and take action that make a practical difference that matters to them.

REFLECTIVE PRACTICE EXERCISE 14.2

Time: 50 minutes
- How do these line up with your values and worldview when you think of people who have mental health problems?
- What are the features in your particular context that support and manifest these principles?
- What features create barriers?
- What attitudes, values and skills do you bring to the situations you face that demonstrate and support these principles? In what aspects do you feel you need more training, skill and support?
- In what ways does the gender of the person affect your inclination to connect with the person?
- How does it affect your sense of personal safety?
- What issues come up for you as you reflect on these things?

A BIO-PSYCHO-SOCIAL PLUS APPROACH TO MENTAL ILL-HEALTH AND RECOVERY

In health care environments, it is especially easy to reduce ethical considerations to clinical factors alone. In mental health, that is easily reduced further to a neuro-biological view of ill-health, especially of chronic conditions. While acknowledging the importance of an understanding of the neurobiological dimension, we propose a model of ill-health, health and recovery called the biopsychosocial plus (BPS+) approach (Skinner & Herie 2014).

➤ Biological – In this model, the biological dimension reaches beyond a narrow focus on the brain to look at other aspects of physiological functioning that are fundamentally important to human wellbeing, including nutrition, sleep hygiene and fitness. Particularly among people experiencing mental ill-health, these areas of functioning are suboptimal and compromise the ability to function as a healthy organism in stressful and adverse environments

➤ Psychological – The psychological dimension concerns itself with the person's mindscape, their emotional needs, strengths and vulnerabilities, and their goals and motivations

➤ Social – The social dimension starts with the proximal interpersonal and familial influences that constitute the lived interactive world in which we all reside, extending beyond that to include the socio-structural factors that are less explicit, but which construct lived experience in deep ways. The model adds two other dimensions to the original tripartite that Engel (1977) proposed: culture and spirituality

➤ Cultural – Culture here includes ethno-racial location, but also the diverse possibilities that shape identity and one's sense of location in the world. Examples are: gay culture (*See* Chapter 7), and micro-cultural identifies related to the wide scope of human experience in places such as the workplace, the home, with peers and at play.

➤ Spiritual – Spirituality (*See* Chapter 23) is an important dimension that is often overlooked in health care that is secular and rationalist. However, the person's sense of connection in an existential way to life, nature, to a creator, to existence – which can be radically particular for each person, even when they appear to reflect stereotypic notions that are commonplace – can be key to both the demoralisation that accompanies chronic ill-health, to the resolve to keeping working at the recovery process, and to the magnanimity that produces mindful acceptance of one's travails as part of the larger reality of community and cosmos, and the journey of living and dying (*See* Chapters 21 and 22).

While each of these dimensions opens a different vector, we see them not as separate, but interconnected, and in many ways interdependent. We use the approach as a pragmatic and rounded way of putting the principles of integrated, holistic care into practice. Like any model, it has its limitations, but the BPS+ model has value in organising the way care is approached, planned and delivered. Its use encourages a comprehensive understanding not just of the problems associated with mental ill-health, but with the pathways that we need to explore collaboratively to find the best solution for a particular person and their particular circumstances.

An important consideration with the BPS+ model is that as much as it facilitates a comprehensive understanding of mental ill-health, it is even more important in drawing attention to the ways that each of these dimensions, individually and conjunctively, open up pathways to care and to recovery. Ensuring that each of these dimensions is considered in making therapeutic responses at all of the stages of change and recovery that are part of the healing journey that results from applying the values of palliative care to build a person-centred, collaborative care plan.

Our experience is in working with a diverse population of individuals experiencing mental health and substance use problems, particularly those with whom these problems co-occur. Our professional expertise is more on the psycho-social intervention side than the bio-medical. We have had the opportunity to work on inter-professional teams where our awareness of the importance of a comprehensive BPS+ approach has been developed and trued. At the same time these experiences have made each of us aware of the scope of our own individual practice, they have enhanced our appreciation of the importance of understanding care and recovery in the context of this 'big picture' approach.

SELF-ASSESSMENT EXERCISE 14.1

Time: 40 minutes
- In the context of the BPS+ perspective, how would you delineate your scope of practice?
- What are the areas that are outside that scope?
- In giving persons access to a comprehensive approach to care, what are the ways that are accomplished in your setting?
- What are some of the gaps you have noticed in providing comprehensive, integrated care?
- What needs to happen to bridge any gaps you have identified?
- What is one thing that you could do right away to make that gap a bit smaller?

Two other essential considerations in an ethics of palliative care for men experiencing mental health problems are the therapeutic relationship and the importance of empathic connection. While we would not go as far as to claim that it is 'all' about the helping alliance, we would say that you cannot get very far without it. The key to an effective relationship, the evidence keeps reiterating, is the ability to connect empathically with the people whom you are working alongside (Miller & Rollnick 2012; Skinner & Cooper 2013). In our experience, to fully embrace this has radical implications not just for the person–therapist relationship, but the relationships we have with everyone involved in the circle of care. What we have learned is that, while level of empathy varies from person to person, the practice of empathy is skillful, and can always be improved. Each of us needs to keep working at it. One crucial way to become more empathic is to seek feedback, and who better to give that feedback than the persons, families and colleagues with whom we work.

A PRACTICAL AND INTEGRATIVE ETHICAL FRAMEWORK: THE CLEOS APPROACH

Working with adult males experiencing mental health problems requires the skillful ability to work alongside real people with real problems in ways that are useful to them. To that end, an ethical framework that is both integrative and practical can help guide and inform the realities of everyday care (Russell & Skinner 2017). The CLEOS model developed by bioethicist Barbara Russell offers a powerful heuristic that is built on a strong conceptual and value base. Drawing on the work of Arthur Frank in particular, Russell asserts that 'how we interact with and treat one another, whether in our day-to-day interchanges, or the process of making a decision, is about ethics' (Russell, 2008, p.10). She calls on practitioners to go beyond reducing ethics to doing tasks such as getting written consents to 'the ongoing work of being ethical' (Russell, 2008, p. 10). She advances a practical approach to ethics, which draws on five key dimensions: clinical, legal, ethical, organizational and systemic (CLEOS).

Examining the situation through a rounded consideration of each and all of these factors makes explicit the relevant issues that are at play, while integrating ethics within the lived reality of everyday practice, rather than being something that is brought in for exceptional situations.

1. Clinical considerations include the therapeutic relationship, the particularities of the person (problems, strengths, needs, goals) and therapeutic options (short-term and long-term risks and benefits, availability, accessibility)
2. Legal aspects include the rules and guidelines of professional colleges, applicable laws and regulations
3. Ethical considerations focus on values and virtues such as respectfulness, generosity, trustworthiness and caring
4. Organisational issues include availability of resources, authority structure, funding sources and workplace culture
5. Systemic factors include the social determinants of health, stigma and discrimination, inequalities in the burden of disease and access to resources, and social priorities (for example, a focus on youth mental health compared to the needs of adults with chronic ill-health, or supportive housing for men without equal consideration of the needs of adult women). It is not that each of these will be equally important in every situation: the model allows the key factors that are in play in a given situation to be identified, so that they are given due consideration.

Employing the CLEOS framework ensures that reflective ethical practice is not just occasional, but a steady activity where the essential questions – what is the right thing to do here, what would be wrong, and why? – are ever present and always invited (Russell 2008).

EXPLORING AN ETHICS OF PALLIATIVE CARE IN MEN'S MENTAL HEALTH – CASE STUDIES FOR REFLECTIVE PRACTICE

By creating an intersectional model of palliative care values and practices, comprehensive therapeutics using the BPS+ approach, and the practical ethical framework that CLEOS provides, we can explore a palliative care ethics for men's mental health by applying the model to illustrative clinical scenarios. This approach is not an end in itself, just a means.

KEY POINT 14.2

The purpose of care is the wellbeing of the person, understood in the full dimensionality of their lives: biological, psychological, social, cultural and spiritual.

These scenarios contain themes that are particularly significant in men's mental health:
➤ substance use disorders
➤ depression and suicide
➤ workplace health
➤ the criminal justice system
➤ homelessness
➤ marginalisation
➤ and severe mental ill-health.

Our own work experience is Canadian, working with diverse populations, in an urban context, particularly with individuals and families experiencing co-occurring mental health and substance use problems. This is reflected in the scenarios that follow.

Case Study 14.1.1 Disabled party guy

Rick is a 56-year-old warehouse worker, a daily drinker for most of his life. He had several alcohol-related demotions during his working life, but was never dismissed because his diligence and energy were highly valued. At 53, he had an accident whilst working a fork lift. The accident left him disabled and forced him to use a wheelchair for the rest of his life. He retired early with a reasonably good pension. His stay in a nursing home became problematic because of his persistent heavy drinking and his inclination for sharing his alcohol with fellow residents. Regular events of mayhem led to frequent threats of eviction, which never led anywhere because he had 'nowhere to go'. Eventually, after numerous efforts, Rick succeeded in finding an apartment that was rent-supported.

Rick keeps a fridge full of beer for anyone in the building who visits. Frequently, his 'drop-in friends' would entice him into drinking more than his usual daily amount. As a community outreach worker for the health team that supports Rick, you have been visiting him regularly. He likes this contact, but when you ask him about his drinking goals, he suspects you are going to tell him to stop altogether, and pre-emptively tells you he has no such ambitions. This allows you to talk about low-risk drinking guidelines. He surprises you when he tells you he will limit his drinking to two or three bottles of beer per day, on a trial basis for two months. Discussion centres around how he can achieve this goal, including controlled-drinking techniques he could use in everyday situations.

Rick is surprised to learn how easy it is for him to reduce his overall consumption. In spite of this he has several setbacks, triggered by frustrating events such as someone having set fire to the Christmas wreath he had hung on his apartment door. He takes this very personally and keeps asking himself who might 'have it in for him'. On another occasion, he got very upset with one of the many 'drop-in' drinking friends. Rick drank so much he had to be taken to hospital by ambulance. The doctor at the hospital tells Rick that he has developed a heart condition so that another heavy drinking bout could be fatal, and strongly recommends abstinence.

Rick takes this news seriously. Though he has not stopped drinking completely, he is able to keep to three bottles of beer per day. This is having consequences for his friendships and social contacts. He no longer fills his fridge with beer, and limits what he offers visitors, admonishing them about the risks of heavy drinking. He has less company, and admits to feeling more socially isolated and feeling down.

To date, you have been keeping infrequent but regular contact with Rick. On this occasion, you wonder if he is clinically depressed. As you talk with him, he becomes tearful and upset, mentioning that now he is not drinking as heavily as he did, he is having flashback thoughts related to his accident, which leave him in a panic. He also feels he has failed at relationships and now is paying the price with little family involvement. He says his life is pointless. His heavy drinking and cavorting with friends helped him get through.

You commiserate with him, reflecting back what you hear him say with such candor. You thank him for his straight talk. You ask him if he would like some help to deal with this. He looks you in the eye and says, "What can you do to help me"?

SELF-ASSESSMENT EXERCISE 14.2

Time: 50 minutes

Take a moment to think about how you would respond directly to Rick's question, and in what direction you would want to guide things.

- What can you do?
- What can be done?
- Your interaction in this meeting shows that your focus on listening respectfully and reflectively has facilitated Rick moving his conversation with you to a deeper level. But it also reveals that Rick has a darker view of his situation, past, present and future, than he has ever shared before. When you look at Rick's situation using the BPS+ approach, what strength and deficits do you see: biologically, psychologically, socially, culturally and spiritually?
- From the CLEOS perspective, what clinical, legal, ethical, organizational and systemic issues stand out for you?
- From an ethical perspective, what duties do you have to Rick now that he has made you privy to his own sense of his predicament?
- From a clinical perspective, seeing Rick now as not just a man with a serious physical handicap who drinks too much, but as someone with underlying issues related to relationships, lack of purpose, demoralization and perhaps trauma?
- What *can* you do?

Case Study 14.1.2 – Commentary

Rick's question is both a challenge and an opportunity. Much depends on how you respond to such a direct question. The risk in responding ineffectively is that Rick feels confirmed in his view that he is trapped in his circumstances. The opportunity is that you can use this to build a stronger collaborative connection with Rick that can lead to palliative improvements in his situation. A direct response, which validates rather than contests his lived experience, is crucial.

You: "That's a good question, Rick. First of all, I want to help. I think your situation sucks. But I see you as a survivor already. You had found a way, but it isn't working for you anymore. I'd like to see if we can find a new way so that things could work better for you, on your own terms. What do you think about that"?

Rick: "I appreciate that, but is there a point to trying . . . for what? I mean, look at me . . ."

You: "There is a point . . . and I look at you and I get the point that this is worth a try".

Rick: "But what is the point . . ."?

You: "Well, you're a pretty smart guy. That's why this sucks so much. You actually get how compromised your situation is compared to most folks. We can use your smarts to make things better for you. It means working on it . . . but maybe you wouldn't mind having something worthwhile to work on just now".

Rick: "Maybe . . ."

continued . . .

'Maybe' can be good enough when working with someone who is demoralised, using palliative values and practices. This exchange shows that the relationship dynamic is a vital part of the process of working on improving his situation. Following up, you present Rick to your community care team at case rounds. The team discusses whether a medication would help Rick's depression. This would be taking a neuro-biological view of what is ailing Rick. The team notes it as an option. The doctor will explore it further when Rick returns to the follow-up clinic in two months, if the matter is not brought up earlier. The team supports your recommendation that you increase your visits to see Rick to bi-weekly rather than bi-monthly, especially since Rick mentioned that he would like more frequent contact. You emphasised to Rick that he could call you whenever he wanted to.

The team asked you about suicide risk, and you mentioned that you did ask him about ideation and any plans. You rate his risk as low, much as it has been since you started seeing him, and that you are actively monitoring it. Instead of medication, which Rick is not keen on, you suggest engaging Rick in peer support with a focus on living with a disability. Rick expressed an interest in learning to become more fluent in online technologies, hoping he can make more social contact that way to compensate for his mobility limitations. You agree to look with him for courses, and point out that in the support group there are members who have a lot of digital savvy who could help him. You mention that you can work with Rick to arrange transportation to the group, which meets once a week. Creating a safe place where Rick could risk sharing his feelings of hopelessness has led to Rick being willing to try peer support, something he avoided in the past. Briefing the group facilitator will ensure that Rick has a smooth entry into the group. Keeping in contact with Rick will allow you to offer support and help problem-solve any issues that may arise. You note that you could even consider using email and other virtual technologies to provide Rick with more frequent, brief contacts as a way of helping him consolidate this change.

KEY POINT 14.3

We use Motivational Interviewing (MI) as our approach to therapeutic communication. It focuses on four basic skills: Open questions, Affirmations, Reflections and Summaries (OARS). But of equal importance is MI's focus on empathy. The spirit of MI is manifest in four principles – partnership, autonomy, compassion and evocation – that guide MI's approach to interpersonal communication in helping relationships (Miller & Rollnick 2012; Skinner & Cooper 2013).

Case Study 14.1.3

Bundled in this response are a number of elements that could be understood using the BPS+ model and the CLEOS framework. This includes a recognition that Rick's solutions are not just clinical ones. Having a peer support group available is one thing, but being able to access it is another. You offer to work with Rick to arrange transportation. You take on the task of connecting with the group facilitator to ensure successful engagement. These are

continued . . .

socio-structural realities that you have the knowledge and skill to navigate. The goal is to enhance Rick's 'social capital'. This term refers to the connections Rick has to other people that give him access to support and resources to meet his needs and his goals (Bourdieu 2000; McKenzie, Whitley & Weich 2002; Cloud & Granfield 2008). This scenario shows the importance of socio-cultural factors in men's mental health and the role that alternatives can play in helping people move to more healthy and sustainable options. One subsequent goal, although you didn't immediately mention it to Rick, is to talk with him about family members he is close to. Can he identify one or two whom he would be willing to involve in his care plan so that they can be invited to be active members of his circle of care?

SELF-ASSESSMENT EXERCISE 14.3

Time: 20 minutes
- As we move on from this scenario, what questions are you left with?
- What insights would you offer if you were part of the care team?
- What one or two key learnings can you take from this that you could apply to your own work?
- Perhaps this case study reinforces some key learnings you have already had in your work: what are they, and how do you apply them in your work?

Case Study 14.2.1 Wounded warrior

Michel is a military veteran, on a disability pension, who works sporadically. He served in Afghanistan, working to help indigenous workers learn policing and community engagement skills. A francophone with good English language skills, he is the son of a Haitian immigrant man and a French-Canadian woman, growing up in a working-class district of Montreal. Prior to his deployment, he had a policing background in Canada, where he developed a reputation working with marginalised populations. He quickly made strong bonds with his colleagues and Afghani students, and before long was asked to go along on their rounds in a provincial centre, to observe and give them feedback. Travelling in convoy, they came under attack. Michel was wounded, and saw comrades killed. He then witnessed the summary execution of an enemy combatant captured when reinforcements arrived to rescue them. His wound affected his mobility, and he was repatriated and given desk duty. He found that work frustrating, showing a shorter fuse and increased bursts of anger. His relationship with his girlfriend, Keiko, became conflicted, and although there were no episodes of abuse, she left, telling her close friends she did not feel safe with Michel any more. For his part, Michel became increasingly erratic, deciding to quit military service. His alcohol and cannabis intake increased significantly. After his discharge, he quickly became homeless, rejecting efforts from friends and family for support and help. He now talks about leaving town in the hope that life might be better someplace else. He suffers from sleep disruption and nightmares, and can't seem to get a handle on what is happening to him. He suspects no one can help him calm his troubled mind.

SELF-ASSESSMENT EXERCISE 14.4

Time: 30 minutes
- What is the picture that emerges when we look at Michel's situation using the BPS+ approach?
- We seem to know more about his problems than his goals and motivations. How could we begin to explore that?
- What pathways to recovery can be identified along each of the BPS+ dimensions?
- What concerns do you have in working with someone both demoralised and marginalised?
- What can be done to build his 'social capital'?
- What can happen when someone begins to feel they have more access to resources and can make choices that are meaningful for them?

Case Study 14.2.2

You had been Michel's support worker with the Veterans' Affairs office. He saw you briefly when he left military service, but you have not seen him since. Now a worker at a shelter is calling, advocating for Michel to get reconnected so that he can access some of supports that military veterans qualify for. You meet with Michel, letting him share his story with you. He tells you that the loss of the relationship with Keiko has been very painful for him. Being together helped him keep a grip on things and believing he had a future. He hopes he can reconnect with her, but is not sure how to go about it. He recognises that he could use some support from the few good friends and family from whom he has become estranged. He wants to stabilise his living situation, but also feels unsafe in the shelters and hostel settings that are now his only resort. He struggles with ambivalent thoughts and feelings: he has trouble accepting that he needs help and cannot really take care of himself at this point, which makes him want to give up, but he also knows he is not the only person who has had this kind of thing happen to him. He states that if it was someone else (he thinks of some of his buddies from his military days and how 'screwed up' they have become), he would be there for them. He admits, "It's way too hard to admit that this is about me and how messed up I have become . . . and then he pauses . . ."

SELF-ASSESSMENT EXERCISE 14.5

Time: 20 minutes
- Michel has just opened 'the can of worms' that is his current life. There are many issues here that need to be addressed. What are your thoughts?
- What feelings come up for you?
- What observations do you have as you hear Michel unload his story?
- What options do you see for him?
- How would you proceed?

Case Study 14.2.3 Commentary

You recognise that his symptoms point to Post-Traumatic Stress Disorder (PTSD – *See* Chapter 11), and there are good programmes that are available that can help Michel manage the symptoms related to that. You realise that in terms of the BPS+ dimensions, there are deficits in each area. He has been living marginally, which means that his nutrition has likely been inadequate and that his sleep has been compromised, not to mention the neurobiological aspects of PTSD symptoms and the effects of alcohol, cannabis and possibly other drugs as he tries to self-medicate, all of which compromise his ability to function biologically. Psychologically, he is subject to intrusive memories and nightmares, as well as depression. Socially, he is marginalised and dislocated from those with whom he has felt connected in the past. Issues related to culture and spirituality are things to explore later. Culturally he is disconnected and dislocated. Spiritually, he is demoralised and not grounded to a belief system that he can draw on.

Case Study 14.2.4

Michel's comment:	"It's just that it's way too hard to admit that this is about me and how messed up I have become".
You:	"You've seen other good guys have this happen to them, and you know you would be totally there for them. But now that it's you with the injuries, it's harder to give yourself the same support".
Michel:	"I feel stuck in a deep hole and all I seem to be able to do is to keep digging".
You:	"Sounds like you'd rather be climbing out of this rather than digging yourself down deeper. And it's hard to ask for help".
Michel:	"That just about says it. I'm stuck, man".
You:	"Given what's been happening to you, it must be hard to believe that not all paths lead deeper down. But I can see some paths that lead out of the space you are stuck in".
Michel:	"Like what? I've too deep in this hole to see the light of day . . ."
You:	"I get it that every move you make ends up making you feel more frustrated. Well, I can think of a number of options, including some that we could do right away to get you in a safer place, as well as some things we would have to work on over time".
Michel:	"What are you thinking of"?

Case Study 14.2.5 Commentary

In this brief exchange, Michel has gone from fatalistic resignation to at least a curious interest in what other options there may be for him. And he is connecting with you. For some persons, you, the helper, represent the first reliable social capital that marginalised persons have access to when they try to change to a more stable situation. Access to your support, advocacy and expertise to develop a careful, gradual, sustainable care pathway shows Michel that his situation can be palliated. Options include hospital admission for stabilisation, withdrawal management and care planning. But you respect that it is Michel's decision to make. He indicates that he wants to think about it, that he feels he can trust the shelter worker who referred him, and that he will go back there to think on things, but would like to see you again as soon as possible. You agree to see him tomorrow on a drop-in basis, though he might have to wait. You indicate that he is eligible for some financial benefits and other social supports that he has not been accessing and you want him to know about that.

In our clinical enthusiasm, we sometimes overload the person with all the good things that we want to give them. But what is the pace that is best for the person? Sometimes, the maximum is not the optimum, especially people with complex issues. A palliative perspective tunes the helper to being astutely person-centred. The goal is not a quick-fix and then you are done, but a sustainable care journey that opens pathways in ways that build the person's self-efficacy and produce practical results that matter to the person. In this case, Michel does return, and initially works on concrete issues that get him housing. He agrees to a mental health assessment that supports a PTSD diagnosis, along with anxiety and substance use problems. He chooses the option to attend a treatment programme on an outpatient basis that builds resiliency skills to reduce his symptoms, with a focus on emotional self-regulation and interpersonal communication skills. He is prescribed a medication that helps stabilise his sleep. You continue to look as his situation from the multifocal lens of BPS+, and with the team you review palliative care issues using the CLEOS framework, focusing on the intersection of clinical factors with the socio-structural and organisational issues that are in play in Michel's situation.

SELF-ASSESSMENT EXERCISE 14.6

Time: 30 minutes

He next asks for help re-engaging people who remain important to him, including his ex-girlfriend, Keiko and his estranged sister.

- From an ethical perspective, what concerns would you have about him doing this?
- What role do you see yourself playing if he were to ask for your help?
- How do we as helpers work with persons to repair and re-establish old connections?
- How would you approach Michel's specific requests to reconnect with Keiko and his sister?

We raise this here for exploration rather than resolution, recognising that addressing one set of problems often means other issues will emerge and can then be addressed as part of the palliative care journey.

CONCLUSION

The data we have presented show that there are burdens to masculinity that can be measured in the mental suffering manifest in suicide, homelessness, substance use problems and chronic mental ill-health such as schizophrenia. Poverty, inequality and the other social determinants of health affect men's lives, just as they do for other populations. Yet it is all too easy to see these problems as primarily neurobiological ones. This points to the need of a renewed therapeutics for men's mental health. A palliative model, which sees these problems not as merely bio-psychological afflictions, but predictable consequences of the socio-structural contexts of men's lives, including developmental and epigenetic stages, offers a more realistic and actionable approach. 'Solutions' draw on the clinical dimension, and will also need to address the effects of dislocation and disadvantage that obtain from class, race, gender and other dimensions of inequality.

An ethic of palliative care takes us beyond a 'just fix it' approach to men's mental suffering. An integrated and comprehensive view of health and wellbeing – and risk and vulnerability – and the way they are present in men's lives, just as they are with other populations, is needed. A question to consider in this newly emerging discourse about men's mental health: are there unarticulated attitudes and ingrained beliefs that men and their mental suffering that create barriers to a renewed palliative therapeutics based on compassion and collaboration? Here, in conclusion, are some considerations that can contribute re-imagining an ethics of palliative care for men experiencing mental health problems.

➤ Severity predicts complexity: take a comprehensive approach that explores the person's challenges and strengths
➤ Complexity is more the norm than the exception: think intersectionality
➤ Family is already involved: identify and include those the person sees as most able to support and help them on their care journey
➤ Be empathic rather than just a problem solver (and problem solve collaboratively)
➤ Work collaboratively: it is a worrisome sign to find yourself working alone, with no clinical collaborators, and without the person participating as actively as is appropriate
➤ It's about the journey, not the destination
➤ Build the person's social capital – what are the resources and supports that give the person more choice and control over the decisions that will improve their life
➤ The moment matters most: connect, understand, proceed.
➤ Clinical work is as much about how we do it, as what we do – and the how is about compassion and empathy.

SELF-ASSESSMENT EXERCISE 14.7

Time: 20 minutes
- As you look at and consider this list, which ones stand out in particular?
- If you were to add one or two that are key for the way you see ethics of palliative care for men's mental health, what would they be?
- What one or two things can you take from this and apply right away to the work you do?
- What one or two key points would you want to share with your colleagues?
- And or with the individuals and families you serve?

REFERENCES

Bourdieu, P. (2000) *The Weight of the World: Social Suffering in Contemporary Society*. Stanford, CA: Stanford University Press.

ChartsBin statistics collector team. (2010) World Female Prisoners (percentage within the Prison Population), ChartsBin.com Available at: http://chartsbin.com/view/t5b (Accessed: 1 November 2017).

Cloud, W. and Granfield, R. (2008) 'Conceptualizing recovery capital: expansion of a theoretical construct'. *Substance Use and Misuse*, 43, pp. 12–13.

Cooper, J. and Cooper, D. B. (2012) 'Embracing palliative care-mental health'. In Cooper, D. B. and Cooper, J. eds. *Palliative Care in Mental Health: Principles and Philosophy*. London, UK: CRC Press.

Engel, G. L. (1977) 'The need for a new medical model: A challenge for biomedicine'. *Science*, 196, pp. 129–36.

Fichtner, J. (2010) 'Male homelessness as an apparent matter of course. Homelessness in Europe'. Spring, 2010, pp. 9–11. Available at: www.feantsa.org/download/homeless_in_europe_spring10_en5953934337965060559.pdf (Accessed: 1 November 2017).

Folsom, D. P., Hawthorne, W., Lindamer, L., Gilmer, T., Bailey, A. et al. (2005) 'Prevalence and risk factors for homelessness and utilization of mental health services among 10,340 persons with serious mental illness in a large public mental health system'. *American Journal of Psychiatry*, 162, 370–6. Available at: http://ajp.psychiatryonline.org/doi/full/10.1176/appi.ajp.162.2.370 (Accessed: 1 November 2017)

Golomb, M., Fava, M., Abraham, M. and Rosenbaum, J. F. (1995) 'Gender differences in personality disorders'. *American Journal of Psychiatry*, 154, pp. 579–82.

Mayock, P. and Bretherton, J. (eds) (2016) *Women's Homelessness in Europe*. London, UK: Palgrave Macmillan UK.

McGrath, J. (2006) 'Data on schizophrenia: data versus dogma'. *Schizophrenia Bulletin*, 32, pp. 195–7. Available at: https://doi.org/10.1093/schbul/sbi052 (Accessed: 1 November 2017).

McKenzie, K., Whitley, R. and Weich, S. (2002) 'Social capital and mental health'. *The British Journal of Psychiatry*, 181, pp. 280–3. Available at: http://bjp.rcpsych.org/content/181/4/280 (Accessed: 1 November 2017).

Miller, W. R. and Rollnick, S. (2012) *Motivational Interviewing: Helping People Change*. New York, NY: Guilford Press.

Moffit, T., Caspi, A., Rutter, M. and Silva, P. (2001) *Sex Differences in Anti-Social Behaviour: Conduct Disorder, Delinquency and Violence in the Dunedin Longitudinal Study*. London, UK: Cambridge University Press.

Niero, M. and Bretan, G. (editors.) (2011) 'Vulnerability and social frailty: a theory of health inequalities'. *Salute e Società*, 10, pp. 9–120.

Ochoa, J. U., Cobo, J., Labad, X. and Kulkarni, J. (2012) 'Gender differences in schizophrenia and first-episode psychosis: a comprehensive literature review'. *Schizophrenia Research and Treatment*. Available at: www.hindawi.com/journals/schizort/2012/916198/ (Accessed: 1 November 2017)

O'Grady, C. P. and Skinner, W. (2012) 'Journey as destination: a recovery model for families affected by concurrent disorders'. *Qualitative Health Research*, 22, pp. 1047–62.

Picchioni, M. M. and Murray R. M. (2007) 'Schizophrenia'. *British Medical Journal*, 335, pp. 91–5. Available at: www.ncbi.nlm.nih.gov/pmc/articles/PMC1914490/ (Accessed: 1 November 2017).

Russell, B. (2008) 'An integrative and – practical approach to ethics in everyday health care'. *Risk Management in Canadian Health Care*, 10, pp. 8–13.

Russell B. J. and Skinner, W. (2017) 'Service provision: ethics in everyday practices in mental health use work', in Cooper, D. B. (ed.). *Ethics in Mental Health-Substance Use*. London, UK: CRC Press.

Segaert, A. (2012) *The National Shelter Study: Emergency Shelter Use in Canada 2005–2009*. Ottawa, CA: Human Resources & Skills Development Canada. Available at: http://homelesshub.ca/sites/default/files/Homelessness%20Partnering%20Secretariat%202013%20Segaert_0.pdf (Accessed: 1 November 2017).

Standing Committee on Public Safety and National Security, House of Commons, Canada (2010) *Mental Health and Alcohol and Drug Addiction in the Federal Correctional System.* Available at: www.ourcommons.ca/DocumentViewer/en/40–3/SECU/report-4/page-5 (Accessed: 1 November 2017).

Skinner, W. and Herie, M. (2014) 'BioPsychoSocial plus: a practical approach to addiction and recovery', in Herie M. and Skinner, W. (editors.) *Fundamentals of Addiction: A Practical Guide for Counsellors.* Toronto, CA: Centre for Addiction & Mental Health.

Skinner, W. and Cooper, C. (2013) *Motivational Interviewing for Concurrent Disorders.* New York, NY: Norton & Co.

Värnik, P. (2012) 'Suicide in the World'. *International Journal of Environmental Research Public Health,* 9, pp. 760–71.

World Health Organization. (2015) Health in 2015: From Millennial Development Goals to Sustainable Development Goals. Geneva: World Health Organization Press. Available at: http://apps.who.int/iris/bitstream/10665/200009/1/9789241565110_eng.pdf (Accessed: 1 November 2017)

Wilkinson, R. and Pickett, K. (2011) *The Spirit Level: Why Greater Equality Makes Societies Stronger.* New York, NY: Bloomsbury Press.

Wilkinson, R. and Marmot, M. (eds) (2003) *Social Determinants of Health: The Solid Facts.* 2nd edition. Geneva, Switzerland: World Health Organization Press. Available at: http://www.euro.who.int/__data/assets/pdf_file/0005/98438/e81384.pdf (1 November 2017)

To Learn More

Beat Stress, Feel Better: www.menshealthforum.org.uk/beat-stress-feel-better?_ga=2.104329923.23366 1551.1509044853-2117959340.1509044853&_gac=1.209447334.1509045532.EAIaIQobChMIp9 vH9_-O1wIVj4NpCh1jYQQjEAAYAyAAEgI6VvD_BwE

Campaign Against Living Miserably (CALM): www.thecalmzone.net/about-calm/what-is-calm/

Canadian men's mental health foundation: https://menshealthfoundation.ca/

Men and Depression: https://headsupguys.org/ and www.beyondblue.org.au/who-does-it-affect/men

Men's Health Forum: www.menshealthforum.org.uk/male-health

Men's Mental Health Australia: http://manup.org.au/

Men and Mental Health: www.nimh.nih.gov/health/topics/men-and-mental-health/index.shtml and https://cmha.ca/documents/men-and-mental-illness/

CHAPTER 15

Specific Needs of the Older Adult

Patrick Ryan and Julie Lynch

INTRODUCTION

The human population worldwide is living longer, leading to a dramatic increase in the number of people living into their 70s, 80s and 90s. The proportion of people aged 65 years and older is steadily increasing in the World Health Organisation (WHO 2011) – European Region. In 2009, this age group represented almost 15 per cent of the population of most European Union countries. By 2050, demographic estimates suggest that more than one quarter of the population of the European Region will be aged 65 years and older (Organisation for Economic Cooperation and Development – OECD 2009). Whilst this is a testament to better education, better health services and better quality of life policies and practises, it also poses a new set of challenges to health service delivery internationally. In accordance with these figures, the number of older adults experiencing mental health difficulties is expected to rise. For example, the number of people experiencing dementia is predicted to double every 20 years, to 81 million by 2040 (WHO, 2011).

SELF-ASSESSMENT EXERCISE 15.1

> **Time: 10 minutes**
> What do you understand by a 'palliative care approach'?

The application of the palliative model outside of the traditional hospice setting has expanded steadily since the turn of the century, with the cornerstones of palliative care (i.e. managing pain and symptom control, spiritual and psycho-social care, person-centred approach, impeccable assessment and access to community services) now widely integrated into the management of life-limiting diseases. For example: chronic obstructive pulmonary disease (COPD – Blackler, Mooney & Jones 2004), heart failure (Selman et al. 2007) and HIV/AIDS (Harding et al. 2005; Selwyn & Forstein 2003). More recently, the potential for its application to mental health care has been recognised, with Trachsel and colleagues (2016) coining the term 'palliative psychiatry'.

In adopting a palliative approach to the care of older adults with mental health difficulties, the practitioner will likely be presented with a unique set of challenges from assessment, through to formulation, diagnosis and treatment. Older individuals often live with illnesses that are preceded by long periods of physical decline and functional impairment. Thus, providing care for this population can be a complex task, requiring ethically complex decision-making, consideration of comorbid conditions, quality of life and wishes regarding treatment. This chapter seeks to highlight such complexities, stimulate debate and guide the deliberations of mental health professionals as they consider the ethical dimensions of care in helping the individual with life-limiting conditions to live life as well as possible, for as long as possible.

TYPICAL WELLNESS PROFILE OF THE OLDER ADULT

Prior to addressing some specific needs of the older adult (including dementia, pain, agitation, restlessness), a discussion around the typical wellness profile and functioning of the older adult will be outlined to provide a backdrop against which difficulties can be appropriately interpreted.

Physical Well-being

In general, the capacity of our biological systems (e.g. cardiac capacity, muscular strength) reaches its peak in early adulthood and declines thereafter. Lifestyle factors in adolescence and adulthood inextricably impact on the rate of this decline as do other variables including gender, cognitive profile and social support. However, contrary to common opinion, the majority of individuals remain fit and able to care for themselves in later life. A small minority of older people become disabled to the point that they need care and assistance with activities of daily living. Age-related decline in physiological systems only becomes clinically and socially relevant when it impacts on societal roles and expectations that feed the pathway to disablement (Grembowski et al. 1993).

Emotional Well-being

Older people are often perceived as lonely, hopeless and sad, to such an extent that older adults themselves who report high levels of satisfaction and happiness, express concerns and beliefs that most of their counterparts are not faring well (Röcke & Lachman 2008).

REFLECTIVE PRACTICE EXERCISE 15.1

Time: 10 minutes
- Consider the above statement
- What are your views regarding older adults? Do you agree? If not, why?

Evidence suggests that such an opinion is widely unwarranted, indicating instead that most older adults enjoy high levels of affective well-being and emotional stability well into their 70s and 80s (Kessler & Staudinger 2009; Scheibe & Carstensen 2010). Emotional experience is reported to improve with age and older adults are better at regulating their emotions, and experience negative affect less frequently than younger cohorts. Emotional improvements have been documented in longitudinal studies as well as cross-sectional studies (Steptoe, Deaton & Stone 2015), supporting the central tenets of socio-emotional selectivity theory (Carstensen, Fung & Charles 2003), which posits that as people age, they accumulate emotional wisdom that leads to selection of more emotionally satisfying events, friendships and experiences.

Cognitive Well-being

Cross-sectional studies typically demonstrate a pattern confirming the stereotypical view of ageing as reflecting general decline in most cognitive abilities (Woods & Clare 2008). Researchers have made a distinction between the fluid and crystallised abilities of older adults, with fluid intelligence (cognitive processes concerned in identifying complex relations among stimulus patterns (Horn & Stankov 1982); proven to decline in older adulthood, while crystallised intelligence (the lifelong cumulative produce of information acquired mainly through interaction with the environment; Horn & Stankov 1982) can continue to strengthen. Although differences in cognitive capacity is evident between the young and elderly in some specific areas, declining cognitive ability does not necessarily translate into impairment of daily activities, and this is of particular relevance when considering quality of life.

REFLECTIVE PRACTICE EXERCISE 15.2

Time: 15 minutes
Relating this to older adults that you work alongside. How often do you ask each person about his or her 'quality of life'?

Age-related decline across a variety of functional domains is part of the human experience and is a norm. However, based on the profile of older adults as a whole, in developed societies, today's elders are healthier and more independent than they were in the past, and there is a trend for older persons to stay in their own homes rather than move in with younger family or to long-term care facilities. Perhaps then there is a need to step back and detach commentary from the stereotypical view that maintains the view of old age as a time of withdrawal into passivity and dependence.

KEY POINT 15.1

Old age can be seen as a time of 'clearance' where people perceive and reflect with a sense of wonder, critique and appreciation of all they have achieved and often develop new capabilities and seek new challenges.

We draw the readers' attention to this stance as a reminder that in adopting a palliative ethos to engaging with older adults, we may first need to question and critique the attitudes and disposition that we bring as practitioners to an older person with psychological difficulties. Evidence teaches us that older adults are generally fit, competent, able and attuned to their needs. Palliation directs that we place them at the centre of any professional interaction as a partner and collaborator. However, society has conditioned us that it is permissible to adopt an authoritative or dismissing stance because we can assume that all physical or psychological distress for an older person is 'just the norm'. The morality and ethical standpoint of each and every professional interaction with an older adult, holds the potential to challenge our fundamental assumptions about a significant proportion of the population.

THE ROLE OF ETHICS IN PALLIATIVE CARE WITHIN MENTAL HEALTH

Applying an ethical framework to a palliative care model within the context of mental health conceptually requires an intersectional approach, whereby existing frameworks of ethical mental health care and ethical palliative care are cross-referenced and where possible, amalgamated. Codes of Ethics in mental health care (e.g. American Psychological Association Ethics Code (2010) mirror many of the ethical principles and values that must be considered when adopting a palliative approach (e.g. National Health and Medical Research Council 2011), as demonstrated in the below Table 15.1.

KEY POINT 15.2

The shared ethical principles and values between the two disciplines highlights that mental health care and palliative care have historically shared common ground, and it has been argued that 'in many aspects, psychiatry itself is a form of palliative care because psychiatric treatments are frequently not curative' (Balon et al. 2016, p. 205).

Thoroughly and meaningfully integrating a palliative approach to the care of persons experiencing mental health difficulties poses several ethical challenges, often focused on issues of capacity, consent and communication difficulties. Some of these issues are further compounded when dealing with older adults specifically, who through the normal process of age related decline have acquired impairment that compromises functions related to these domains. In addition, adopting a palliative approach within mental health care will inevitably require active treatment to run concurrently alongside a palliative approach, something that may be unfamiliar or contrary to service ethos and or staff expectations. However, the advancement of mental health advocacy groups has created a space for shared decision making in mental health management. Similarly, as services for older adults expand from traditional medical and nursing only approaches to include other professions, so has the opportunity for the individual to become more involved in decision making that directly impacts on their experience of service delivery.

The risk of suffering deterioration in mental capacity and thus the ability to understand and interact effectively with the world around us is one of the most significant worries for older people and their families. Although the essential components and issues involving capacity and consent are the same as those that occur with other groups such as those with a learning disability or with acquired brain injury, the longitudinal and progressive manner in which these can occur in later life requires a tailored response to each case. Initial acknowledgement of the impairment in capacity is often the most difficult step as families and carers often have observed early symptoms but want to protect their loved ones. Equally, individuals themselves will have noted impairment but do not wish to burden family members with worry. So, a collusion of well-intended silence is created, which inhibits the possibility of full involvement of all stakeholders in

Table 15.1 Ethical principles

Ethical Principles in Mental Health*	Ethical Principles in Palliative Care**
Beneficence and Non-Maleficence Psychologists strive to benefit those with whom they work and take care to do no harm. In their professional actions, psychologists seek to safeguard the welfare and rights of those with whom they interact professionally and other affected persons . . .	*Beneficence* Requires that the person's changing needs and preferences about care and treatment options and sites of care are recognised, regularly reviewed and acted upon, so that the person may live as comfortably as possible in this final phase of their advanced chronic or terminal condition, with their inalienable human dignity always respected.
Fidelity and Responsibility Psychologists establish relationships of trust with those with whom they work. They are aware of their professional and scientific responsibilities to society and to the specific communities in which they work. Psychologists uphold professional standards of conduct, clarify their professional roles and obligations, accept appropriate responsibility for their behavior, and seek to manage conflicts of interest that could lead to exploitation or harm. Psychologists consult with, refer to, or cooperate with other professionals and institutions to the extent needed to serve the best interests of those with whom they work.	*Fidelity and Responsibility* (not named as an Ethical Principle in Palliative Care)
Integrity Psychologists seek to promote accuracy, honesty, and truthfulness in the science, teaching, and practice of psychology . . .	*Clinical Integrity* Refers to the importance of respecting all of a person's values, needs and wishes in the context of health care. It thus requires continuity and integration of the best available care and treatment in order to bring genuine benefit to the person with an advanced chronic or terminal condition, and in a way, that is just to all concerned.

continued . . .

Table 15.1 Ethical principles

Ethical Principles in Mental Health*	Ethical Principles in Palliative Care**
Justice	*Justice*
Psychologists recognize that fairness and justice entitle all persons to access and benefit from the contributions of psychology and to equal quality in the processes, procedures, and services being conducted by psychologists . . .	Requires that those who are ill and all other people involved in their care – families, carers, and even the wider community – are treated fairly and that limited resources are used responsibly and wisely.
Respect for People's Rights and Dignity	*Respect for Persons*
Psychologists respect the dignity and worth of all people, and the rights of individuals to privacy, confidentiality, and self-determination. Psychologists are aware that special safeguards may be necessary to protect the rights and welfare of persons or communities whose vulnerabilities impair autonomous decision making . . .	Requires that people's wishes be respected and that they be helped to participate in decisions about their treatment or care, to the extent that they are informed, willing and able.

* American Psychological Association (2010) Ethical Principles of Psychologists and Code of Conduct.

** National Health and Medical Research Council (2011) An ethical framework for integrating palliative care principles into the management of advanced chronic or terminal conditions.

key decisions particularly in the areas of end-of-life care and legal responsibilities pertaining to guardianship.

KEY POINT 15.3

Upholding palliative principles, a preference for a functional rather than a diagnostic approach to the evaluation of mental capacity is useful.

Being diagnosed with dementia does not in itself automatically imply that someone is unable to make a decision and professionals can play an important role in ensuring that the dignity of the older person is not lost in a process of infantilisation. Education on the nature and course of mental capacity across physical and psychological deterioration is of great value in maintaining the place of the individual in the centre of the care matrix. Uncomfortably, there is clear recognition of the fact that some people make unwise decisions and they should be free to do so (as they are in earlier parts of their lives with, for example, alcohol use, gambling, risky sexual behaviour) provided the decision does not impact on the wellbeing of others.

SPECIFIC NEEDS OF THE OLDER ADULT

There are several health presentations that offer a useful platform to highlight ethical implications and challenges that may arise when adopting a palliative approach to mental health care and treatment of older adults. Specifically, dementia, depression, restlessness and agitation as well as being distressing in and of themselves, create difficulties for the individual, practitioners and carers alike. These are often outside of the normal parameters of decision making that fundamentally challenge attitudes around best practice, needs of older adults, rights of individuals, organisational policy and practise and societal social, legal and religious norms.

DEMENTIA

What is Dementia?

Dementia is a chronic, degenerative, life-limiting illness that affects mental capacity and communication. Deficits in cognitive abilities are usually accompanied by behavioural disorders leading to a progressive loss of the person's autonomy in common daily activities (Caltagirone et al. 2001). Dementia is caused by a range of underlying neuropathological processes, the most common of which is widely known as Alzheimer's disease (31%), with others, including vascular dementia (22%), Lewy body disease (11%) and fronto-temporal lobar degeneration (7.8%) (Stevens et al. 2002). The prevalence of dementia increases with age (from 1 in 1000 at age 40–65 years to 1 in 5 over age 80 years) and the disease course that dementia typically follows is one of prolonged and progressive disability (Murtagh, Preston & Higginson 2004). The level of baseline function is often low as the disease primarily affects older adults who have already acquired much other co-morbidity (Murray et al. 2005). Dementia is therefore associated with complex needs and people experiencing dementia have been shown to have palliative care needs equal to those of cancer patients (Hughes, Robinson & Volicer 2005).

Specific ethical challenges arise in relation to the care of individuals experiencing dementia, some of which include respecting autonomy and assessing capacity to consent to treatment, communication issues (where speech becomes disabled or incoherent), ensuring the overall well-being of individuals as well as their family/carers (See Chapter 16), making decisions about pain management, and withholding and withdrawing treatment (Golan & Marcus 2012; Jaworska 2009). Dementia shares a common pathological aetiology as other neurodegenerative disease, such as, Parkinson's Disease, Motor Neurone Disease and Huntington's Disease, thus the ethical implications and issues that arise are generalisable to other conditions.

Pain in Dementia

Research has consistently demonstrated that pain experienced by dementia patients is under recognised and under treated (Scherder et al. 2005; Zwakhalen et al. 2006).

KEY POINT 15.4

Palliative care when used as a service delivery model emphasises impeccable assessment as well as the importance of pain management and relief to improve quality of life.

In the context of dementia this can pose a challenge to the practitioner as for the most part, pain assessment is reliant on self-reporting. People experiencing dementia can struggle with communication skills as the disease progresses, and may experience progressive difficulty in expressing thoughts and emotions. Similarly, when older adults experiencing mild to moderate dementia report pain, it has been observed that they cannot recall symptoms from earlier times and may not be able to integrate pain symptoms over time. Thus, more frequent assessment is often required to adequately identify and assess the severity of pain, leading to greater demand on often over-stretched resources.

Applying a palliative approach to the care of people experiencing dementia necessitates the regular use of other pain assessment tools that utilise direct observation and validated observational pain scales, such as the Abbey Tool (Abbey et al. 2004), as well as increased use and observation of nonverbal communication such as facial expressions or vocal sounds. Close attention should also be paid to mood disturbances, functional decline and changes in behaviour that may reflect increasing levels of pain. Gathering information from a variety of sources can allow the practitioner to compare and contrast data related to the experience of pain so that a reliable consensus on diagnosis can be reached.

KEY POINT 15.5

The practitioner must be comfortable in not being the sole expert in the decision-making process but fulfilling the role of a repository to which various data sources can be directed and cross-referenced to make a best practice clinical judgement on what a person in care is experiencing.

Eating and Swallowing in Dementia

Difficulties with eating and swallowing commonly develop in persons experiencing advanced dementia, bringing into question the use and administration of clinically assisted artificial nutrition and hydration, such as a nasogastric tube (through the nose into the stomach) or a percutaneous endoscopic gastrostomy (invasive surgical procedure with the tube passed into stomach through abdominal wall). The decision to use internal tube feeding is an emotive one as it carries numerous medical risks and is influenced by a variety of complex ethical issues, the most considerable of which is whether life in advanced dementia should be artificially prolonged and what is considered to constitute 'euthanasia', i.e. that by withholding food and fluids, death will likely be hastened (Sampson 2010). However, food has an emotional, symbolic and social importance that should not be underestimated, and the human contact provided by the act of feeding assistance may be of therapeutic benefit not just to the individual but as a meaningful and tangible act for carers as they begin to come to terms with the end-of-life for their loved one (*See* Chapters 21 and 22). Providing the person wants to, and enjoys eating. The individual will let you know if he or she does not. Good, ongoing observation of body language including facial expression is a determinant.

Decisions pertaining to the commencement or continuation of clinically assisted nutrition and hydration require careful consideration of its burdens and benefits in the context of the specific goals of care for the person experiencing dementia, including the ill-health trajectory, expected clinical outcomes and the preferences and values of the person experiencing dementia or substitute decision maker (McCarthy et al. 2016). Applying a palliative approach to this aspect of dementia guides towards 'helping people live as long as possible', but comes into conflict with 'helping them to live as well as possible', as by using a tube the probability of causing a poorer quality of life through either increased risk of infection or increased irritability related to a nuisance factor, is increased. As in any such dilemma, best practice directs towards ensuring that all perspectives are as comprehensively informed as is practically possible and personal, familial, social and legal frameworks are used to make a decision that causes the least harm, produces the most benefit and is within extant laws and ethical frameworks.

> **KEY POINT 15.6**
>
> Decision-making processes are not designed to bring clear and directive answers for professionals or families – they are designed to ensure that rash, single perspective and single dimension decisions are avoided.

Behavioural and Psychological Issues in Dementia

Over 90 per cent of people experiencing dementia are affected by behavioural or psychological difficulties at some point over the trajectory of the disease, the experience of which can be distressing both for the individual and their family or carers. The management of these symptoms is complex and requires a structured approach. Difficult behaviours such as aggression or agitation can often indicate unmet needs that cannot be verbally communicated, such as undetected or untreated pain.

Kitwood (1997), with his philosophy of person-centred care, defined the psychological needs of people experiencing dementia as comfort, occupation, identity, inclusion and attachment. On identity and inclusion, a long-standing tradition within Western philosophy strongly identifies personhood with intellectual abilities of various kinds, i.e. the use of language, the capacity to think rationally, to make moral decisions, etc. This consequently feeds into the commonly held perception that dementia is a condition that destroys the identity of the affected individual, and thus encourages the withdrawal of others' regard.

Developments in dementia care emphasise the intrinsic value of an individual, regardless of his or her ability to communicate and engage with others and a palliative approach encourages meeting the psychosocial and spiritual needs of the person, even when the usual attributes that communicate their identity have been compromised. The role of the professional is critical in this scenario as families often struggle with relating to their loved one when their perception of that person has fundamentally changed. This is often seen where previously sanguine, easy-going people develop challenging behaviour tendencies and family members report that 'this is not the person I knew'. Professionals can act as a buffer between the person experiencing dementia and their families so that feelings of guilt, shame or grief do not become the lens through which the end-of-life relationship is seen.

Autonomy and Capacity for Decision Making in Dementia

In Western culture, autonomy has a variety of different meanings, including self-rule, self-determination, freedom of will and independence (Agich 2003). In medical ethics, respect for the autonomy of the individual is considered a principle of fundamental importance. In dementia care however, several ethical challenges can arise for the professional while attempting to balance respect for the person and their autonomy, with the individual's safety and well-being.

Although dementia typically involves a slow deterioration of cognitive capacities, which may suggest an inability to make decisions, the law assumes that all adults, including those experiencing dementia, have capacity unless there is contrary evidence.

KEY POINT 15.7

There are four 'abilities' that are taken into consideration when assessing an individual's capacity to make decisions:
1. understanding
2. appreciation
3. reasoning
4. and expression of choice.

It is important to iterate that capacity is not an all-or-nothing concept and that the person can make a decision about preference related to daily care or activities but perhaps not make a decision about a complex treatment choice or changes to living will (*See* Chapter 8). A responsible capacity assessment should prevent two potential mistakes: first, the unjustifiable overruling of autonomy in order to safeguard a person's well-being, and second, the unjustifiable respecting of autonomy at the cost of the person's well-being (Berghmans 2001). The concept of justifiability is neither tangible nor concrete and in each individual case needs to be discussed, not with the objective to arrive at a dogmatic conclusion, but rather to create an environment where a practical resolution can be agreed between all interested stakeholders.

To ensure the rights of the person experiencing end-stage dementia are respected and protected, the Irish Hospice Foundation (in its guidance document for palliative care for the person experiencing dementia) proposes the notion of 'relational autonomy'. This draws attention to the embodied nature and social interdependence of human beings – our embeddedness in a family or a cultural context (Kissell 2004). Congruent with a palliative approach, a relational autonomy-centred perspective obliges health professionals to focus on the experiences of the person receiving care and on what matters most to them. It proposes that practitioners need to:
➤ be attuned to the way in which people make sense or meaning out of the world
➤ help the person to express themselves
➤ meet the person where they are in themselves and in their environment of care
➤ recognise and meet the needs of carers.

The guidance document emphasises that even though a person's decision-making capacity may be impaired, their autonomy can still be promoted through adherence to their advance plans or directives, and continued respect for their current wishes where possible (McCarthy et al. 2016). Developments in neuroscience suggest that people experiencing dementia retain emotional and practical abilities long after they have suffered severe cognitive losses. This implies they may continue to hold ethical values and core preferences, which should be respected (Jaworska 1999).

When applying a palliative model, it can be reasonably assumed that people experiencing dementia are encouraged to live at home or at a place of their choosing. The issue of autonomy in this instance is particularly challenging as the potential to be at risk for difficulties with nutrition, personal hygiene, drug management, getting lost, financial fraud and social isolation is heightened. So, trying to support people experiencing dementia to be cared for at home can create ethical dilemmas of how to balance autonomy with the need for maintaining safety and wellbeing. The problems with such a dilemma are further exacerbated by the real politic of limited resources available to manage associated risk in the home. Many identifiable risks can more than adequately be managed with appropriate levels of support. But such support incurs a human resource cost that many health care providers or indeed families simply cannot sustain. Despite decades of rhetoric in relation to person centred care, deinstitutionalisation and social role valorisation; creating the structures and supports for meaningful and thoughtful home care based on palliative principles often seems as remote as ever, irrespective of what condition is being managed. Thus, the ideals inherent in the palliative approach are subsumed in the prevailing climate of viewing health problems solely through the perspective of risk and health and safety legislation, which offers little scope for the individual to maintain control or influence over the latter stages of their lives.

DEPRESSION IN OLDER ADULTS

Depression is subsumed within a larger group of 'mood disorders', and is ascertained by the presence of such criteria as:

> ➤ depressed or irritable mood
> ➤ loss of interest or pleasure in usual activities
> ➤ changes in appetite and weight
> ➤ disturbed sleep
> ➤ motor agitation or retardation
> ➤ fatigue and loss of energy
> ➤ feelings of worthlessness or excessive guilt
> ➤ suicidal thinking or attempts
> ➤ difficulty with thinking and concentration.

(American Psychiatric Association, 2013)

Depression affects about one in ten people over 65 years of age, making it the most common mental health disorder in later life (Anderson 2000).

The assessment of psychological problems in later life is complex in that older adults have longer histories of interaction with the environment, a greater probability of having experienced various diseases followed by prescribed medications, a greater number of personal losses as well as an increased likelihood of comorbid physical and mental disorders. All of these factors should be taken into account when assessing older people presenting with emotional problems and symptoms.

KEY POINT 15.8

The assumption that depression is simply a correlate of being old should be challenged as there is little evidence to support this and more importantly because this stance is in itself ethically flawed.

It takes one variable – depressed mood – and links it to one putative cause – ageing. This is a lazy approach that undermines the ethos of palliative care as it reduces the need for a comprehensive, methodical and carefully analysed set of information before a clinical judgement is made.

Moreover, it highlights that practitioners need to continue to grapple with what is known and not known about ageing populations as empirically based models for depression continue to evolve for older populations. The area is fraught with societal assumptions and not aided by the fact that empirical knowledge remains behind the rapid expansion of older cohorts in the general population.

The question of age-appropriate diagnoses is one of substantial interest and remains open to debate (Nordhus & Pallesen 2003). Accurate diagnostic criteria for older people, based on research that actually reflects their demographic profile will potentially lead to better diagnosis and eventually better treatment. Palliative care with its emphasis on impeccable, person-centred assessment can guide professionals in terms of best practice. The experience and presentation of depression in older adults may differ from that of younger adults, so it does not follow that instruments developed for younger cohorts are valid for older people. Clinical assessment through psychological tests or rating scales should be based on measures that have been validated in an older sample. Clinicians should carefully review the manual for the tests they use, and, if necessary, seek out expertise to determine if evidence for reliability, validity and relevant norms for older people are available. Otherwise, extreme caution should be adopted in interpreting responses or scores and in how these are reported to the individual and their families.

Other issues to consider are how physical changes and medication use impact on psychological well-being. As with other cohorts in the general population, physical ill-health can mask psychological problems and psychological problems can mask physical ill-health. Thus, the nature and complexity of mental and physical problems among older adults demands a multi-dimensional assessment, ideally involving an inter-disciplinary team of professionals (Woods & Lamers 2016); an approach reflected in the holistic ethos of palliative care.

AGITATION AND RESTLESSNESS

In the literature, agitation and restlessness are often referred to as 'delirium', which is defined as an altered level of consciousness characterised by reduced attention and memory, perceptual disturbances (hallucinations and or delusions), incoherent speech and altered sleep/wake cycles (Weissman, Anbuel & Hallenbeck 2010). It is sometimes referred to as terminal agitation, terminal restlessness and end-stage restlessness. Causes of delirium in the elderly include:

➤ constipation
➤ urinary retention

> spiritual distress
> dyspnea (shortness of breath)
> uncontrolled pain
> infection but specific causation may never be determined as it may be a result of interaction between various precipitating factors and or by the shut-down of different body systems during the dying process.

(Blanchette 2005)

If part of a presenting profile, it can have serious consequences on an older person's quality of life as it compromises effective communication between the individual and their loved ones during a critical time of impending permanent separation. For families and carers, it can result in painful memories that are carried forward into the bereavement process.

The presence of delirium at the end-of-life interferes with the assessment and management of other physical and psychological problems (*See* Chapters 21–23). It impedes the ability of professionals to formulate clear plans and make decisions that fully integrate the person's wishes and thus, can undermine adherence to a comprehensive palliative ethos of care.

Indeed, the presence of delirium poses a significant challenge in the adoption of a palliative approach, as palliative goals of care may preclude intrusive investigations or treatments that are required to detect or address etiologic factors of delirium. Where possible, goals of care should be established in all instances. These goals could be:

> a desire to live as long as possible
> to maintain functional abilities
> comfort
> to achieve important life objectives
> or to relieve the burden on loved ones.

Establishing goals of care for an older adult experiencing delirium approaching the end-of-life involves careful consideration of the medical, psychosocial and cultural characteristics of the person, as well as the laws governing the determination of capacity and consent to treatment.

Just as in issues pertaining to consent and capacity, this is not a straightforward process, further compounded by the reality that goals can change from day-to-day with fluctuations in the person's clinical condition. To ensure fidelity to the palliative ethos, professionals must adopt an attitude and disposition that enhances where possible an individualised approach to determining the appropriate intensity of investigation and treatment of delirium. In order to provide compassionate, respectful and person-centred care of the individual and his or her family, six core recommendations were developed (Brajtman et al. 2011):

1. Person-centred care of the older individual experiencing delirium at the end of life should be based on a thorough understanding of her or his life history (i.e. the psychosocial, relational and spiritual narrative) in addition to current clinical status and prognosis
2. There is a need to consider the person's family: their strengths and needs, what role they may play in the care of the older individual at the end of life who is at risk for or has delirium, and how the delirium experience affects their own well-being, both

pre- and post-bereavement. 'Family' should be understood broadly to include all individuals who are close to the individual or client in knowledge, affection and care, regardless of biological relationship

3. Terminally ill individuals who are at risk for or have end-of-life delirium – and their families – should be encouraged to connect with what is sacred or spiritual in their lives, if desired and appropriate

4. At the time of first contact with the older individual at the end of life, goals of care should be clarified with the individual (or their proxy if the older individual lacks capacity). Continuous reassessments should be ongoing and documented throughout the course of their care, and the significance of involving the family in this process should not be underestimated

5. In caring for older adults at the end of life, the clinician is encouraged to follow accepted guidelines that are consistent with the principles and philosophies of quality end-of-life care

6. Adequate training and education of all members of the intra- inter-professional health care team in how best to prevent, detect and treat delirium, as well as how best to communicate with and support those affected by delirium, is crucial.

PROMOTING AN ETHICAL PALLIATIVE CARE ENVIRONMENT – KEY TRANSFORMATIONAL QUESTIONS

A key player in the advancement of a palliative approach in mental health care giving will be the practitioner in the context of the service provider. In times of acute and chronic stress, individuals, families and carers will often turn to a professional service or practitioner to provide some sense of stabilisation while difficult health news is being dealt with. Therefore, it is imperative that practitioners have, through a process of reflection and critique of their attitudes to issues outlined in this chapter, adopted a clearly articulated stance on how best to work alongside older adults who have conditions that may adversely impact on their ability to live a life that resonates with dignity and respect. The practitioner does not work in isolation from the ethos of the work environment and reflexive questioning represents an organisational learning tool for both systemic and individual transformation. To that end the Australian National Health and Medical Research Council (2011) developed a series of questions for practitioners to assist with the type of reflection that would lead to enhanced use of palliative principles in chronic or terminal conditions. They have been adopted here to show their relevance to both providers and practitioners, and to open them towards action oriented reflection.

Key questions for the service provider to guide that process of reflection may include:

➤ How can an analysis of need be conducted that can establish whether a palliative approach to care alongside symptomatic treatment of the advanced chronic or terminal condition would enhance the life of an individual?

➤ What processes ensure that the person has reasonable access to all information and options relating to their care, treatment and management and access to other health professionals or health care settings?

➤ What support services or community groups are available to provide further assistance to the person in addition to medical, nursing and allied health care?

➤ How will it be determined if the primary focus of treatment changes from cure to relief of symptoms?

➤ How can the person's autonomy be preserved even if their physical and psychological independence has been reduced or lost?

➤ Has spiritual and or cultural support been made available to the person? (e.g. hospital/health service religious personnel, volunteer visitors)?

➤ Has the person been afforded opportunities to express their wishes clearly (regarding all aspects and/or limitations of care)?

➤ How is it concluded that this person is being cared for in the most appropriate setting to meet their expressed wishes and needs?

➤ If professionals are not available for one-on-one time with the person, has consideration been given to alternatives such as a friend or regular volunteer visitor?

➤ Who is the best person to facilitate discussions about a change in care focus?

Key questions for the individual practitioner to guide that process of reflection may include:

➤ How can I integrate a palliative care approach into the care of this person?

➤ Am I offering realistic options for care and treatment?

➤ How do I know that I am explaining the likely outcomes of care in a way this person and their family can understand?

➤ How have I provided for the person's emotional, physical, spiritual, social and cultural well-being?

➤ How will I deal with a person's stated wishes (or an advance directive) when I reasonably consider that those wishes are not in the person's best interests or not in keeping with best clinical practice?

➤ How do I ensure that I am sufficiently aware of the palliative and any condition-specific needs of this person?

➤ How have I involved the person and their carers/family in reviewing their care plans at key times during their care?

➤ How do I establish that I am taking enough time to hear what the person and their family consider to be a burdensome intervention or an unacceptable outcome?

➤ Who have I identified as others who can assist me in supporting this person's autonomy and respecting their human dignity?

➤ How do I go about enlisting their support and how do I use this support to bring added value to the work that I do?

CONCLUSION

What this chapter has outlined is that older people do not necessarily have to be ill or distressed. When they are, there is need for attention to attitudes that lead to a diminution of the dignity of the older person by side-lining their right to influence and control decisions that are being made about their minds, bodies and lives; that the complexities of well-being in older adulthood cannot be reduced to a simple, linear technical formula or diagnosis; that the palliative care approach in tandem with other established approaches can assist practitioners in handling the multi-factored interactions that influence decision making; that ethical concerns and dilemmas are a normal constituent in dealing with many of the health issues that significantly impact on older adults; and that the principles of palliative care can be employed in conjunction with ethical decision-making frame-works so that the breadth and depth of issues that are causing concern are delineated clearly and methodically before a resolution is agreed to.

REFERENCES

Abbey, J., Piller, N., De Bellis, A., Esterman, A., Parker, D., et al. (2004) 'The Abbey pain scale: a 1-minute numerical indicator for people with end-stage dementia'. *International Journal of Palliative Nursing*, 10, pp. 6–13.

Agich, G. J. (2003) *Dependence and Autonomy in Old Age: An Ethical Framework For Long-Term Care.* New York: Cambridge University Press.

American Psychiatric Association. (2013) *Diagnostic and Statistical Manual of Mental Disorders* (5th edition.) Washington, DC: American Psychiatric Association. Available at: http://dsm. psychiatryonline.org/doi/book/10.1176/appi.books.9780890425596 (Accessed: 28 September 2017)

American Psychological Association. (2010) *Ethical Principles of Psychologists and Code of Conduct.* Available at: www.apa.org/ethics/code/ (Accessed: 28 September 2017)

Anderson, I. (2000) 'Selective serotonin reuptake inhibitors verses tricyclic anti-depressants: A meta-analysis of efficacy and tolerability'. *Journal of Affective Disorders*, 58, pp. 19–36.

Balon, R., Motlova, L. B., Beresin, E., Coverdale, J. H., Louie, A. K. and Roberts, L. W. (2016) 'A case for increased medical student and psychiatric resident education in palliative care'. *Academic Psychiatry*, 40, pp. 203–6.

Berghmans, R. L. (2001) 'Capacity and Consent'. *Current Opinion in Psychiatry*, 14, pp. 491–9.

Blackler, L., Mooney, C. and Jones, C. (2004) 'Palliative care in the management of chronic obstructive pulmonary disease'. *British Journal of Nursing*, 13, pp. 518–21.

Blanchette, H. (2005) 'Assessment and treatment of terminal restlessness in the hospitalized adult patient with cancer'. *MEDSURG Nursing Journal*, 14, pp. 17–23.

Brajtman, S., Wright, D., Hogan, D. B. Allard, P., Bruto, V. et al. (2011) 'Developing guidelines on the assessment and treatment of delirium in older adults at the end of life'. *Canadian Geriatrics Journal*, 14, pp. 40–50.

Caltagirone, C., Perri, R., Carlesimo, G. and Fadda, L. (2001) 'Early detection and diagnosis of dementia'. *Archives of Gerontology and Geriatrics Supplement*, 33, pp. 67–75.

Carstensen, L., Fung, H. and Charles, S. (2003) 'Socioemotional selectivity theory and the regulation of emotion in the second half of life'. *Motivation and Emotion*, 27, pp. 103–23.

Golan, O. G. and Marcus, E. L. (2012) 'Should we provide life-sustaining treatments to patients with permanent loss of cognitive capacities'? *Rambam Maimonides Medical Journal*, 3. e0018. Available at: www.rmmj.org.il/userimages/160/1/publishfiles/177article.pdf (Accessed: 29 September 2017)

Grembowski, D., Patrick, D., Diehr, P., Durham, M., Beresford, S. et al. (1993) 'Self-efficacy and health behavior among older adults'. *Journal of Health and Social Behaviour*, 34, pp. 89–104.

Harding, R., Karus, D., Easterbrook, P., Raveis, V., Higginson, I. and Marconi, K. (2005) 'Does palliative care improve outcomes for patients with HIV/AIDS? A systematic review of the evidence'. *Sexually Transmitted Infections*, 81, pp. 5–14.

Horn, J. and Stankov, L. (1982) 'Auditory and visual factors of intelligence'. *Intelligence*, 6, pp. 165–85.

Hughes, J. C., Robinson, L. and Volicer, L. (2005) 'Specialist palliative care in dementia'. *British Medical Journal*, 330, pp. 57–8.

Jaworska, A. (1999) 'Respecting the margins of agency: Alzheimer's patients and the capacity to value'. *Philosophy and Public Affairs*, 28, pp. 105–38.

Jaworska, A. (2009) 'Advance directives and substitute decision-making'. *Stanford Encyclopedia of Philosophy*. Available at: https://plato.stanford.edu/entries/advance-directives/ (Accessed: 29 September 2017)

Kessler, E. M. and Staudinger, U. M. (2009) 'Affective experience in adulthood and old age: The role of affective arousal and perceived affect regulation', *Psychology and Aging*, 24, pp. 349–62.

Kissell, J. L. (2004) 'The moral self as patient', in Purtilo, R. B. and Henk, A. M. J. ten Have, M. D. (eds.). *Ethical Foundations of Palliative Care for Alzheimer Disease.* Baltimore: The John Hopkins University Press, p. 133.

Kitwood, T. (1997) 'The experience of dementia'. *Ageing Mental Health*, 1, pp. 13–22.

McCarthy, J., Campbell, L., Dalton-O'Connor, C., Andrews, T. and McLoughlin, K. (2016) *Palliative Care for the Person with Dementia: Guidance Document 6 Ethical Decision Making*. Ireland: Irish Hospice Foundation.

Murray, S. A., Kendall, M., Boyd, K. and Sheikh, A. (2005) 'Illness trajectories and palliative care'. *British Medical Journal*, 330, pp. 1007–11.

Murtagh, F. E., Preston, M. and Higginson, I. (2004) 'Patterns of dying: palliative care for non-malignant disease'. *Clinical Medicine*, 4, pp. 39–44.

National Health and Medical Research Council. (2011) An ethical framework for integrating palliative care principles into the management of advanced chronic or terminal conditions. National Health and Medical Research Council. Available at: https://dr892t1ezw8d7.cloudfront.net/wp-content/uploads/2015/11/Ethical-Framework-for-Integrating-Palliative-Care-Principles-.pdf (Accessed: 29 September 2017)

Nordhus, I. H. and Pallesen, S. (2003) 'Psychological treatment of late-life anxiety: an empirical review'. *Journal of Consulting and Clinical Psychology*, 71, pp. 643–51.

Organisation for Economic Co-operation and Development. (2009) *Factbook: Economic, Environmental and Social Statistics*. Paris: Organisation for Economic Co-operation and Development Publishing.

Röcke, C. and Lachman, M. E. (2008) 'Perceived trajectories of life satisfaction across past, present, and future: profiles and correlates of subjective change in young, middle-aged, and older adults', *Psychology and Aging*, 23, pp. 833–47.

Sampson, E. L. (2010) 'Palliative care for people with dementia'. *British Medical Bulletin*, 96, pp. 159–74.

Scherder, E., Oosterman, J., Swaab, D., Herr, K., Ooms, M., Ribbe, M. et al. (2005) 'Recent developments in pain in dementia'. *British Medical Journal*, 330, pp. 461–4.

Schiebe, S. and Carstensen, L. L. (2010) 'Emotional aging: recent findings and future trends'. *The Journals of Gerontology, Series B: Psychological Sciences and Social Sciences*, 65, pp. 135–44.

Selman, L., Harding, R., Beynon, T., Hodson, F., Coady, E. et al. (2007) 'Improving end-of- life care for patients with chronic heart failure: "Let's hope it'll get better, when I know in my heart of hearts it won't"'; *Heart*, 93, pp. 963–7. Available at: www.ncbi.nlm.nih.gov/pubmed/17309905 (Accessed: 29 September 2017)

Selwyn, P. A. and Forstein, M. (2003) 'Overcoming the false dichotomy of curative vs palliative care for late-stage HIV/AIDS: "Let me live the way i want to live, until i can't"'; *Journal of the American Medical Association*, 290, pp. 806–14.

Stevens, T., Livingston, G., Kitchen, G., Manela, M., Walker, Z. and Katon, C. (2002) 'Islington study of dementia subtypes in the community'. *British Journal of Psychiatry*, 180, pp. 270–6.

Steptoe, A., Deaton, A. and Stone, A. (2015) 'Subjective wellbeing, health and ageing', *Lancet*, 385, pp. 640–8.

Trachsel, M., Irwin, S. A., Biller-Andorno, N., Hoff, P. and Riese, F. (2016) 'Palliative psychiatry for severe persistent mental illness as a new approach to psychiatry? Definition, scope, benefits, and risks', *BMC Psychiatry*, 16, p. 260.

Weissman, D., Anbuel, B. and Hallenbeck, J. (2010) *A Resource Guide for Physician Education* (4th Edition). Milwaukee, WI: Medical College of Wisconsin.

Woods, R. and Clare, L. (2008) *Handbook of Clinical Psychology of Aging* (2nd edition). New York: John Wiley & Sons Ltd.

Woods, B. and Lamers, C. (2016) 'Psychological problems of older people', in Carr, A. and McNulty, M. (eds.). *The Handbook of Adult Clinical Psychology: An Evidence Based Practice Approach* (2nd edition). London: Routledge, pp. 918–50.

World Health Organisation. (2011) Palliative care for older people: better practices. Available at: www.euro.who.int/__data/assets/pdf_file/0017/143153/e95052.pdf (Accessed: 29 September 2017)

Zwakhalen, S. M., Hamers, J. P., Abu-Saad, H. H. and Berger, M. P. (2006) 'Pain in elderly people with severe dementia: a systematic review of behavioural pain assessment tools'. *BMC Geriatric*, 6, pp. 3. Available at: https://bmcgeriatr.biomedcentral.com/articles/10.1186/1471-2318-6-3 (Accessed: 29 September 2017)

To Learn More

The European Association for Palliative Care. (2013) *Recommendations on palliative care and treatment of older people with Alzheimer's disease and other progressive dementias.* www.eapcnet.eu/LinkClick. aspx?fileticket=SouPo-_uNLw%3D

McCarthy, J., Campbell, L., Dalton-O'Connor, C., Andrews, T. and McLoughlin, K. (2016) *Palliative Care for the Person with Dementia: Guidance Document 6 Ethical Decision Making.* Ireland: Irish Hospice Foundation. http://hospicefoundation.ie/healthcare-programmes/dementia-palliative-care/guidance-documents-dementia/

National Health and Medical Research Council. (2011) *An ethical framework for integrating palliative care principles into the management of advanced chronic or terminal conditions.* https://dr892t1ezw8d7.cloudfront.net/wp-content/uploads/2015/11/Ethical-Framework-for-Integrating-Palliative-Care-Principles-.pdf

Ryan, P. and Coughlan, B. J. (2011) *Ageing and Older Adult Mental Health: Issues and Implications for Practice.* Routledge: London.

CHAPTER 16

Listening to the Family's Pain

Lottie Morris

> Therapy is enhanced if the therapist enters accurately into the patient's world. Patients profit enormously simply from the experience of being fully seen and fully understood.
>
> (Yalom 2001, p. 18)

INTRODUCTION

Holistic care is a cornerstone of the palliative care philosophy, as described by the World Health Organisation's (2017) definition of palliative care: 'Palliative care is an approach that improves the quality of life of patients and their families . . . through the prevention and relief of suffering by means of early identification and impeccable assessment and treatment of pain and other problems, physical, psychosocial and spiritual'.

Therefore, involving the family and other significant individuals within the individual's system is key. Indeed, it is also increasingly acknowledged that, as well as being a crucial resource for the individual in need of palliative care, families are, in a sense, 'patients' in their own right. Families' needs are routinely assessed and recognised – both formally via structured assessments, and informally through a culture of viewing their needs as equal to those of the individual. As much as palliative care intends to alleviate the person's pain and suffering and maximise their quality of life, the same is true for their families.

In a palliative care context, it is recognised as inevitable that the family will usually experience distress in relation to their loved one's ill health and death. In mental health settings, while carer distress is acknowledged, it is less common for services to be organised formally to offer support to family members.

FAMILIES' EXPERIENCES OF PAIN ACROSS PALLIATIVE CARE AND MENTAL HEALTH SERVICES

Family Experiences

Loved ones, families and friends are arguably the most important source of emotional support in people's lives. Even where relationships have been historically tense or difficult, when a loved one develops a mental health problem or a life-limiting condition, this can be a great source of distress to those in their support system. Those providing emotional support will themselves experience grief, loss, fear, identity and role change, stigma and stress. Any small difficulties within family relationships may well become magnified, when a family member has mental health problems or palliative care needs. While this is understandable, it can cause a great deal of emotional pain and anguish: at the very time families need each other's emotional support the most, the stress of ill-health may limit family members' capacity to be emotionally available to each other.

The impact of mental health difficulties on family members has been acknowledged for decades, as illustrated by Table 16.1, copied from an article in *The Lancet* from 1963 (Grad & Sainsbury 1963).

Figure 16.1's concentric circles summarise some of the typical concerns or difficulties that family members encounter in palliative care and mental health contexts, and the significant overlap between the two.

It is well known that distress in caregivers of people with mental health difficulties and those with palliative care needs is high. Given that 'mental health problems'

Table 16.1 Effects of mental health difficulties on family members

Effect on	% families		
	Some disturbance	Severe disturbance	Total burden
Health of closest relatives:			
Mental	40	20	60
Physical	28	0	28
Social and leisure activities of family	14	21	35
Children	24	10	34
Domestic routine	13	16	29
Income of family	14	9	23
Employments of others than the patient	17	6	23

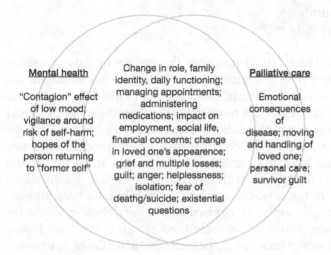

Figure 16.1 Family concerns in palliative care and mental health contexts

themselves are, according to the biopsychosocial model, usually caused by significant psychosocial stressors, it is not surprising that 'psychiatric morbidity' has been found to be as high as 52 per cent in family and friends of palliative care patients (Rumpold et al. 2015). Indeed, this is also likely to be the case in caregivers of people experiencing mental health difficulties. Oldridge and Hughes (1992) found anxiety, depression and insomnia to be twice as high for this group, compared with the general population.

In line with the above definition of palliative care, which explicitly incorporates care for families, most palliative care services operate services for family members, including bereavement support following the death of a loved one. Appointments are frequently conducted with family members present, and carer assessments are commonly undertaken, to identify any psychosocial needs. In mental health services, provision for family members is not routinely available and may only become available if a family member develops their own 'mental health problem', possibly contributed to by the stress of caregiving. While this is likely to be influenced by funding and commissioning agreements, it is also influenced by the culture, training and beliefs of the professionals working within the organisation. For example, professionals who have been trained in systemic (i.e. family therapy-based) approaches may be more likely to invite family members to appointments than those who have been trained in more individualised approaches to care. This type of professional would view the 'problem' as within the system as opposed to within the individual themselves.

National Guidelines on Care Provision for Families

In 1999, the UK's Department of Health (DoH) Published Caring about Carers: A National Strategy for Carers. This was then reviewed in 2010, leading to the publication of Recognised, Valued and Supported: Next Steps for the Carers Strategy. The key priorities of this more recent document are:

➤ Supporting people with caring responsibilities to identify themselves as carers at an early stage
➤ Involving carers in care planning
➤ Providing personalised support to enable carers to:
  – Fulfil their educational and employment potential
  – Have a family and community life
  – Remain mentally and physically well

A recent report from the King's Fund (2015) describes the impact of cuts to mental health services on safety and quality of care; for example, only 14 per cent of individuals reported receiving appropriate care in a crisis. In this climate of cuts, it is easy to see how difficult it is for already stretched services to offer formal assessment and support to family members, in line with the recommendations from the DoH's Carers' Strategy. However, where staffing levels and inpatient beds in mental health services are lower than required, family members are likely to be greatly affected by this. In particular, the pressure on inpatient beds means that people with increasingly complex presentations are now being cared for in the community, often mostly by family members. Indeed, family members are arguably a hugely under-recognised and under-valued resource for people using mental health services. Indeed, now more than ever, it is vital that family members are well-supported as they will increasingly bear the 'burden of care' as pressure on mental health services rises.

Case Study 16.1 – Listening to David's pain

David was a 46-year-old man with a diagnosis of schizophrenia and learning difficulties. David had always lived at home with his parents and has a very close relationship with his mother in particular. He received support from the Community Mental Health Team (CMHT) in the form of weekly home visits from a support worker and monthly meetings with his psychiatrist. His schizophrenia had been well controlled for several years, through the use of medication and a course of Cognitive Behavioural Therapy (CBT) for Psychosis, and Relapse Prevention work. David's mother, Mary, had been diagnosed with breast cancer several years ago. In the last twelve months, the cancer had unfortunately metastasised to her liver and bones. Mary was referred to the Palliative Care Service by her oncologist, and upon completion of a family-based needs assessment, David was referred for psychological support by the family's Clinical Nurse Specialist (CNS). Support was requested in relation to his role of caring for his mother, and also in relation to anticipatory grief.

Fortnightly psychological support sessions were arranged through the Palliative Care Service, in collaboration with David and the CMHT. David's goal for these sessions was to have time and space where he could open up and express his feelings as (a) he recognised a tendency to bottle up his emotions, which he had learnt could sometimes lead to an increase in stress levels and put him at risk of relapse; and (b) so that he could be emotionally available to make the most of his relationship with his mother, in her last few months of life. These sessions involved the professional taking a curious stance, and drawing heavily on active listening skills to assist David towards his goal of expressing his feelings.

These sessions continued for a few months into the bereavement phase. While David understandably found the loss of his mother extremely painful due to the very close nature of their relationship, it seemed as though he was experiencing a 'normal' as opposed to complicated grief reaction. Therefore, he was discharged from the palliative care psychological support service and continued to have weekly visits from his support worker. This was, again, arranged in collaboration with professionals in the CMHT to allow for continuity of approach. The support worker and David agreed to put time aside in their sessions where David could continue to share his emotions. David and his father shared, towards the end of the psychological support sessions, that they believed that the opportunity to express emotions and be listened to had enabled David to cope well and create some treasured memories with his mother in her last months of life. Mary had identified the family home as her preferred place of death, and died peacefully at home, with support from the Hospice at Home service. David and his father provided much of the care for Mary during her last months of life, in line with her wishes. They also discussed how they felt David may have been at risk of a relapse of schizophrenia, if he had not had an opportunity to express his feelings. David particularly appreciated how his feelings had been validated and normalised by the therapist.

THE VALUE OF LISTENING IN PALLIATIVE CARE AND MENTAL HEALTH SETTINGS

Research suggests that family members tend towards feeling un-involved in care planning, despite the guidance from government (Cree et al. 2015) and the fact that they are experts by experience. Even in mental health teams that are highly committed to providing information to family members and involving them in care planning, they report that their emotions are not acknowledged (Lavis et al. 2015). Repeatedly, when asked, the individual and family members alike rate listening skills as one of the most desirable qualities in their health and social care professionals (e.g. Griffiths et al. 2012).

As a clinical psychologist, I am sometimes shadowed by medical or nursing students during psychology appointments. During these sessions, I tend to ask the person or family to tell the student what qualities they value most in health and social care professionals. Without exception, every single person has said something along the lines of "taking time to listen to me". Moving into a palliative care context from mental health, I have been struck by my colleagues' reasons for working in this field. Many report that it is because, in this context, they are afforded the time to get to know patients and their families, and spend time with them. In other contexts, care can feel rushed and task-focused. Here, there is a culture of listening as an intervention in itself, which is valued by the organisation (and of course, the individual and family) as much as more traditionally 'medical' tasks. Families of people using palliative care or mental health services are frequently highly distressed, for a range of reasons. In such circumstances, listening is a powerful tool, which can be used to bear witness to the person's suffering:

➤ come alongside them
➤ develop a helpful relationship
➤ facilitate catharsis
➤ enable the person to 'let go' of emotions and make sense of the situation
➤ and hopefully alleviate their suffering somewhat.

While there is much debate in the scientific literature about the 'active ingredients' of psychotherapy, listening skills appear in nearly every modality (with the recent exception of computerised and app-based self-help therapies). The therapeutic alliance, to which listening is key, is thought to be fundamental to success in all of the below approaches to helping people in distress:

➤ Systemic approaches – curiosity is a key component of systemic approaches, alongside taking a position of 'not knowing'. Questions are used in this approach to explore the person's perspective, and to enquire about strengths, resources and significant others within their system. The therapist pays particular attention to the language used and, in some family therapy clinics, there might also be a 'reflecting team' of other professionals who are also listening, in order to provide a range of different hypotheses or perspectives.
➤ Humanistic approaches – according to this approach, pioneered by Carl Rogers (1951), the therapist can foster growth in the individual through empathic enquiry, openness, and a non-judgemental, accepting attitude towards the person seeking support. It is hypothesised that, by creating a safe and supportive atmosphere where the person feels valued and listened to, they will themselves be able to achieve resolution.

➤ Psychodynamic approaches – these approaches tend to place emphasis on using the therapeutic relationship to help the person to gain insight into their conscious and unconscious thoughts, feelings and actions. The concept of 'catharsis' is thought to come from psychoanalytic theory, whereby the emotions associated with traumatic events can be released or expressed.

➤ Cognitive behavioural approaches – listening skills are viewed as fundamental in cognitive behavioural approaches. Socratic questioning and guided discovery (i.e. asking questions which draw the individual's attention to relevant information which they might not be focusing on) is used heavily. Careful listening goes hand-in-hand with these questions, in order to inform the therapist's response.

➤ Narrative approaches – these approaches promote the power of storytelling as a means to 'externalising' the 'problem' (i.e. locating the problem as existing outside of the person). In this form of therapy, the therapist listens closely to the person's language as they tell their story, listening out for any hints of strengths, resources and abilities. The aim is to assist the person to move away from 'problem-saturated talk' and realise their own agency and competence in the face of their difficulties.

➤ Trauma-focused approaches – most approaches to post-traumatic stress-type reactions incorporate some form of 'reliving' or talking about the traumatic event(s) in detail, with the therapist drawing on active listening skills, amongst others. Given that memory processes are likely to be influenced in traumatic situations, importance is placed on supporting the individual to develop a coherent account of the trauma.

It must be noted that the approaches outlined above are intended to highlight the importance of listening, rather than providing a comprehensive overview or exhaustive list of different approaches. Across therapeutic modalities, it is agreed that effective listening skills are essential to the therapeutic relationship. Importantly, it has been found that expressing thoughts and feelings can reduce the high levels of physiological arousal that are typically associated with family members' distress (Mendolia & Kleck 1993); this is something that an effective listener is well-placed to facilitate.

EFFECTIVE LISTENING SKILLS

Active listening skills are fundamental for all health and social care professionals working in mental health and palliative care contexts. Both settings have goals of alleviating suffering and enhancing quality of life. To begin to help people, the professional must demonstrate an interest in the person's life, giving them their full and undivided attention. Brennan's seminal (2004) text, *Cancer in Context*, proposes that emotional support seems to consist of two key components: empathy and validation. Empathy can be defined as using listening skills to attempt to understand how it feels to be in the other person's shoes, and conveying this understanding through words and body language. Validation is also conveyed through non-judgemental listening, alongside words and gestures to communicate to the person that their thoughts and feelings are understood and also understandable, given their particular circumstances. Key components of active listening are outlined below, drawn from Jenkins and North (2008).

If there is a hypothesis that a family member is experiencing emotional distress, consider carefully the timing and the setting of eliciting a conversation about this:

➤ Ensure that you have time to listen properly. Ideally, set aside at least half an hour and make the person aware of the amount of time you have at the start of the conversation. If the conversation arises unexpectedly and you are short of time, it may be helpful to use a phrase such as, "I can hear how upset you are and how distressing this is for you. I'd really like to put aside a good amount of time to talk through this properly. I only have ten minutes now, which doesn't feel nearly long enough. Could we arrange another time to discuss this in detail so I can support you"?

➤ Consider privacy: is the person's family around? Does the person want to discuss this in front of their family? Systemic approaches introduce a concept called 'talking about talking' (e.g. Stott & Martin 2010, p.94), which usually occurs close to the start of a therapeutic interaction. This may include asking the person who they would like to include in the conversation, and how they feel more generally about the idea of talking about their problems.

➤ Try to ensure that the setting you are in is comfortable, inviting and free from interruptions and distractions.

➤ On a practical note, family members of people approaching the end of their life often find it difficult to attend appointments due to their caring responsibilities. It is likely that this is also sometimes the case for families of people with mental health difficulties. In such scenarios, it may be helpful to explore care arrangements so the family member is able to attend an appointment, as they may feel unable to talk candidly and openly within their home, for fear of being overheard.

Non-verbal Elements of Active Listening

➤ Consider how close you are to the individual. While you may wish to be close enough to encourage the person to feel supported, be aware of the other person's personal space. Notice their body language and be alert to any cues that suggest you are either too close or too far away.

➤ Ensure that you are at the person's eye level. Ideally, you should both be sitting down on seats of a similar height to address power imbalance within your relationship. Be aware of the furniture that is commonly used in medical settings, whereby the professional sits in a higher, fancier chair! This is not a good start to making someone feel comfortable about opening up.

➤ Ensure that you make good eye contact with the person, but avoid excessive eye contact, which is likely to make the person feel uncomfortable.

➤ Whether or not you touch someone who is distressed is a personal choice. A guiding principle from Jenkins and North (2008) is, 'if in doubt, don't'. If you do choose to touch someone who, for example, is crying, it is suggested that you lightly place your hand on theirs rather than an embrace or an arm around the shoulder. This way, if the person finds it uncomfortable, it is easier for them to disengage.

➤ It is often the case that, as soon as someone's eyes well up, the professional will notice this and pass some tissues. This may inadvertently communicate that the professional has a desire for them to stop crying, or is not comfortable being with their distress. It can be useful to wait a few seconds before passing the tissues, to subtly send a message that you are comfortable with their tears.

➤ Ensure that your undivided attention is fully on the person. To avoid obviously looking at the clock or your watch, it can be helpful to position yourself somewhere in the room where a clock is naturally in your eyeline.

➤ Use non-verbal encouragers, such as nodding, and congruent facial expressions.

Verbal Elements of Active Listening

➤ Consider the tone and volume of your voice. In general, match it to that of the person you are listening to. While a soothing tone and slower pace of speech might convey empathy, balance this with remaining true to yourself as it is important to come across as genuine.

➤ Avoid the use of medical or mental health-based jargon, which is likely to alienate the person and contribute to a power imbalance within the therapeutic relationship.

➤ Judiciously use verbal encouragers, such as "go on", "mmmm".

➤ Importantly, allow silences. Oppawsky (2016) proposes that silence is a helpful aspect of a listening interaction, as it allows the person time to truly experience their feelings, and to think more deeply about the topic in question.

➤ Consider the use of a short summary, in the form of a therapeutic letter following the appointment. This can be particularly useful for people with memory problems, and also for helping family members to feel that their concerns have been heard and appreciated.

ACTIVE LISTENING SKILLS, DRAWN FROM ROGERIAN, PERSON-CENTRED COUNSELLING PRINCIPLES

Carl Rogers (1957) proposed a hypothesis that the following 'core conditions' predict therapeutic change, independently of the particular therapeutic approach being used:

➤ Unconditional positive regard – a deep and genuine sense of caring for the person through affirmation, validation and warmth

➤ Empathic understanding – ability to understand what the person is feeling, and to communicate this understanding

➤ Congruence – genuine; bringing one's real self into the interaction, rather than trying to present a 'blank canvass'.

Rogers (1980, p. 115) stated: 'It is that the individual has within himself or herself vast resources for self-understanding, for altering his or her self-concept, attitudes and self-directed behaviour – and that these resources can be tapped if only a definable climate of facilitative psychological attitudes can be provided'. Decades of research (Kirschenbaum & Jourdan 2005) have been found to support this hypothesis, although the main criticism has been one of causality: perhaps people rate these attributes as better where therapy has been successful. In addition to the above core conditions for therapeutic work, the below principles are also critical to active listening:

➤ The use of open questions encourages people to talk. Open questions are those that elicit a detailed response, as opposed to closed questions, which elicit a yes or no response. For example, "Are you having a tough time of it at the moment?" is a closed question, as it elicits a yes or no response, thus running the risk of closing down opportunities for discussion. "What's it been like for you, since your brother was diagnosed with X?" is an open question, inviting more of an in-depth response.

➤ As the person responds to questions, the listener should be looking and listening carefully for emotional content, and consider commenting on this, in a warm, empathic manner. For example, "I noticed you just welled up as you were talking about X"; or, "It sounds like you feel really guilty whenever you take some time for yourself".

➤ Enter the conversation with a genuine spirit of curiosity: give yourself permission to step away from any ideas of needing to know the answer in advance. Often, coming alongside the person and sharing in their uncertainty can be very validating for the person. Your role is to listen and facilitate emotional expression, not to solve the problem for the person.

➤ Use reflection to show you are following what the person is saying, either by repeating back an important phrase that they said, for example, Family member: "Things just feel so hopeless at the moment, the number of appointments we have to attend with different people is just taking over my life". Professional: "taking over your life"

➤ Or by paraphrasing, for example, Family member: "I feel like I have to be here all the time, watching out in case anything happens. People keep telling me to look after myself, to take some time out, even just have a bubble bath, but I'd feel so guilty" Professional: "It feels really hard to give yourself permission to take a break".

➤ Similar to paraphrasing, use summarising to help make sense of what the person has told you, at carefully chosen points throughout the session. This can be particularly helpful after a long description of multiple stressors, by helping the person to feel that they have been understood. For example: Professional: "So can I just summarize to check I've understood you correctly? It sounds like you are juggling a lot at the moment. You're feeling a huge sense of loss about your husband being so unwell, and in addition, you understandably feel very angry and let down about the manner in which the diagnosis was made. On top of that, you're trying to maintain routine with collecting your grandson from school, but it's all becoming quite a struggle. Is that right?"

➤ Listen out for metaphors and analogies that the family member uses to describe their experience. Exploring these metaphors can be very helpful in facilitating exploration of the matter at hand. In addition, it can be helpful to tentatively offer metaphors you have heard other people use, while listening to the family's distress. This can often help the family to feel understood, and as though they are not alone in their experiences. For example, "Have you read the Harry Potter books? I'm just wondering something . . . some people have said to me that the word 'schizophrenia' is a bit like 'Voldemort' in Harry Potter. Instead of saying 'Voldemort', people were so frightened, that they would call him 'He Who Must Not Be Named' instead. I'm wondering if it feels like that with the word 'schizophrenia' "?

Below are some ideas for questions to open up discussion about family members' distress. It is usually a good idea to start by 'talking about talking', to begin the process of offering support. It may be useful to normalise the process of offering support to family members, as unfortunately, a taboo still exists around seeking or accepting psychosocial support, in many portions of society:

➤ We tend to offer support for family members as we know how concerning all of this can be. People can feel worried or stressed or alone at times like this. How would you feel about putting aside some time to talk about how this is affecting you?

➤ When and where would be most convenient for you? Who, if anyone, would you like to join us?

➤ What do you think about the idea of talking?

➤ If talking was helpful, how would you know it had been helpful?

If the person whom the family member is caring for has high-level care needs:
➤ Is there any practical support you'd need, to be able to attend an appointment?

During the appointment, again acknowledge that families cope with loved ones' health and mental health needs in many different ways, therefore normalising in advance and giving permission for the family member to be candid:
➤ What's it been like for you, since X became unwell?
➤ How have you been feeling, in yourself, over the last couple of weeks?
➤ What are the main difficulties you face, in caring for X?
➤ How do you feel your family has been managing?
➤ So you're the main support person now . . . how's that affected your role within the family?
➤ How has all of this affected your relationship with X?
➤ Who are you most worried about, in the family?
➤ Is there anyone else around who you talk to about all of this?
➤ What things do you or others do to help you cope with this?
➤ What's kept you going through this, so far?
➤ What are you most proud of about how you've coped as a family?
➤ How are you finding it, talking about all of this with me today?

In certain cases, the person's responses to your questions may cause concern, in which case consider in collaboration with the family member referral to a specialist service. Examples of matters that may indicate a need for referral (Brennan 2004) to a more specialist service (e.g. family therapy service, psychologist, social worker) include:
➤ If the family seem to be unable to care adequately for the person experiencing mental health problems or there is risk of family breakdown due to conflict
➤ If the family member identifies unmet health or social care needs
➤ If the family member appears to be suffering with mental health difficulties above and beyond what might be considered carer distress within the 'normal' range (i.e. the level and duration of distress is causing impairment in daily functioning)
➤ If the family's distress is such that it is interfering with their loved one's recovery or care
➤ If there is conflict between the family member(s) and the professionals.

SELF-ASSESSMENT EXERCISE 16.1 – SEE ANSWERS ON P. 235

Time: 20 minutes
List five barriers and five facilitators to effective listening.

BELIEFS AND URGES ABOUT FIXING PROBLEMS WITHIN THE CARING PROFESSIONS

Most health and social care professionals enter this field because they have a strong desire to help people. This is undoubtedly a worthy and useful attribute that we would all hope our professionals hold. However, in the context of listening to the family's emotional and spiritual pain where a relative has serious mental health difficulties or is dying, this idea of helping can be constraining rather than helpful, depending on how 'helping' is understood by the professional.

In the prevailing medical model of 'mental health problems', ideas around 'curing' or 'fixing' problems abound. Indeed, many models of psychotherapy are also structured around language of 'treatment' and using binary cut-off points on various measures to indicate whether someone's distress is, or is not pathological. Conforming to this medical approach has been hugely beneficial in terms of enabling a plethora of research to be conducted into the various forms of psychotherapy. As a result, psychotherapy is now more widely and freely available than ever before. The down-side to this is that many models of therapy commit the professional to ideas of using techniques to 'fix' people or 'cure' them of their distress.

In the case of family grief about the impending death of their loved one, or a sense of losing their loved one to the grips of mental health difficulties, ideas around fixing and curing are likely to constrain the professional, putting them at risk of sharing in the person's hopelessness. In this context, it is helpful and liberating (and most importantly, beneficial to the family member receiving support) to abandon a 'fixing' mind-set, in favour of 'coming alongside' the person; 'bearing witness to their suffering'; 'walking with them for a portion of their journey'.

What we as professionals want to achieve is often different to what the family members want us to do. Our own urge may be to use techniques to somehow make the pain go away. The family members most often wish to be heard, understood, to have their experiences validated, to feel as though they have an ally, and possibly to have a sounding board. The function of therapy in these cases is therefore to be purely one of listening and validating, in order to provide the family member with time to express their emotions. It is important to put boundaries on 'listening', according to individual services' capacity to mitigate the risk for a dependent relationship developing. It can be helpful to use humour judiciously when discussing this, for example: "There is some flexibility in how many appointments I can offer to talk about this, but funnily enough, most people don't want to see me forever! How about we do X?"

'JUST' LISTENING

During my work in palliative care, my colleagues and I have noted a repeated theme arising. This issue occurs so often that it has been given a name: 'just' listening. We have all been trained in a range of sophisticated psychological models of supporting people. While effective listening skills are key to each of these models, they include multiple techniques, which can be drawn upon to facilitate therapeutic change. From our trainings, we hold beliefs that listening is essential, but not always sufficient for positive outcomes. We hold fears that 'just' listening may encourage rumination, awfulising, and negative attention biases, well-known maintaining factors in multiple mental health difficulties. However, for family members of people using mental health and palliative care services, often the main emotions they encounter are grief and loss. For these emotions in particular, effective listening skills are possibly the most powerful tools we have at our disposal. Grief and loss are not pathological, nor is anxiety in the context of witnessing a loved one's suffering. People consistently report feeling listened to at their time of need as highly beneficial. Whilst further research into the most effective ways of supporting relatives is clearly required, our practice-based evidence strongly suggests that listening is an efficient and effective approach, with many people requiring only one session.

We have come to the conclusion that, while techniques from a range of psychological approaches are very useful if used judiciously, for many family members experiencing pain in relation to their loved one's suffering, 'just' listening is more than sufficient.

REFLECTIVE PRACTICE EXERCISE 16.1

> **Time: 15 minutes**
> - What is effective listening?
> - How will this help you, in practice?
> - How will this help the individual and family in practice?

In your professional role, practice using effective listening skills. Notice how it feels to really listen, resisting the urge to offer solutions. Notice any thoughts that come up while you are listening (e.g. "I should be offering an intervention"; "This seems hopeless, what can I do to help?"). Notice these thoughts and quickly bring your attention back to listening to the person. Notice how this influences your relationship with the person. Notice how it affects the direction and content of the session.

CONFIGURING SERVICES TO PROVIDE SUPPORT FOR FAMILY MEMBERS

Given the financial and social pressures faced by mental health services, it is likely that the burden on family members is increasing exponentially. Demand for mental health services is increasing and it seems unlikely, given the global economic climate, that funding is going to increase within the next decade. While the burden for family members is increasing, this means that relatives are providing a large proportion of mental health service delivery for free. They are keeping people out of hospital; they are probably providing informal therapy in the form of listening and advice giving; and they are certainly often providing a highly vigilant risk-management service.

It is clear from the research literature that family members of people experiencing mental health difficulties have far higher levels of anxiety, depression, stress and distress than those in the general population (e.g. Oldridge & Hughes, 1992). They are therefore, at considerable risk of burnout, characterised by emotional exhaustion, depersonalisation (i.e. a cynical and uncaring attitude towards the person they care for) and an inadequate sense of accomplishment (Maslach 2001). If family members themselves become mentally unwell or burnt out, this will undoubtedly have significant ramifications for mental health services. It is therefore worthwhile for service managers to consider investing in support for families and caregivers in the same way that palliative care services do. In palliative care, family support is an integral part of the service and is enshrined in the values and mission statements of palliative care services. Indeed, from a systemic perspective, it is essential to consider people within the wider system in which they live and to directly include members of the system in the intervention.

It is well known that for initiatives to succeed in health settings, there must be both top-down and bottom-up processes. Therefore, in terms of providing support to family members in mental health settings, lessons can be learnt from palliative care settings. Examples of top-down artefacts that demonstrate organisations' support for family members include:

> ➤ Information Technology (IT) or filing systems, which include files for family members
> ➤ family policies
> ➤ family member support groups
> ➤ training for staff in supporting family members
> ➤ carer assessments being routinely conducted
> ➤ services being commissioned and rewarded financially for demonstrating their support of family members.

Evidence of bottom-up factors relating to support for family members would include a culture existing amongst professionals whereby holding an appointment with a family member is as valued as an appointment with a person experiencing mental health difficulties. Indeed, if the 'problem' is located within the system rather than within the person, then it stands to reason that if the health of the system is restored, results from the intervention are likely to be more effective and long lasting.

It has been demonstrated in palliative care contexts that looking after family members is as much of a sound financial investment, as it is an ethical obligation. The recommendation about caring for family members is not a new one, and is recommended in the 2010 (DoH) Carers Strategy. While it is easy to see how the current economic climate makes it difficult for mental health services to implement this, it is highly likely that investing in this area would pay for itself.

REFLECTIVE PRACTICE EXERCISE 16.2

Time: 50 minutes
- What is the culture in your organisation, in relation to listening to family members' concerns?
- What evidence is there, in your organisation, of structures, systems and policies (e.g. family members' or carers' groups, carer assessments, IT systems, targets) that support listening to family members?
- How do you go about including the family in 'patient work' at present?
- How might you improve your own and your organisation's ability to listen to families' pain more routinely?
- Identify a senior professional who is in a position to influence and to make changes needed. TAKE ACTION!

THE ETHICS OF LISTENING IN A MENTAL HEALTH CONTEXT

The experiences of severe and life-limiting mental and physical illnesses are deeply personal and individual. Telling one's own story or narrative about this has benefits in addition to catharsis or emotional expression. By speaking about the experience and being listened to, people are able to make sense and make meaning of what has happened to them. They can develop a coherent explanation of events, and find a way to integrate this into their broader life story and belief system (Brennan 2004). It is clear to see, therefore, that listening is a vital resource in a mental health context.

In mental health contexts, it could be said that a curative (as opposed to symptom management) culture prevails – and rightly so: most people enter into treatment with the aim of 'cure'. However, it is important to consider how 'cure' is defined, in the world of mental health services. Many services use symptom-based questionnaires and outcome measures to monitor how people are responding to treatment. This presents a risk that professionals and individuals become so caught up in trying to 'get rid' of unpleasant symptoms, that listening to the person's distress or taking a curious interest in their hopes and dreams for life inadvertently becomes neglected.

Indeed, this may mirror a process that often takes place during the goal-setting phase of therapy, whereby the person seeking help articulates goals around symptom reduction, e.g. "I want to feel less anxious/depressed"; "I want to stop these panic attacks". Therapists across modalities will usually explore this further, to move the goal away from symptom elimination, and towards actions, values and quality of life, e.g. "So, if you were less depressed, what would you be doing differently"; "If your panic attacks were better, what difference would that make to your life?". Moving away from goals based on symptom cure then frees up both the person and the professional to consider how the person can maximise their quality of life.

It could be the case that using a listening approach as opposed to a technique focused on 'getting rid of' unpleasant emotions may liberate the health and social care professional to attend more closely to the family's pain. If the clinician's goal is to listen to the family's pain rather than trying to make it go away, this could, paradoxically, be more helpful than trying to 'fix' it. For example, Acceptance and Commitment Therapy (ACT, a form of Cognitive Behavioural Therapy (CBT), focusing on using mindfulness skills to help people to 'make space for' emotions in order that they can pursue a valued direction in life) proposes that attempts to control or get rid of emotions are futile. The metaphor of quicksand is used to illustrate this: when you fall into quicksand, your instinct is to struggle to climb out. However, the more you struggle, the deeper you sink into the quicksand. The solution is, despite your urges to struggle, you should lie still, spreading your body weight over a large surface area so that you float. The same can be said for emotions: struggling against them is not effective and takes us away from doing the things that really matter to us in life. ACT proposes that people drop the struggle and instead, allow feelings to be there (Harris 2009), whilst focusing on taking actions towards a valued and fulfilling life.

There are parallels here at the level of service delivery: perhaps listening to family members' pain allows the professional to drop the struggle with trying to fix the person's difficult emotions, and enables the professional to behave in a way that is congruent with the values that initially brought them into the profession. By accepting thoughts of wanting to apply a particular technique or say something astute, and instead acting on values of compassion, warmth, empathy and kindness, this can set the conditions for the most powerful of interventions; one we all have at our disposal: listening.

REFLECTIVE PRACTICE EXERCISE 16.3

Time: 30 minutes
- What are your values as a professional?
- What kind of helper do you want to be?
- How do you want to be remembered by your colleagues and those individuals you are caring for?
- What sort of attributes do you hold dear?

> KEY POINTS 16.1

➤ People who use palliative care and mental health services do not exist in a vacuum: systemic approaches strongly advocate involving and supporting families.

➤ Families are an under-recognised and under-valued source of care and support in people's lives.

➤ Family members providing emotional support are likely to experience grief, loss, fear, role change and stress.

➤ National policy documents recommend that services are configured to include families in care planning, and to provide emotional support to them.

➤ Effective listening skills are key to nearly all empirically grounded psychotherapeutic approaches.

➤ Active listening is a powerful tool at the disposal of all health and social care professionals, which is rated as highly beneficial by family members.

➤ It may be common for health and social care professionals to feel an urge to 'fix' problems. While problem solving is very useful, in cases where there is no obvious short-term solution, listening can be an effective intervention, through validating the person's experience.

➤ Service managers and commissioners should consider reviewing the extent to which their organisation is designed to provide support to family members, from both an ethical and economic perspective.

REFERENCES

Brennan, J. (2004) *Cancer in Context.* Oxford: Oxford University Press.

Cree, L., Brooks, H. L., Berzins, K., Fraser, C., Lovell, K. and Bee, P. (2015) 'Carers' experiences of involvement in care planning: a qualitative exploration of the facilitators and barriers to engagement with mental health services.' *BioMed Central Psychiatry*, 15, 1–11. Available at: https://bmcpsy chiatry.biomedcentral.com/track/pdf/10.1186/s12888-015-0590-y?site=bmcpsychiatry.biomed central.com (Accessed: 26 August 2017)

Department of Health. (DoH – 1999) *Caring About Carers: A National Strategy for Carers.* London: Department of Health.

Department of Health. (2010) *Recognised, Valued and Supported: Next Steps for the Carers Strategy.* London: Department of Health.

Grad, J. and Sainsbury, P. (1963) 'Mental illness and the family'. *The Lancet*, 281, pp. 544–7.

Griffiths, J., Speed, S., Horne, M. and Keeley, P. (2012) ' "A caring professional attitude": What service users and carers seek in graduate nurses and the challenge for educators'. *Nurse Education Today*, 32, pp. 121–7.

Harris, R. (2009) *ACT Made Simple.* CA: New Harbinger.

Jenkins, K. and North, N. (2008) *Psychological Assessment Skills: A Training Course for All Health and Social Care Staff Working in Cancer Services.* Salisbury: Macmillan.

Kirschenbaum, H. and Jourdan, A. (2005) 'The current status of Carl Rogers and the Person-Centred Approach'. *Psychotherapy: Theory, Research, Practice, Training*, 42, pp. 37–51.

Lavis, A., Lester, H., Everard, L., Freemantle, N., Amos, T. et al. (2015) 'Layers of listening: qualitative analysis of the impact of early intervention services for first-episode psychosis on carers' experiences'. *British Journal of Psychiatry*, 207, pp. 135–42.

Maslach, C. (2001) 'What we have learned about burnout and health'. *Psychological Health*, 16, pp. 607–11.

Mendolia, M. and Kleck, R. E. (1993) 'Effects of talking about a stressful event on arousal: does what we talk about make a difference'? *Journal of Personality and Social Psychology*, 64, pp. 283–92.

Oldridge, M. and Hughes, I. (1992) 'Psychological well-being in families with a member suffering from schizophrenia'. *British Journal of Psychiatry*, 161, pp. 249–51.

Oppawsky, J. (2016) 'Silence is a counselling skill'. *The Journal of the American Association of Integrative Medicine*, Available at: (Accessed: 26 August 2017)

Rogers, C. R. (1951) *Client-Centered Therapy*. London: Constable.

Rogers, C. R. (1957) The necessary and sufficient conditions of therapeutic personality change. *Journal of Consulting Psychology*, 21, pp. 95–103.

Rogers, C. R. (1980) *A Way of Being*. Boston: Houghton Mifflin.

Rumpold, T., Schur, S., Amering, M., Kirchheiner, K., Masel, E. K. et al. (2015) 'Informal caregivers of advanced-stage cancer patients: every second is at risk for psychiatric morbidity'. *Supportive Care in Cancer*, 24, pp. 1975–82.

Stott, J. and Martin, E. (2010) 'Creating contexts for talking and listening where older people feel comfortable and respected'. In: Fredman, G., Anderson, E. and Stott, J. eds. *Being With Older People: A Systemic Approach*. London: Karnac, pp. 87–112.

The King's Fund. (2015) *Briefing Paper: Mental Health Under Pressure*. Available at: www.kings fund.org.uk/sites/files/kf/field/field_publication_file/mental-health-under-pressure-nov15_0.pdf (Accessed: 26 August 2017)

World Health Organization. (2017) *WHO definition of palliative care*. Available at: www.who.int/ cancer/palliative/definition/en/ (Accessed 31 August 2017)

Yalom, I. D. (2001) *The Gift of Therapy: Reflections on Being a Therapist*. London: Piatkus.

To Learn More

Blanchard, G. G. (1997) 'The crisis of cancer: psychological impact on family caregivers'. *Oncology*, 11: 189–94.

Brennan, J. (2004) *Cancer in Context*. Oxford University Press: Oxford.

Girgis, A., Lambert, S., Johnson, C., Waller, A. and Currow, D. (2013) 'Physical, psychosocial, relationship, and economic burden of caring for people with cancer: a review'. *Journal of Oncology Practice*, 9, 197–202.

Withnell, N. and Murphy, N. (2012) *Family Interventions in Mental Health*. Open University Press: England.

ANSWERS TO SELF-ASSESSMENT EXERCISE 16.1 – *SEE* P. 229

➤ Barriers: inadequate time; clock-watching; lack of privacy; interruptions; distractions (e.g. TV on); practical issues such a family member not being able to spare time to attend appointment; invading personal space; excessive or inadequate eye contact; filling silences; offering platitudes (e.g. "look on the bright side", "it could be worse"); jargon; putting on an act; closed questions

➤ Facilitators: personal space; good eye contact; reducing power imbalances (e.g. consider height and positioning of chairs); silences; allowing someone time to cry; nodding; congruent facial expressions; congruent tone of voice; verbal encouragers (e.g. "go on", "mmhmmm"); unconditional positive regard; validation; warmth; empathy; congruence (being yourself rather than trying to act like a therapist); open questions; looking and listening for emotions; curiosity; reflection and paraphrasing; summarising; metaphors.

CHAPTER 17

Substance Use

Jacqueline Talmet and Charlotte Francis Champion de Crespigny

INTRODUCTION

No-one sets out to develop alcohol or other drug (AOD) problems or dependence. Alcohol and other drugs (AODs) are used to feel good, have fun or for a specific purpose such as alleviation of distressing mental ill-health symptoms, traumatic memories or to manage physical pain.

Some people who use AODs will develop long-term, severe dependence where change is often difficult or impossible. The philosophy and practices of palliative care can be used to provide treatment and supportive interventions to severely dependent people and or their family members or significant others. This may include a situation where a severely dependent person is terminally ill (*See* Chapter 22 and 23).

The palliative care approach to caring for all individuals consists of 'total' active person-centred care by the intra- inter-disciplinary team, throughout ill-health where a curative treatment is not an option. It consists of symptom management (*See* Chapter 9), addressing physical, psychological, spiritual and social needs and extends into bereavement. The focus is not only on the individual but also those people whom the individual identifies as family. The goal of palliative care is to promote quality of life and 'comfort care'. Relief of suffering is the overriding ethic of palliative care. All health professionals can adopt and provide this approach, whatever the person's ill-health needs.

What is not recognised is that AOD treatment and interventions are not often associated with being a palliative strategy. However, this is the case and it will become evident in the topics and in case scenarios used to highlight the use of palliative care practices, provision of care and its outcomes. This chapter will identify:

➤ Strategies of palliative care in AOD specialist treatment settings
➤ Barriers, dilemmas and special considerations, which often impact negatively on the severely dependent persons health care experience and treatment outcomes
➤ Components of assessment, care planning, palliative treatment and interventions
➤ Continuity of treatment when a person who is receiving medication-assisted treatment for opioid dependence (MAT: OD) is admitted to or discharged from hospital
➤ What needs to happen for palliative care to receive recognition as a legitimate approach in AOD service settings.

ALCOHOL AND OTHER DRUGS (AOD) PALLIATIVE CARE STRATEGIES

Palliative care provision is a legitimate component of the continuum of care for people experiencing severe AOD dependence. In this setting, it is not necessarily about managing end-of-life although it may be. It is about using the strategies of palliative care to respond to the needs and maintain the quality of life of people who for any reason are not able to enact change.

In this setting, a range of strategies are deployed to address all concurrent comorbidities to maintain the person in an optimal state until they are ready for change and or recovery or to support a person long term and or to the end-of-life.

This approach recognises the person's long and often difficult journey prior to referral to a specialist AOD service as well as the time required to, achieve stabilisation, treat and/or manage severe dependence and to obtain differing levels of recovery. Common examples where the need for a palliative approach might be established include:

➤ The severity of dependence where the fear of change inhibits or makes sustained change difficult or unachievable despite a high level of commitment and the person working hard to reduce their use or to obtain or maintain abstinence (*See* Case Study 17.1 John pp. 248–249)

➤ Repeated attempts and difficulty in sustaining change leading to a person's decision that they cannot or do not wish to engage in treatment and are amenable to receive continued support. In this instance, the person makes this decision in full knowledge of the consequences to their health, well-being, quality of life and life expectancy (*See* Case Study 17.2 Julie. pp. 250–251)

➤ A person has severe iatrogenic opioid dependence and is increasingly seeking higher doses of opioid medications when there is no current identifiable or justified need for these medications

➤ A person living with dependence who has a terminal illness.

BARRIERS

People experiencing severe dependence have the same needs and rights to access the same range of services including palliative interventions as any other person receiving health care.

However, despite the need for compassion and equity of access to services, people often experience discrimination, are stigmatised and negative labelled, and receive inadequate care.

This leads to people refusing to attend health services even when they are critically ill and impacts negatively on the willingness or decision to engage, agree to or adherence to treatment requirements and early opting out. These factors often result in negative treatment outcomes, increased morbidity, needless suffering or early death.

Past negative experiences may result in people feeling stressed or fearful when attending health services and to responding in ways aimed at self-protection. People commonly report anxiety and anger arising from:

➤ Failure to provide or provision of inadequate medication doses to avoid or ameliorate withdrawal symptoms. In alcohol dependence, it is an act of cruelty that can lead to complicated withdrawal including seizures, hallucinosis or life-threatening delirium tremens. This experience is exceedingly traumatic and never forgotten.

➤ Altering, discontinuance or failure to administer their daily MAT: OD dose.

➤ Under medicating pain or fear of its re-emergence when there is currently good pain relief. This arises when professionals label legitimate requests as 'drug seeking'. People receiving MAT: OD report, being ignored, withholding of prescribed doses or of medication orders not being actioned and experiencing traumatic unrelieved pain.
➤ Negative professional response when the person does not meet expectations of abstinence or change and acceptance of treatment options to reach this goal when this is not the person's goal.

Being welcoming, kind, respectful, culturally sensitive, non-judgemental and encouraging will assist engagement, allay fear and anxiety and assist the person to make decisions about their care. It will also assist in rapport building, development of trust and engagement and retention in treatment, which is the primary consideration when providing any health service.

Encouraging people to discuss their fears and providing information around how their dependence, or MAT: OD may affect pain management. Providing reassurance that care plans will include noting the need and frequency of pain relief and or withdrawal medications will be communicated to the entire care team, will allay fear and anxiety and build trust and confidence that the service will meet their needs.

Encouragement to report inadequate care will empower the person to raise concerns and be reassured the service is taking their concerns seriously.

DILEMMAS

Health professionals may encounter ethical dilemmas in hospital or other residential settings, particularly where a person:
➤ Wishes to continue illicit or legal drug use onsite where this is inappropriate or banned may cause earlier death, or result in a vulnerable person being discharged
➤ Seeks to use cannabis in jurisdictions where this is illegal to assist with pain relief or where this may impact on others
➤ Requests for pain relief are beyond the daily opioid or MAT: OD or other drugs of dependence dosing limits or the frequency noted in service procedures
➤ Requests for administration of high or additional doses, which will induce intoxication, toxicity or induce overdose
➤ Requests euthanasia in jurisdictions where it is illegal
➤ Is intoxicated on presentation, which has implications for informed consent. Advanced care directives may need to be considered or consent sought from next of kin
➤ Asks a health professional for support in exploring their spirituality when the professional does not hold beliefs, or, to practise their spirituality where this is at variance with the professional's beliefs or is forbidden in that country.

Consideration of expected dilemmas and the development of guidelines to communicate accepted responses and enact common practices will promote appropriate care and provide professionals with confidence and support to respond in a supportive way. This is particularly important when working with AOD dependent people who have a wide peer network and share information about the practices of professionals.

Prescribing regular or rescue pain relief medications for people in community settings may raise concerns about the potential risk to the community from medication diversion, particularly when a nominated carer is also opioid dependent. Diversion risk can be difficult to judge and navigate when seeking to ensure adequate pain relief, including when the person is on MAT: OD and has hyperalgesia. Strategies such as limiting unsupervised doses and weekly or daily pick up of doses or weekly rescue medications from a community pharmacy can reduce diversion risk.

SPECIAL CONSIDERATIONS

Multiple Comorbidities, Multi Pharmacy and Illicit Drug Use

People experiencing dependence often have a range of complex bio psycho comorbidities that require poly pharmacological treatment and at times the prescription of more than one drug of dependence or central nervous system (CNS) depressant.

Poly Pharmacy can affect the efficacy of medication treatment due to 'pharmacokinetic and pharmacodynamic drug interactions'. [These may include] 'additive effects, potentiation, synergism and antagonism'. [In addition, there may be risks for increased side-effects] 'drug toxicity, intoxication, overdose, adverse drug reactions, cross tolerance and poly drug dependence', (de Crespigny & Talmet 2012, p. 2).

Commonly used methadone and combined buprenorphine and naloxone medications in MAT: OD treatment and or illicit AOD use add further complexity and additional needs for considering these effects. With ongoing medication review at the time of initial assessment and when prescribing new medications, an addictions specialist physician can assist in the monitoring and management of these effects, potential drug interactions and impact on treatment efficacy.

CONCURRENT MENTAL ILL-HEALTH

A person experiencing comorbid severe mental ill-health may be prescribed medications to provide symptomatic relief or may use illicit or other prescribed drugs to reduce or enhance the symptoms of mental ill-health or to create a euphoric state. Some examples include:

➤ The use of high doses of benztropine prescribed to control extra pyramidal effects to obtain euphoria, which may also cause death. Daily or weekly pick up of doses can limit potential for misuse

➤ Destabilisation of mental health conditions arising from high dose amphetamines and or cannabis use, particularly when a drug is used for a specific purpose related to mental health symptoms, such as:

   – Use of amphetamines to prevent downward mood swing in bipolar disorders. Engaging in a discussion around the unwanted downward mood shift and the development of plans for early identification and interventions (EI&I) can prevent the need for self-medication with amphetamines

   – Increasing cannabis use to re-establish auditory hallucinations (which need further investigation when they are not a symptom of mental ill-health) when they have always been present, and the person feels lost without them. This follows their unwanted removal by antipsychotic medications. Negotiation around wanted and unwanted symptoms of mental ill-health, review of medications and or dose and engaging with the person to obtain the wanted medication effect may assist in treatment adherence, reducing cannabis use and the severity of both dependence and mental ill-health.

➤ High-risk poly drug use and dependence may increase the severity of mental ill-health symptoms and impede treatment. Engaging and supporting the person in a discussion about concerns for safety will open the dialogue where encouragement and support can be provided to either seek AOD treatment or reduce drug use. It may be helpful to initially focus on the drug causing the most harm to mental health (often amphetamines). Seeking consultancy or referral to a specialist AOD services may also assist.

LOSS OF HOPE AND SELF-EFFICACY BELIEFS

Loss of hope for recovery from severe dependence, multiple relapses, limited effectiveness of pain relief medications and/or feelings of powerlessness over pending terminal ill-health outcome, can all impact negatively on the person's beliefs about the ability to achieve change or recovery and or loss of interest in living.

Encouragement, accurate positive feedback around reaching goals, installing hope and skills building will enhance beliefs that change, recovery and/or improvement is possible. Where this is not possible, being open to and drawing on the person's spirituality and or religious beliefs can assist in developing peace, strengths and sense of life's meaning and knowing for the future (*See* Chapter 23).

SELF-ASSESSMENT EXERCISE 17.1

Time: 20 minutes
- Consider your experiences working alongside people experiencing severe dependence. Does your experience fit with what has been outlined? What might you add?
- What would you do to address the circumstances raised in your professional practice?
- What guidelines might you implement and what would be their content if you wanted to maintain the person in treatment?

ASSESSMENT

Screening for AOD problems or dependence and when indicated, 'assessment' [of their significance and potential impact on the options and needs for care and treatment,] 'is required in all health care settings irrespective of the persons need for health care', (Adapted with permission from de Crespigny & Talmet 2012, p. 30). In undertaking assessment, the use of street jargon is best avoided as drug terms and slang names are used interchangeably across different communities and may result in obtaining an inaccurate drug history.

Content of Assessment

The assessment provides an opportunity for engagement in discussion about past negative experiences, allaying anxiety and providing information about what will occur and to plan for what the person can do if a negative experience occurs.

The assessment obtains information that will assist in planning interventions and includes obtaining information about:

> Past and current AOD use:
> – 'type of drug used' (illicit, prescribed or OTC)
> – the purpose medications or illicit drug use is fulfilling

> Age and time of first use (e.g. days, weeks, months, years)
> 'Dose, pattern and frequency of use'
> 'Date and time of last use' to predict the likely time of withdrawal onset for each drug of dependence and its severity
> Method of use (injected, swallowed, smoked, snorted), perceptions of harms associated with use and or route of administration and to identify high-risk practices
> Needs for harm reduction education
> History of past and current AOD treatment
> History of past 'withdrawal syndrome' to predict severity of dependence likely severity of withdrawal and possible complications including 'withdrawal seizures' or delirium tremens
> History of mental ill-health, current treatment and medications, wanted and unwanted effects on mood or symptoms and their purpose. History of self-harm and risk of harm to or from others
> Physical assessment and urine drug screen, blood tests for liver function, hepatitis B, C and or human immunodeficiency virus – HIV infection) with pre- and post-test counselling and informed consent.

(Adapted with permission from de Crespigny & Talmet 2012, pp. 37 and 178)

SELF-ASSESSMENT EXERCISE 17.2

Time: 30 minutes
- Consider how you undertake assessment with a person who attends your health service
- Look at the components of AOD assessment and how it might apply to your everyday practice
- Consider any changes you would like to make to what occurs now
- Consider how these could be implemented.

INTERVENTION PLANNING

Treatment and intervention planning alongside people experiencing severe AOD dependence seeks to address all issues identified in the comprehensive assessment. The plan is developed in collaboration with the care team, the person and welcomes in accordance with the person's wishes the involvement of family, partners, carers and or significant others. It is helpful if the person and all carers (*See* Chapter 16) receive a copy of the plan and plans for relapse management to enable understanding of what to do in these circumstances.

Considerations in planning care include the person's readiness, willingness and ability for change, level of dependence, needs for treatment and, current evidence-based practice and AOD treatment guidelines and:

➤ The need for congruency between the professional's and the person's treatment goal.
➤ The utility of withdrawal as it is not a stand-alone or effective treatment in alcohol or opioid dependence, but is useful in stabilising uncontrolled AOD use
➤ Identifying a palliative approach to treatment and interventions where change is not immediately possible or is unlikely in the long term and or where the person is terminally ill
➤ Where a person is competent, discussing their advanced care directives might provide an opportunity to refresh their memory or to have them reviewed and or amended. These are communicated to the treating team and documented in the clinical record.

In addition to addressing severe dependence, the plan may also need to address AOD sequelae including where the person may have:
➤ Severe alcohol dependence where breath alcohol levels regularly reach 0.35–0.4mgl (milligrams per litre of blood) without intoxication. There may also be alcohol-related liver disease or brain injury, oesophageal varices, spontaneous bleeding due to low platelet count and a risk for Wernicke's encephalopathy if malnourished or Wernicke Korsakoff's Syndrome (See Case Study 17.1 John pp. 248–249)
➤ Blood borne virus and liver failure from chronic hepatitis C and or acquired immune deficiency syndrome (AIDS) from human immunodeficiency virus (HIV) infection
➤ Health problems relating to a drug's action that can occur with single or occasional use such as methamphetamine related cerebro-vascular accident (CVA)
➤ Intoxication related accidental injury
➤ Intentional or accidental overdose due to high dose or concurrent use of CNS depressants
➤ Increasing opioid dependence severity arising from long-term treatment like a painful injury or musculoskeletal condition or, when evidence based pain relief guidelines are not followed, (See Case Study 17.3 Myra and May pp. 252–253)
➤ Experienced a long history of severe dependence and other comorbidities that may have led to:
   – Loss of employment
   – Decreased physical fitness or mobility
   – A lifestyle where obtaining AODs is the primary activity
   – Criminology to purchase drugs and current pending legal matters
   – Reduction in life skills and capacity for attention to self-care and activities of daily living such as cleaning, nutrition, and financial issues, which may lead to homelessness
   – Social Isolation

The family and partners (See Chapter 16) of people experiencing severe dependence may also have had a lengthy journey where events may have resulted in the loved one being shunned or lost to family contact. This may include:
➤ Unsuccessfully assisting the person to address their drug use and frustration when they do not understand the nature of dependence, why AOD use continues despite the presence of harm and that relapse is to be expected
➤ Experiencing stress when the loved one is incarcerated for drug related crime

➤ Providing care for chronic conditions and sadness when the condition deteriorates
➤ Grief for the loss of the loved one as they were before commencing AOD use
➤ Violence towards family members
➤ Initiation of younger siblings into AOD use
➤ Extreme stress for the loved one's welfare when drug dealers threaten violence for non-payment of debts. This results in requests to provide money, which may create financial difficulties but is paid to prevent the threatened harm.

KEY POINT 17.1

As in a palliative care setting, the ethic of care is on the family, as well as the individual receiving treatment.

Referral to AOD services might be indicated for management of severe iatrogenic or drug dependence for people who are not in the end-of-life stage of their ill-health or where the aim is stabilisation and or long-term recovery. AOD professionals may need to provide consultancy, advocacy, training and support to health services for assessment, investigation of pain and its management, withdrawal and counselling strategies.

The needs for family support may include, assisting the family to re-establish or maintain contact with the dependant person, supporting the family member to assist their loved one throughout the journey, not just whilst they are terminally ill, or in the event of death and further providing support during the grief period, (*See* Case Study 17.2 Julie pp. 250–251).

TREATMENT

Most AOD treatment and interventions are aimed at palliative care. That is to maintain the person at their optimal state until they are either ready for change or at the end-of-life. (*See* Chapter 21).

Intervention and treatment responds with immediacy or timeliness to changes in the person's presentation. Alcohol and other drug (AOD) treatment and other palliative interventions, such as, harm reduction are used to provide the required care.

A person receiving treatment may be able to attain recovery in the longer term or be in a terminal phase of life and or may be at continual risk of sudden death from drug related sequelae. Treatment strategies may include:

➤ MAT treatment for AOD dependence. This treatment includes MAT: OD for severe opioid dependence where methadone, buprenorphine and naloxone combined and on occasion, other pain relieving medications are used to stabilise drug use to one daily dose of long acting analgesia. This manages dependence, provides chronic pain relief and prevents withdrawal. Following relapse, re stabilisation may be required
➤ MAT: OD for chronic pain management may also include the use of:
  – complimentary treatments including massage, TENS (transcutaneous electrical nerve stimulation), acupuncture or exercise
  – non-opioid alternatives to augment analgesia such as paracetamol or non-steroidal anti-inflammatory drugs (NSAIDs)

- residential commencement and stabilisation of MAT: OD treatment, usually when withdrawal from other drugs of dependence is wanted by the person and is clinically indicated or community based stabilisation is not helpful.

➤ Referral to a substance use specialist for consultation advice on the management of:
- hazardous patterns of poly drug use
- chronic pain associated with iatrogenic dependence
- medical sequelae arising from AOD use
- complex comorbidities and multi-pharmacological management
- advice about managing analgesia in the person with diagnosed chronic pain established hyperalgesia and severe dependence treatment with MAT: OD

➤ Ongoing monitoring progress, outcomes and follow up for all AOD sequelae may include referral for treatment of oesophageal varices, urine drug screens or periodic blood profiles to monitor progress or scans to indicate the need for hepatitis C treatment

➤ Admission to specialist withdrawal services or hospital, which may be the first step in stabilisation on MAT, or to reduce the level of dependence. This occurs when moderate to severe withdrawal is predicted requiring medication management or where there is a history of withdrawal seizures, alcohol hallucinosis or the life-threatening withdrawal complication of delirium tremens

➤ Admission to respite care, hospital or AOD service may occur to:
- provide live in re-stabilisation
- improve physical or nutritional status or during hygiene remediation of the person's living environment
- treat acute or chronic disease or give the person a break from their current situation or when they are unwell
- support carers through giving opportunities for holidays or a rest to prevent exhaustion
- create the environment to encourage and enhance motivation for change, enable decision making, to amend treatment plans.

➤ Provision of counselling and supportive interventions and its content will depend on the person's needs. It may be needed to guide the person through treatment or interventions processes, provide support for change or assist in preventing relapse and maintaining the person in treatment. Moreover, it may be to provide support for and educate the person and family about what will occur as the condition deteriorates and there is progression towards end-of-life or to plan and implement change when it becomes possible due to decreased severity of dependence and/or changes to the persons AOD goals.

➤ Person and family education depends on needs and might include:
- Education about their condition, the drugs being used, risks, dependence, adaptive behaviours and available intervention and treatment options available will assist in selecting preferred options

- Lifestyle advice including activities, nutrition, hydration and sleep
- Relapse prevention information and skills development
- How to manage the side effects of MAT: OD medications.

➤ Harm reduction information is aimed at preventing 'AOD related harm' by providing education to reduce the risks related 'to, the drug, dose, duration and frequency of use, method of administration' and 'poly drug use', and:
- the varying purity of illicit drugs
- reduction in tolerance and potential overdose following periods of abstinence
- 'preventing overdose due to concomitant use of more than one CNS depressant drug
- 'always using clean injecting equipment (tourniquets, spoons, needles, syringes, alcohol swabs, water and filters) to avoid blood borne virus (BBV) infection' and prevent the injection of foreign bodies
- choosing less risky methods of use such as oral or nasal administration
- 'safer and sterile injection techniques to avoid vein damage', or infections that can cause abscesses or septicaemia.

(Adapted with permission from de Crespigny & Talmet 2012, pp. 5 & 6)

➤ Vaccination – Influenza in vulnerable people, hepatitis B immunisation for injecting drug users not already exposed to the virus, and other preventable diseases
➤ Provision of thiamine for high risk or binge drinking and or poor nutrition.
➤ Referral to mental health services for collaborative management of mental health and AOD comorbidity
➤ Intra- inter-disciplinary and agency liaison and case conferencing including participation of the person, family, partners or significant others in accordance with the individual's wishes and carers. This serves to coordinate and manage care and seamless transition across services, monitor health status and acts as an early warning system for increased risks, physical deterioration, need for review and or respite management.
➤ Addressing social problems, which may include referral to NGO services to address:
- Housing and or homelessness
- Legal matters and or imprisonment, which has poorer health outcomes
- Financial matters relating to drug debt and/or under or unemployment
- Isolation, alienation from family
- The lack of fun activities such as interests or hobbies
- Friendship group comprising people who use AODs.

ACUTE PAIN MANAGEMENT

When providing care, it is important to note that pain relief is to maintain comfort and that 'pain is a natural antagonist to opioid induced respiratory and CNS depression' (de Crespigny & Talmet 2012, p. 226).

Keeping in mind that requests for increased pain relief may be required due to tolerance and hyperalgesia in a person experiencing a long opioid dependence history and can assist in making clinical decisions to maintain comfort.

'The respect and belief of the person's reports of pain' [and] 'treating' [acute] 'pain aggressively' [acknowledges that] 'treating dependence' [is not a priority during the acute pain period] (de Crespigny & Talmet 2012, p. 227).

When there are concerns regarding the nature or severity of pain, objective 'assessment can provide for evidence of pain which will decrease the chance of' [over medication and] 'support administration of opioid analgesia', (de Crespigny & Talmet 2012, p. 226).

SMOOTHNESS TRANSITION FOR PEOPLE RECEIVING MEDICATION ASSISTED TREATMENT FOR OPIOID DEPENDENCE (MAT: OD)

Seamless transition across community and hospital services is important to ensure continuity of dosing, maintenance of dose stability and to prevent extraneous drug use. It requires intra- inter-agency communication at specific points in the person's transition.

There is a prominent misconception that the MAT: OD dose provides adequate pain relief and provision of further medication is unnecessary. On admission to hospital, the health professional on being advised of MAT: OD treatment contacts the medication private prescriber, AOD service or dispensing pharmacy to obtain or provide information about:

➤ Admission: confirm 'the date, time' and 'amount' of last dose and when the next dose is due
➤ Needs for pain relief in addition to MAT: OD treatment
➤ Where the person gets their medication, e.g. at the AOD service or community pharmacy
➤ The medication being used e.g. methadone or buprenorphine or other e.g. Fentanyl
➤ 'Dose (recorded in mgs)'
➤ 'Number of unsupervised doses usually provided per week and whether the person has any in their possession. If so, forward them to the hospital pharmacy. These doses are not used in hospital and are not returned to the person on discharge. The treatment service or doctor is advised of the number of doses retrieved so the person is not identified as diverting doses'.

(Adapted with permission from de Crespigny & Talmet
2012, pp. 206 & 207)

On discharge the hospital team:
➤ Notifies the AOD service, GP and/or pharmacy of the person's impending discharge and when they will receive the last dose at the hospital
➤ 'Advises of any medications such as opioids or benzodiazepines given during hospitalization' [as] 'they may show up on routine urine drug screening' [which may affect access to or the provision of unsupervised doses] (Compton, Athanasos & de Crespigny 2006 in de Crespigny & Talmet 2012, p. 228)
➤ 'Provides details of any short-term analgesia (opioid or otherwise) provided on discharge', (Compton, Athanasos & de Crespigny 2006 in de Crespigny & Talmet 2012, p. 228)

➤ 'Arranges' for 'MAT: OD prescription from the AOD service' or prescriber to be at the persons dosing pharmacy prior to discharge. 'The person is informed' of 'any arrangements' made (de Crespigny & Talmet 2012, p. 207).

CHRONIC PAIN AND IATROGENIC DEPENDENCE

Dependence may arise from the long-term use of prescribed drugs of dependence for severe injuries, multiple surgeries or pain from cancer treatments or the relief of chronic pain. In this instance dependence occurs when medications are taken at the prescribed dose (iatrogenic dependence) and are required for a specific purpose.

Iatrogenic dependence can also occur when prescribing is not in keeping with evidence-based guidelines for the management of a particular chronic condition. For example, use of benzodiazepine medications to treat long-term anxiety, opioid analgesia for the treatment of migraine headache (*See* Case Study 17.3 Myra and May, pp. 252–253).

Medication treatment for chronic pain depends on the condition and the evidence-based medication treatment for those conditions. For example, best practice treatment of the pain associated with chronic diabetic peripheral neuropathy and post-surgical neuralgia includes newer generation anticonvulsants such as gabapentin and tricyclic antidepressants (Hawley 2017, p. 476).

A range of non-prescription medications are considered good practice in addition to MAT: OD and include the use of over the counter (OTC) paracetamol, aspirin, NSAIDS and a range of non-medicated strategies such as exercise, TENS, martial arts, massage, reflexology or counselling.

As drug use increases in an effort to control pain and becomes out of control, the risk of overdose becomes a real possibility and service provision should seek to preserve life through controlling access to unsupervised MAT: OD doses and other opioid treatment medications.

Where service provision is not evidence based and/or the person has experienced harm (including dependence), care planning should include liaison with and the provision of information and collegial support with the health professional involved to support changes to practice. Should this be refused, notification to the professional seniors of the employing agency, pharmaceutical oversight or professional registration authorities can enable investigation of concerns and result in directives for action. In this, the professional identifying the problem is fulfilling their legal obligation to act to protect the person, the family and the community.

Where the person has a terminal ill-health or disease that will shorten life expectancy in the short to medium term, and the person is on the highest dose allowed under the jurisdiction MAT: OD procedures and the dose is not relieving pain, discussion, advocacy and referral to specialist palliative care services can reduce needless suffering. In this instance collaboration between AOD and specialist palliative care services aim to provide seamless support of the person and family.

SELF-ASSESSMENT EXERCISE 17.3

Time: 15 minutes
What barriers might hinder specialist palliative care provision? Note down your answers.

What Can Hinder AOD Palliative Care Service Provision?

People experiencing severe dependence require a range of services, some of which may be provided across other government sectors. Health care and other government funded services are expensive and cost containment needs to occur and this is usually through service inclusion criteria. The positive outcome of this type of funding ensures the provision of health services to those at most need, or for specified illnesses, disability, population or age group. The negative outcome is that some people cannot access the range of services they need as the criteria excludes them from receiving a service. This, therefore, is a valid reason why each service provider aims to offer the palliative care approach within the current service provision. Not necessarily involving specialist palliative care services but using this approach within their own speciality.

Service policies and procedures also impact on service provision and access. For example, the policy of three follow ups and discharge if the person does not contact results in exclusion of people with chaotic lifestyles related to severe dependence and/or other comorbidities who are most in need.

Alcohol and other drugs (AOD) and other health professionals may need to advocate for palliative care services to be provided by AOD skilled professionals for people experiencing severe dependence and/or are terminally ill and in need of community based assistance. These services would then be provided by professionals who know the person and their needs and whom they trust. Residential beds could be attached to withdrawal services or be standalone depending on the need for this type of service within the jurisdiction. These services would:

➤ Ensure fundamental human needs are met in a therapeutic and supportive environment
➤ Use the principles and strategies of palliative care in addition to the range of AOD treatment and interventions, which have a palliative function
➤ Have funding for brokering the range of services and/or packages of service delivery required by the person living in the community
➤ Search for best practice evidence and undertake research to develop new knowledge and skills for palliative AOD nursing care in both of its forms
➤ To care for people experiencing AOD people approaching end-of-life
➤ People experiencing severe dependence requiring long term-support, including family support
➤ Ensure people avoid any negative judgements, attitudes or neglect from health professionals or services at a time when they are most vulnerable.
➤ Allow for education of health professionals.

(Adapted with permission from de Crespigny 2012, p. 21)

Case Study 17.1 – John

John, aged 53 years was referred by his general practitioner (GP) due to alcohol-related liver disease and decreased platelet count. John reported drinking 40 standard drinks daily and a history of high-risk alcohol use over a 38-year period. John reported he began

continued . . .

drinking whilst in the Navy, which he joined at age 18 years and that he had been 'medically' discharged due to an anxiety disorder. John denied any difficulties in the Navy. John's advised his major concern was 'liver damage' and his goal was to maintain abstinence.

John had recently undergone withdrawal and reported never having a day without consuming alcohol since joining the Navy. A comprehensive assessment identified a high severity of dependence evidenced by the severity of the withdrawal episode, drinking to stupor, significant memory issues, poor nutrition and no family. John was living in a caravan park where boredom and social isolation were significant factors. John's dissatisfaction with his drinking, seeking to undergo withdrawal and his commitment to maintain change demonstrated a real commitment to change.

A plan for weekly sessions with the health professional to discuss relapse prevention, strategies for managing memory loss, options for social support and activities to substitute time usually spent drinking was developed in conjunction with John. The plan also included periodic medical reviews to monitor physical health. John refused referral to a residential rehabilitation service and accepted referral to a non-governmental organisation (NGO) service activities group. John began volunteering at a home delivery meal service and a local group, which maintained gardens as he enjoyed gardening.

Over the first eight weeks, John attended twice a week and made significant progress. This period was followed by an ongoing cycle of admission for withdrawal and relapse within two days following discharge. Relapse was treated by the health professional as a symptom of severity of dependence and as a normal part of the recovery process and as an opportunity for learning, further engagement and to plan further assistance. This pattern highlighted the severity of John's dependence and that he was struggling to maintain change.

When relapses continued, a palliative care approach was implemented. This included continued AOD service support, encouragement and self-efficacy building, and initiation of access to his GP and hospital admission for respite or to improve physical condition. The AOD professional arranged home meal delivery and a volunteer home visitor to assist with cleaning, shopping, provide support and social contact. This volunteer advised the AOD service when John was becoming unwell which allowed for early intervention and hospitalisation.

Following six months of palliative intervention, a case conference identified John's case scenario was similar to that of teenage boys who had been sexually abused. This had already been raised with John and denied. The AOD professional asked again about the Navy and what had occurred, and John reported he was raped within two weeks of being placed on a destroyer. John had never disclosed this incident to anyone and reported other symptoms, which indicated post-traumatic stress disorder (PTSD – *See* Chapter 11) for the first time.

John, with his consent, was referred to a veteran's service for management of PTSD and was admitted to a veteran's hospital for three months for medical and mental health treatment. Following discharge, John was referred back to the AOD health professional and GP for ongoing support. John maintained abstinence following discharge and the original intervention plan was reaffirmed by John and implemented. John continued to receive support, achieved his goal of abstinence and was discharged three years later with the door being left open for return at any time.

SELF-ASSESSMENT EXERCISE 17.4

> **Time: 40 minutes**
> - What was the benefit to John arising from the professionals' assertive follow up?
> - What might have been the outcome if John was stigmatised for 'not co-operating' with treatment and no follow up occurred following relapse?
> - Would John have ever disclosed he had been sexually assaulted if the service had not assertively engaged with him and gained his trust? If this had not occurred, would John have revisited his Naval history and achieved recovery?
> - What was the purpose of Johns alcohol use?
> - What palliative strategies were utilised in providing John's care?

Case Study 17.2 – Julie

Julie's mother Dawn aged 78, contacted the AOD service with concerns about her daughter's alcohol use. Dawn advised her daughter was refusing to seek help, and that she did not know what to do but wanted to support her daughter. Dawn advised of Julie's:

➤ daily drinking to point of intoxication
➤ increasing severity of hepatic disease arising from Hepatitis C infection
➤ visits to Dawn's home intoxicated or physically unwell
➤ drinking friends and her concerns about them

Dawn was offered ongoing support, and was given strategies to ensure her safety by asking Julie not to come to her home intoxicated, and how she could provide support through inviting her for a coffee or meal. Dawn was also provided with advice on how she could encourage and support Julie to attend the service and offered to provide support at her home. Dawn had a number of close friends and did not need any other assistance.

After several weeks, Dawn contacted the service advising Julie was prepared to meet the AOD professional. A home visit to Dawn was undertaken and time was spent seeking to engage with Julie. Information was obtained by eliciting Julie's story and concerns.

Information was provided about the range of treatment services available, that Julie would make the decisions and the service would support her with the decision made. Questions were answered. Positive feedback was provided regarding past successful MAT: OD treatment completion and 15 years of opioid abstinence. Julie was invited to advise of any concerns she may have about attending the service and received reassurance and encouragement. Confidentiality was explained. The AOD health professional offered to meet with Julie at Dawn's home if this would help. Julie opted to attend the AOD service.

During the first attendance, Julie gave her history of past heroin use, needle sharing and hepatitis C infection and subsequent liver disease. Julie's reported current alcohol consumption averaging 30 standard drinks (each has 10 grams of pure ethanol) per day. Julie reported she was not feeling well. She had recently seen her GP who had advised of blood results indicating liver damage and a liver scan had shown significant cirrhosis.

continued . . .

Julie advised she could not see herself reducing or ceasing alcohol consumption and was provided with information about the harmful nature of alcohol consumption in hepatitis C related liver disease and the risks of earlier death with continuing consumption and the additional risks for Wernicke's encephalopathy related to poor nutrition.

At a follow up visit, Julie was provided with harm reduction information and an initial supply of thiamine with the recommendations for continued use. Julie accepted the offer of multi service support that could occur without her being 'required' to change her alcohol consumption. Julie agreed to receive periodic contact from the AOD professional and was advised that should she change her decision, the AOD service would make treatment available to her at any time. The supports arranged included:

➤ GP – monitoring and management of health status with GP determination of needs for respite or acute medical ward admission
➤ Emergency room attendance at any time if feeling unwell
➤ AOD professional to liaise with Julie's service providers and to provide:
  - ongoing support for Dawn
  - occasional community support for Julie and during admissions to encourage change and assist with referrals for further support as required

➤ Making arrangements for:
  - a pharmacy to provide medications in blister packs at no additional charge and for notes to take daily liquid medications at a particular time
  - daily meal delivery from a voluntary NGO service
  - home support from an NGO volunteer with cleaning, shopping and socialisation two mornings per week. Arrangements were made with this service provider to advise of changes in Julie's health status to enable timely step up care admissions

➤ Dawn invited Julie for lunch, coffee or a meal at her home or out when it was possible.
➤ Dawn was provided with support and skills to support Julie.

The aim of service provisions was to provide palliative care for Julie to maintain her dignity and the best quality of life possible whilst she underwent an end-of-life process when she was not immediately terminally ill. Here, Julie exercised her right to self-determination in refusing treatment and was supported in her decision without judgement by all services involved.

Prior to her death 18 months later, Julie continued to consume alcohol and consumption reduced as her ill-health progressed. All services remained engaged and continued to provide support until Julie's death. The AOD professional throughout this time, provided support to Dawn to:

➤ Assist acceptance of Julie's decision
➤ Build resilience to enable her to withstand the stressors impacting on her
➤ Assist to navigate her feelings around Julie's decision to not change
➤ Assist her to navigate through the health system when Julie was ill.

The AOD professional attended Julie's funeral to support Dawn and continued to provide support for some months during bereavement. When Dawn was ready, the AOD professional left the door open for her to recontact at any time.

SELF-ASSESSMENT EXERCISE 17.5

> **Time: 20 minutes**
> THINK physical, psychological, social and spiritual
> • Why would an AOD professional seek to support Julie and her mother when Julie did not wish to change?
> • Given the outcome, was this approach helpful for Julie and Dawn? How and why might this have been the case?

Case Study 17.3 – Myra and May – Comparison of Migraine Treatment And Outcomes

Myra

Myra was a 30-year-old woman who in the past year had been having visual disturbance on a weekly basis, which had developed into severe headache and vomiting. Headaches were occurring two to three times per week. Myra became concerned that "something was wrong" and attended her GP who diagnosed migraine and prescribed a short acting compound analgesic containing panadeine and codeine. Myra took these each time a headache developed. After a period of time, Myra began using over the counter compound analgesia for other pain as single non-opioid preparations "did not work". Myra needed to increase the dose to two tablets to remediate her pain. Myra also shared her prescribed medications with others.

Some months later, Myra presented to her GP in distress and was given an intramuscular short-acting opioid, which quickly relieved the pain. This treatment was then sought with increasing frequency as the oral compound analgesic became more ineffective.

Over time, the prescribing practitioner became concerned about the number of times Myra was presenting for oral and intramuscular injections for pain relief injections and raised concern with Myra. The monitoring body for prescriptions identified continuing prescriptions for Myra and wrote to the prescriber advising of concern and requesting changes to practice.

Myra was not concerned at this as she had other prescribers she attended infrequently in the past and who she could now see from time to time. Myra's use of locum services increased.

Eventually the monitoring body advised all prescribers in the jurisdiction that Myra was not to be provided with pain relief medications. Myra arrived at an AOD service in withdrawal and refused to address drug use and was stabilised on MAT:OD as part of a palliative care strategy under a special authority from the prescription monitoring service. Myra continually sought unsupervised doses, which were refused because of risk of overdose. Myra later died of an overdose, which occurred by her taking an unsupervised dose in conjunction with illicitly obtained prescribed opioids and over the counter analgesia containing codeine.

continued . . .

May

May was a 28-year-old woman who presented to her GP reporting visual disturbance twice a month over the last year with no other symptoms. Over the last two months this had increased to four times per month where a mild headache occurred around 20 minutes following visual disturbance onset, which was associated with her menstrual cycle. May did not experience vomiting. May was concerned that "something was wrong". The GP advised the symptoms were likely due to onset of migraine and referred May for neurology assessment. The plan was to take aspirin (evidence based practice). The neurologist confirmed the diagnosis of classic migraine and recommended treatment with migraine preparations to treat episodes plus use of high dose aspirin. May was not able to tolerate aspirin so 1gm of paracetamol was used with positive effect. On seeing her GP, May was given information about migraine, non-medication strategies to manage an attack in addition to pain relief and the advice to never allow anyone to prescribe opioids for migraine as it would result in seeking this treatment, which often leads to dependence. May was advised she was welcome to attend the clinic when she had a migraine for tea and sympathy, which was never needed. May took her medication at onset of the visual disturbance and added paracetamol at the first indication of headache. On many occasions, headache was prevented.

Three years later, the incidence and severity of migraine increased. Following neurology re-assessment, an evidence-based medication to prevent migraine was added to the treatment regime. This was effective in reducing the frequency and severity with moderate to severe headaches reduced to one or two per year with two milder attacks per month, which were easily managed.

May was able to manage her condition with limited medical input on an ongoing basis. Over a 20-year period, May used an over the counter combination of paracetamol and codeine analgesia on two occasions. May lived to the age of 88 years.

SELF-ASSESSMENT EXERCISE 17.6

Time: 40 minutes
- What is the evidence-based treatment for Myra? Was Myra's treatment in keeping with evidence-based treatment of migraine?
- Was this treatment helpful? What was the outcome? Why was this the case?
- Who had the better outcome? Why?
- Does non-compliance with evidence-based practice pose a threat to the community?
- Were there threats to the community arising from this prescriber's practice?
- What would you do if you identified non-evidence based treatment of an individual?
- What were the differences in management between Myra and May?

CONCLUSION

The provision of palliative care services and/or using a palliative approach to people experiencing severe AOD dependence is a humanitarian strategy, particularly when they are also living with other multiple complex problems (*See* Chapter 8). It is useful when individuals are unable to change and as an intervention strategy to support a person where service provision is aimed at long-term engagement for change where this is possible.

There is a need for AOD and all health services to address fundamental human needs to maintain dignity and quality of life and for special purpose services to have some flexibility in who receives assistance. Failing this, there needs to be specific funding to broker services for people experiencing severe dependence that fall between the gaps of service criteria to ensure assistance is available to everyone with needs. Whichever format of service delivery, to ensure equity of access to people experiencing severe dependence, there needs to be formal systems and processes established which guide service delivery.

REFERENCES

Compton, P., Athanasos, P. and de Crespigny, C. (2006) *Opioid Tolerance and the Effective Management Of Acute Pain*, at Drug and Alcohol Nurses of Australiasia Conference. Sydney, in de Crespigny, C. and Talmet, J. eds (2012) *Alcohol, Tobacco and Other Drugs: Clinical Guidelines for Nurses and Midwives.* Version 3 Drug and Alcohol Services of South Australia, the University of Adelaide School of Nursing, Adelaide, South Australia. Available at: https://digital.library.adelaide.edu.au/dspace/bitstream/2440/73718/1/hdl_73718.pdf (Accessed: 12 October 2017).

de Crespigny, C. (2012) *Drug and Alcohol Nursing: Courage through Complexity.* Drug and Alcohol Nurses Association Oration. Available at: www.danaonline.org/wp-content/uploads/2011/04/DANA-oration-2012.pdf (Accessed: 12 October 2017).

de Crespigny, C. and Talmet, J. eds. (2012) *Alcohol, Tobacco and Other Drugs: Clinical Guidelines for Nurses and Midwives.* Version 3. The University of Adelaide School of Nursing and Drug and Alcohol Services of South Australia, Adelaide, South Australia. Available at: https://digital.library.adelaide.edu.au/dspace/bitstream/2440/73718/1/hdl_73718.pdf (Accessed: 12 October 2017) AND Available at: www.sahealth.sa.gov.au/wps/wcm/connect/ATOD+Clinical+Guidelines+for+Nurses+and+Midwives+V3+2012-DASSA-April2014.pdf?MOD=AJPERES

Hawley, P. (2017) 'Fast facts and concepts: nontricyclic antidepressants for neuropathic pain'. *Journal of Palliative Medicine*, 12. Available at: www.mypcnow.org/blank-yniiy (Accessed: 12 October 2017)

To Learn More

de Crespigny, C. (2012) *Drug and Alcohol Nursing: Courage through Complexity.* Drug and Alcohol Nurses Association Oration. www.danaonline.org/wp-content/uploads/2011/04/DANA-oration-2012.pdf

de Crespigny, C. and Talmet, J. eds. (2012) *Alcohol, Tobacco and Other Drugs: Clinical Guidelines for Nurses and Midwives.* Version 3. The University of Adelaide School of Nursing and Drug and Alcohol Services of South Australia, Adelaide, South Australia. https://digital.library.adelaide.edu.au/dspace/bitstream/2440/73718/1/hdl_73718.pdf AND www.sahealth.sa.gov.au/wps/wcm/connect/ATOD+Clinical+Guidelines+for+Nurses+and+Midwives+V3+2012-DASSA-April2014.pdf?MOD=AJPERES

Mundt-Leach, R. (2014) 'End of life and palliative care of patients with drug and alcohol addiction, Mental Health Practice', 20, 17. https://search.proquest.com/openview/1f4e32ba9ac345a858161e0e523b3792/1?pq-origsite=gscholar&cbl=2042234

Reisfield, G. M., Paulian, G. D. and Wilson, G. R. 'Fast facts and concepts #127. Substance use disorders in the palliative care patient'. www.mypcnow.org/blank-iicww

CHAPTER 18

Futility in Anorexia Nervosa

Cynthia M.A. Geppert

PRE-READING EXERCISE 18.1

Time: 30 minutes
- Read the case scenario below about Jane carefully
- Consider your response to Jane's situation
- How would you feel as Jane's parents about her condition?
- What would you do as her health care professional?

Case Study 18.1

Jane is a 29-year-old who was beginning her second year of nursing school before she had to drop out due to medical complications of chronic anorexia nervosa (AN). Jane was first diagnosed with AN when she was 15. During the ensuing 14 years she has been in residential treatment programmes five times, been hospitalised twice and even had force feeding at the age of 17 when her weight dropped to 35 kgs. Jane has had intermittent motivational interviewing, cognitive-behavioural therapy and has been on fluoxetine for many years with unsuccessful trials of antipsychotic medication. Even if she briefly gained weight under duress Jane has never been able to maintain the increase voluntarily, usually losing it through excessive cycling and swimming. This is Jane's third, and the school has now said, final, chance to become a nurse. Jane is exceptionally bright and hard working and did quite well during her classroom year of nursing school. However, each time she attempts the clinical rotations her body mass index (BMI) hovering around 14 leaves her too weak, tired and confused to complete her nursing training. Jane lives with her mother, a homemaker, and her father who is a dentist; the couple have placed a second mortgage on their home to pay for Jane's care. Jane is the youngest of four children, all of whom have done well for themselves, marrying and entering professions. They believe Jane has been 'babied too much' and her parents should throw her out of the house and make her work. Jane has never been married and all her high school friends now have lives of their own and little time or patience for her. Jane spends her days exercising and trying to read but is unable to concentrate. Her psychiatrist has diagnosed her with obsessive compulsive traits and major depressive disorder. Jane's current therapist has suggested to Jane and her parents that there are few evidence-based treatments left that Jane has not failed, and that it might be time to consider palliative care focusing on quality of life.

INTRODUCTION

Anorexia nervosa has among the highest mortality rates of all mental illnesses (Steinhausen 2002) and as the case scenario opening this chapter shows, a high morbidity, as well as being emotionally and financially exhausting for families of individuals who struggle for decades with the disease. DSM-5 criteria for the disorder are listed in Table 18.1.

There are numerous serious medical complications of the condition including osteoporosis and cardiac failure. However, it is the psychological suffering of depression, obsessive-compulsiveness, anxiety, guilt and fear that are the most terrible burden of AN. Anorexia nervosa with its usual onset in adolescence can rob promising young people, despite their often high intelligence, of any hope for a career or relationships. Recently, some eating disorder experts and ethicists have suggested that a palliative approach to the care of people experiencing a type of AN known as 'severe and enduring' should be considered in select cases. Those who object to this approach argue it is an inappropriate application of the already flawed medical criteria of futility to a psychiatric ill-health that, while it may currently be treatment refractory, is not end-stage as is a metastatic cancer. This chapter will first briefly describe the criteria for severe and enduring AN (SE-AN) and then present an overview of the ethical concept of futility as used in medicine. The arguments for and against futility as an ethically justifiable and clinically meaningful designation for SE-AN will be presented. Finally, further directions for further research and policy development are outlined.

SEVERE AND ENDURING ANOREXIA NERVOSA (SE-AN)

The category of severe and enduring anorexia nervosa and its cognates of 'chronic', and 'intractable' AN is an emerging and not fully coalesced classification in eating disorder scholarship. In a 2018 literature review of what they called 'particularly durable forms of the condition in research and clinical contexts' Broomfield et al. found inconsistencies in definition, criteria and terminology (Broomfield et al. 2017). Duration of ill-health and previously failed treatment are the two criteria most frequently utilised to identify a case of SE-AN. The average duration of ill-health found in the literature is seven years at a minimum, but from an unknown incidence point. What meets the bar for treatment failure though is far less solidified. 'Previously failed treatment attempts are the second

Table 18.1 DSM-5 Criteria for Anorexia Nervosa

A. Restriction of energy intake relative to requirements, leading to significantly low body weight in the context of age, sex, developmental trajectory, and physical health. *Significantly low weight* is defined as a weight that is less than minimally normal or, for children and adolescents, less than minimally expected.

B. Intense fear of gaining weight or of becoming fat, or persistent behavior that interferes with weight gain, even though at a significantly low weight.

C. Disturbances in the way one's body weight or shape is experienced, undue influence of body weight or shape on self-evaluation, or persistent lack of recognition of the seriousness of the current low body weight.

American Psychiatric Association. (2013) Diagnostics and Statistical Manual of Mental Disorders (DSM-5), Washington DC, American Psychiatric Association.

most commonly used criterion. But what needs to be made clear, however, is what is an adequate treatment as well as what type of treatment needs to be attempted' (Broomfield et al. 2017). Heuristically though, SE-AN is useful in that it calls clinical attention to a group of individuals who have a long-standing and heretofore treatment resistant form of AN for which an emphasis on quality of life rather than curative modes may be more ethically appropriate.

The authors and other scholars are not unaware of the potential adverse effects of SE-AN as a heuristic that indirectly may convey the message of futility and negatively impact the possibility of recovery (Dawson, Rhodes & Touyz 2014).

It is concerning that a term that may imply an incurable ill-health is currently the most commonly used adjective when referring to people experiencing SE-AN. Whether such people are incurable or not, it is crucial that researchers and clinicians agree on whether it is helpful, or even appropriate, to label these individuals with a term that has such negative connotations. What should be of prime importance is whether this label will affect any hopes of recovery (Broomfield et al. 2017).

Futility

Futility has proven to be even harder to define than SE-AN. The ancient etymology of futility is more revealing than its modern translations. Used as an adjective as in, Jane is a 'futile' case, the word is derived from the Latin, futilis, futtilis, 'vain, worthless'. More symbolically, futile carried a connotation in Latin of 'pouring out easily, being easily emptied'. Many scholars have tried to come up with a watertight (no pun intended!) scientific definition leading the American Medical Association Council on Ethical and Judicial Affairs, to opine, 'Futility is an essentially subjective but realistically indispensable judgment. A fully objective and concrete definition of futility is unattainable' (1999, p. 937).

REFLECTIVE PRACTICE EXERCISE 18.1

Time: 15 minutes
- When you hear the word futility what are your first thoughts and feelings?
- Can you recall episodes of medical care where there were ethical conflicts around futility?
- Are there individuals with a mental ill-health encountered in your practice for whom further treatment might be futile?

Types of Futility

More useful for our purpose is identifying three main types of futility as listed and considering whether any of the three apply to Jane's circumstances.

KEY POINT 18.1

There are three major types of futility: physiologic, quantitative and qualitative.

Dr Thaddeus Pope, probably the world's expert on medical futility explains the three types of futility (Pope 2012).

1. Physiologic futility – is considered ethically inappropriate because it is physiologically ineffective in achieving the desired medical goal. For example, cardiopulmonary resuscitation (CPR) cannot be successfully performed on a person who has suffered a complete rupture of the heart muscle. In such a circumstance, the physician, based on their medical expertise, makes a clinical judgement that CPR need not be administered even if the surrogate or family requests it be performed because it is a scientific impossibility that it will restore circulation. As the dramatic nature of the example suggests, there are few situations in medicine where physiologic futility judgements are applicable, underscoring the lack of certainty regarding prognosis in medicine that bedevils futility in practice. Clearly in the scenario that opens the chapter Jane does not meet criteria for this type of futility.

2. Quantitative Futility – is also a medical judgement but one that is derived from research into similar cases. For example, physicians study the use of dialysis in individuals who require vasopressors to maintain their blood pressure and find that it is rarely successful. Based on their observations, physicians set a threshold below which they determine that the use of dialysis is so unlikely to be effective that it is ethically inappropriate to offer it. Usually that threshold is set at 1 per cent, that is if dialysis could be performed on only 1 of the last 100 individuals whose blood pressure required chemical support, then it need not be provided even if a surrogate requested it. The ethical justification is that there is a low likelihood, 1 per cent or less, that the intervention will achieve the individual's goal of maintaining kidney function or put differently, preventing death from renal failure. As opposed to physiologic futility, this is a more ethically problematic concept as there will always be individuals and their surrogates and families who believe a 1 per cent chance dialysis will work in the face of certain death and is worthwhile. These persons will also likely protest that the determination of whether that it should be their decision, not the health care professionals, whether that small possibility is worth a try (Pope 2012). The professionals caring for Jane might well ground their recommendation in quantitative futility with the backing of the empirical literature on treatment refractory SE-AN as well as Jane's personal history of failed interventions.

3. Qualitative futility – as the most professional driven type is the most ethically paternalistic of the three. This type of futility asks not whether the individual's medical outcomes can be attained but whether those goals of care are ethically worth pursuing (Pope 2012). This is clearly a value judgement, not a medical judgement, and as such, if the professional makes it, it is prone to bias and subjectivity. However, if it is the individual's decision, then it is an expression of autonomy and professionals should strongly consider whether paternalism or compassion is most ethically appropriate. The more clinical version of qualitative futility holds that a treatment can be refused when its burdens outweigh its benefits, such as a third-round of chemotherapy for advanced cancer when that medication is highly toxic. A more humanistic version, posits that an intervention is futile when it cannot provide a person with a minimum quality of life; again, as the person, not the professional, defines it. For example, if a professional was to refuse to repair the hip fracture of an individual experiencing advanced dementia this could be suspect as a personal

prejudice or a micro allocation resource decision. But if their surrogate and family choose home hospice instead of surgery, they are likely sparing their loved one the pain of the operation and aftercare and the dismay of being in the hospital. It is this last type of futility, which appears to be relevant to Jane's situation.

Futility in Psychiatric Ill-Health Brief Literature Review

As suggested in the Reflective Practice Exercise 18.1, many mental health professionals, especially those who work with the seriously mentally ill and persons with substance use disorders have likely at some point believed that further treatment for a person had little hope. However, they would probably not have framed this treatment resistance in terms of futility. The first published association of futility and psychiatric ill-health, was with AN, in 1994 in the *American Journal of Hospice and Palliative Care* (O'Neill, Crowther & Sampson 1994; Williams, Piere & Sims 1998) This was followed in 1998 by a point-counter point in the *British Medical Journal*, (Russon & Alison 1998). In 2010, American eating disorder experts published the first paper to use the actual word futility in their ethical analysis of a case history not unlike Jane in which the individual eventually died in the hospice (Lopez, Yager & Feinstein 2010). This author published a target article entitled 'Futility in anorexia nervosa: a concept whose time has not yet come', in 2015 (Geppert 2015), and as is the custom of the journal, seven scholar commentaries were published in response, (Bruni & Weijer 2015; Mackenzie 2015; McKinney 2015; Paris & Hawkins 2015). Since that time there have been a number of other articles addressing palliative and hospice care in psychiatric ill-health as well as several book chapters (Westmoreland & Mehler 2016).

Arguments Against Futility in SE-AN

There are technical philosophical and linguistic criticisms of the futility concept that are outside the scope of this clinical ethics-oriented chapter. There are also complex legal aspects to the question of futility in AN that also cannot be entertained here. The primary arguments found in the literature that will be outlined here are regarding incorrect classification of SE-AN as an end-stage medical disease; and the inherent cognitive and affective impairments characteristic of SE-AN that preclude the exercise of rational and voluntary choice.

The Medical Argument

Psychiatric ethicist Ronald Pies (2015), has criticised the idea that there are known pathophysiologic indicators that constitute an 'end-stage' or terminal phase of a psychiatric ill-health analogous to those found in cancer or heart failure, which have established classification of disease progression, which inform recommendations for palliative and hospice care. In his words, 'Yet, when writers refer to "end-stage" AN, they cannot point to a well-established temporal gradient of psychopathology that would allow one to say confidently, "This is the end of the process"' (Pies 2015). Pies and this author have argued that while in cirrhosis or renal failure, there is real demonstrable damage to vital organs. Such end-organ damage certainly can be the manifestation of starvation in AN, but this does not mean such metabolic failure will occur as organic progression of the condition with or without treatment, such as in the case of actual end-stage liver or kidney disease (Geppert 2015).

KEY POINT 18.2

The medical argument examines whether or not end-of-life care in mental and physical ill-health are parallel.

The Capacity Argument

A review of Tables 18.1 and 18.2, which contain DSM-V and ICD10 diagnostic criteria for anorexia nervosa finds that both require that the individual has distorted thinking and disordered emotions regarding her experience of her own body, weight and appearance. ICD10 (Table 18.2) is more explicit in its description of these sensations, ideas and emotions as abnormal, that is as a dis-order: 'There is a body-image distortion in the form of a specific psychopathology whereby a dread of fatness persists as an intrusive, overvalued idea, and the patient imposes a low weight threshold on himself or herself' (ICD-10, online)

When paired with the poor insight that so frequently afflicts persons experiencing anorexia nervosa, these overvalued ideas, even if they do not reach delusional proportions, have the potential to seriously impair the ability of the individual experiencing SE-AN to exercise the higher order components of decisional capacity: reasoning and appreciation. It is these cognitive and volitional deficits that so frequently make AN very difficult to treat and render it sadly so fixed a condition in many persons (Adoue et al. 2015). Compounding the diminished executive function demonstrated in some neuropsychological research, is the well-documented adverse effect of starvation on rational thinking and emotional

Table 18.2 ICD-10 Criteria for anorexia nervosa

A. Body weight is maintained at least 15% below that expected (either lost or never achieved) or Quetelet's body-mass index is 17.5 or less. Prepubertal individuals may show failure to make the expected weight gain during the period of growth.

B. The weight loss is self-induced by avoidance of 'fattening foods' and one or more of the following: self-induced vomiting; self-induced purging; excessive exercise; use of appetite suppressants and/or diuretics.

C. There is body-image distortion in the form of a specific psychopathology whereby a dread of fatness persists as an intrusive, overvalued idea and the individual imposes a low-weight threshold on him- or her-self.

D. A widespread endocrine disorder involving the hypothalamic-pituitary-gonadal axis is manifest in women as amenorrhoea and in men as a loss of sexual interest and potency. (An apparent exception is the persistence of vaginal bleeds in anorexic women who are receiving replacement hormonal therapy, most commonly taken as a contraceptive pill.) There may also be elevated levels of growth hormone, raised levels of cortisol, changes in the peripheral metabolism of the thyroid hormone, and abnormalities of insulin secretion.

E. If onset is prepubertal, the sequence of pubertal events is delayed or even arrested (growth ceases; in girls the breasts do not develop and there is a primary amenorrhoea; in boys the genitals remain juvenile). With recovery, puberty is often completed normally, but the menarche is late.

ICD-10 Criteria for Anorexia Nervosa. Available at: http://apps.who.int/classifications/icd10/browse/2016/en#F50.8 (Accessed: January 18, 2018).

stability (McCormick et al. 2008). The high comorbid rate of depression and completed suicide in anorexia also require an even higher bar for treatment refusal (Portzky, van Heeringen & Vervaet 2014). Because these subtle impairments are not usually and persuasively detected through standard cognitive batteries or judicial proceedings, the individual may appear to be rational despite massive internal coercion (Gutheil & Bursztajn 1986).

KEY POINT 18.3

The capacity argument examines whether an individual experiencing SE-AN has capacity to make reasoned, voluntary decisions.

THE ARGUMENTS IN FAVOUR OF FUTILITY IN ANOREXIA NERVOSA

Those who favour a palliative approach to selected SE-AN cases, rightly do not argue 'for futility' just as many pro-choice advocates would not present their positions as 'for abortion'. Among the most compelling statements of this position is the internationally renowned eating disorder expert Dr Joel Yager:

> Despite years of (ineffective) vigorous treatment during which patients, families, professional caregivers and all manner of special treatment centres and consultations have done their best, a few patients with severe and enduring anorexia nervosa continue to experience life as an ongoing, unrelenting terrible, painful ordeal and through these experiences accrue at least significant circumstantial evidence to support their beliefs that they're not likely to get any better. For practitioners, keeping individuals alive who experience life as unrelenting states of chronic torment – even patients with psychiatric disorders – is not necessarily virtuous – or ethical.
>
> (Yager 2015)

This poignant passage is articulating a position based on the ethical theory (*See* Chapter 2) of virtue ethics and care ethics. Compassion for suffering and the obligation to do no harm are the ethical values that are given primacy. Palliative care and eventually hospice are the only viable humane options when all forms of active treatment have repeatedly failed leaving the individual in perpetual anguish. This is as Lopez, Yager & Feinstein have said a treatment of 'last resort' not an option for the adolescent who is only recently diagnosed with anorexia nervosa or the individual who despite the resistance to therapy often integral to the condition is responding to treatment with not just weight gain but improvement in overall functioning.

SELF-ASSESSMENT EXERCISE 18.1

Time: 105 minutes
- Review the major ethical theories introduced in Chapter 2
- Choose two theories and apply them to the ethical dilemma of futility in AN
- After you read the following section of this chapter, compare your application of the theories to that presented below

ETHICAL THEORY AND PALLIATIVE CARE FOR SE-AN

Contrary to this utilitarian ethos, Pies points out that from a deontological perspective futility and hospice care could be considered a form of the individual (and I would add) family abandonment, the understandable expression of frustrated, thwarted and depleted familial and professional caregivers (Pies 2015). Note that from a utilitarian view this could even be ethically defensible as the burdens of the SE-AN for all involved have so outweighed not just any empirical benefit but also any realistic hope of the same. Yet this may be an unfair criticism of the palliative proposal rightly understood. Just as in the provision of palliative care for life-limiting medical conditions, this is essentially a quality of life argument that is grounded in virtue and care ethics. The palliative approach does not eschew active treatment, but instead of directing or even enforcing it, offers such care in accordance with the persons' wishes and values. Moreover, like traditional palliative care for other advanced disorders, individuals are free to change their mind about the treatment trajectory at any time and resume aggressive treatment.

Thus, it is unfair to characterise a palliative approach, even endorsing a futility judgement regarding the prognosis of SE-AN as equivalent to physician-assisted suicide or euthanasia. Yager, emphasises that if an individual experiencing SE-AN is acutely suicidal then the full panoply of legal and medical mental health interventions may need to be employed (Yager 2015). It is presumed that the person experiencing SE-AN wishing to forego further active treatment does not so much wish to die as to stop the agony of the battle with such an implacable foe. It is equally unjust to presume those who oppose futility to lack empathic imagination of the terrible plight of individuals experiencing SE-AN. However, a paradox seldom found in medical ill-health remains. Unlike other truly end-stage conditions, for example, chronic obstructive pulmonary disease or even in the neuropsychiatric realm dementia, the course of the disease is inexorable and there is no known way to reverse it. In contrast, until the final terminus of multi-organ failure efficacious treatment is known but cannot be received precisely because the person refuses it based on their own distorted anorexic cognitions. While several commentators have argued that failing to seriously offer end-of-life options to SE-AN is stigmatising (Campbell & Aulisio 2012), the converse can also be argued, that not requiring the same standard of capacity to refuse life-sustaining treatment because AN is a psychiatric disorder may also be discriminatory.

KEY POINT 18.4

Several of the major ethical theories introduced in Chapter 2 may be utilised in the analysis of futility in SE-AN.

Autonomy and Capacity Claims Supporting Palliation of SE-AN

Not unexpectedly there is also a difference of opinion between proponents and opponents of a palliative approach to the capacity of individuals experiencing SE-AN to participate in decisions. There are two versions of this claim. The first, and strongest, is that in my physician-father's words, "never say never and never say always in medicine". Just as a minority of persons at the end-of-life may not experience terminal delirium but remain lucid, so it is improbable to believe that there are not some individuals experiencing

SE-AN who retain capacity to refuse further active treatment. Especially if these decisions are made before the individual is extremely malnourished. The second iteration would concede that while such persons may not have decision-making capacity in strict neuropsychological testing terms, they can express their deepest emotional and volitional values to cease suffering and struggling to eat and gain weight and that ethically these should be respected. Draper records several cases of older women experiencing SE-AN who elected hospice whom she believes had decision-making capacity (Draper 2000). McKinney's recommendation that such a decision should reflect not the disorder of SE-AN alone, but the emotional acceptance of the individual of their death, as well as the views of the family are profound and construct the lineaments for a decision-making model (McKinney 2015).

INVOLUNTARY TREATMENT

McKinney has underscored that the most difficult question for those who argue against a palliative approach and who contend that there is no place for futility judgements in AN; it is what to do with the Janes of the eating disorder specialty. The obvious, and for many ethically intolerable, alternative is involuntary treatment including forced feeding. Almost all eating disorder specialists and many ethicists agree that involuntary treatment can be ethically justified for young people with rapid deterioration early in the ill-health course. For these individuals, none of the putative criteria for severe and enduring are met and there is no evidence to suggest even forced feeding will not be successful at least in the immediate goal of saving life.

Compelling adults who have fought the disease for a lifetime to be restrained and fed through a nasogastric tube is very hard to defend especially when its ability to alter the fatal long-term trajectory is in doubt. While there is some consensus that involuntary treatment may be in the short-term beneficial, and even well received, the longer-term benefit is disputed (Schreyer et al. 2016). Yet even here a case can be made if there are reasonable clinical indicators that the individual may respond, and such violating intervention may contribute to meaningful recovery. Similarly, when a person clearly lacks decision-making capacity and there are empirical grounds for believing treatment may lead to sufficient insight for the individual to voluntarily participate in care. These last two conditions, while exceedingly rare in SE-AN, are not completely without precedent. Dawson tells the story of eight women experiencing chronic AN who recover against the odds (Dawson, Rhodes & Touyz 2014).

HOPE AND THE FUTURE

As with so many debilitating and longstanding disorders, mental and physical, much of the disagreement between those who propose and oppose a palliative approach or even an outright judgement of futility differ on their view of the future and the content of hope. At the time of this writing, a search on PubMed located several promising new therapies for SE-AN, leading to the equally trenchant question. How is it determined that all further treatment is in vain? (Hay & Touyz 2015). Yet another querying of the same database found several new papers developing the concept and practice of palliative care in psychiatry (Trachsel et al. 2016). Who should decide when enough is enough or tell an individual or their family they need to go farther? Most importantly, what if, as some research suggests, treatment of disordered eating behaviour and weight gain are in fact key to improvements in quality of life even in SE-AN? (Bamford et al. 2015).

Factors beginning to be explored in research on SE-AN may illuminate the answers to these conundrums that both sides must fairly and carefully consider.

➤ The voice of the individual experiencing SE-AN (Conti, Rhodes & Adams 2016)
➤ The role of the surrogate decision maker in SE-AN (Bruni & Weijer 2015)
➤ Decision making frameworks for futility/palliative ethical analysis and moral deliberation (McKinney 2015)
➤ Contextual factors such as financing, family support
➤ More holistic measures of decisional capacity in SE-AN
➤ Legal mechanisms for ensuring due process for all stakeholders (Mackenzie 2015).

SELF-REFLECTION EXERCISE 18.2

Time: 60 minutes
- Return to the pre-reading exercise that opened the chapter
- Reread the case of Jane
- Respond again to the questions posed
- Have your responses changed after reading the chapter? In what way? What do you think explains the change in your thinking?

CONCLUSION

The one lesson the author aims to communicate in this brief overview of the ethical debate regarding futility and palliation in SE-AN is that absolutes on either pole of the spectrum are least likely to be ethically justifiable. There will always be persons whose unique narratives and clinical circumstances constitute valid exceptions to the arguments that qualitative and quantitative futility judgements are inappropriate in SE-AN or those who contend there should be a wider exploration and application of palliative approach and hospice care for persons experiencing SE-AN. The march of science may well open a new path between these two camps but until then sheer humility, if not humanity, must recognise that there will be individuals who despite heroic and Herculean efforts on the part of all involved, succumb to this terrible disorder and once a person meets true physiologic futility criteria hospice care is the only viable ethical decision. At this early stage of an exceedingly complicated debate, this and profound empathy for Jane and those like her and a commitment from professionals to continue the work of understanding how we can best help them bear or lift their enormous burden.

REFERENCES

Adoue, C., Jaussent, I., Olie, E., Beziat, S., van Den Eynde, F., Courtet, P. and Guillaume, S. (2015) 'A further assessment of decision-making in anorexia nervosa'. *European Psychiatry*, 30, pp. 121–7.

American Psychiatric Association. (2013) *Diagnostics and Statistical Manual of Mental Disorders (DSM-5)*, Washington, DC: American Psychiatric Association.

American Medical Association. (1999) 'Medical futility in end-of-life care: report of the Council on Ethical and Judicial Affairs'. *Journal of the American Medical Association*, 281, pp. 937–41.

Bamford, B., Barras, C., Sly, R., Stiles-Shields, C., Touyz, S. et al. (2015) 'Eating disorder symptoms and quality of life: where should clinicians place their focus in severe and enduring anorexia nervosa'? *International Journal Eating Disorders*, 48, pp. 133–8.

Broomfield, C., Stedal, K., Touyz, S. and Rhodes, P. (2017) 'Labeling and defining severe and enduring anorexia nervosa: A systematic review and critical analysis'. *International Journal Eating Disorders*, 50, pp. 611–23.

Bruni, T. and Weijer, C. (2015) 'A misunderstanding concerning futility'. *American Journal of Bioethics*, 15, pp. 59–60.

Campbell, A. T. and Aulisio, M. P. (2012) 'The stigma of "mental" illness: end stage anorexia and treatment refusal'. *International Journal Eating Disorders*, 45, pp. 627–34.

Conti, J., Rhodes, P. and Adams, H. (2016) 'Listening in the dark: why we need stories of people living with severe and enduring anorexia nervosa'. *Journal of Eating Disorders*, 4, p. 33.

Dawson, L., Rhodes, P. and Touyz, S. (2014) ' "Doing the impossible": the process of recovery from chronic anorexia nervosa'. *Qualitive Health Research*, 24, pp. 494–505.

Draper, H. (2000) 'Anorexia nervosa and respecting a refusal of life-prolonging therapy: a limited justification'. *Bioethics*, 14, pp. 120–33.

Geppert, C. M. (2015) 'Futility in chronic anorexia nervosa: a concept whose time has not yet come'. *American Journal of Bioethics*, 15, pp. 34–43.

Gutheil, T. G. and Bursztajn, H. (1986) 'Clinicians' guidelines for assessing and presenting subtle forms of patient incompetence in legal settings'. *American Journal of Psychiatry*, 143, pp. 1020–3.

Hay, P. and Touyz, S. (2015) 'Treatment of patients with severe and enduring eating disorders'. *Current Opinion Psychiatry*, 28, pp. 473–7.

ICD-10 Criteria for Anorexia Nervosa. Available at: http://apps.who.int/classifications/icd10/browse/2016/en#F50.8 (Accessed: 18 January 2018)

Lopez, A., Yager, J. and Feinstein, R. E. (2010) 'Medical futility and psychiatry: palliative care and hospice care as a last resort in the treatment of refractory anorexia nervosa'. *The International Journal of Eating Disorders*, 43, pp. 372–7.

Mackenzie, R. (2015) 'Ms X: a promising new view of anorexia nervosa, futility, and end-of-life decisions in a very recent English case'. *American Journal of Bioethics*, 15, pp. 57–8.

McCormick, L. M., Keel, P. K., Brumm, M. C., Bowers, W., Swayze, V. et al. (2008) 'Implications of starvation-induced change in right dorsal anterior cingulate volume in anorexia nervosa'. *International Journal Eating Disorders*, 41, pp. 602–10.

McKinney, C. (2015) 'Is resistance (n)ever futile? a response to "futility in chronic anorexia nervosa: a concept whose time has not yet come" by Cynthia Geppert'. *American Journal of Bioethics*, 15, pp. 53–4.

O'Neill, J., Crowther, T. and Sampson, G. (1994) 'A case study: anorexia nervosa. Palliative care of terminal psychiatric disease'. *American Journal of Hospice and Palliative Care*, 11, pp. 36–8.

Paris, J. J. and Hawkins, A. (2015) ' "Futility" is a failed concept in medical decision making: its use should be abandoned'. *American Journal of Bioethics*, 15, pp. 50–2.

Pies, R. W. (2015) 'Anorexia nervosa, "futility," and category errors'. *American Journal of Bioethics*, 15, pp. 44–6.

Pope, T. M. (2012) 'Medical futility', in Hester, D. M. and Schonfeld, T. L. (eds.) *Guidance for Healthcare Ethics Committees*. Cambridge: Cambridge University Press.

Portzky, G., van Heeringen, K. and Vervaet, M. (2014) 'Attempted suicide in patients with eating disorders'. *Crisis*, 35, pp. 378–87.

Russon, L. and Alison, D. (1998) 'Does palliative care have a role in treatment of anorexia nervosa? Palliative care does not mean giving up'. *British Medical Journal*, 317, pp. 196–7.

Schreyer, C. C., Coughlin, J. W., Makhzoumi, S. H., Redgrave, G. W., Hansen, J. L. and Guarda, A. S. (2016) 'Perceived coercion in inpatients with anorexia nervosa: associations with illness severity and hospital course'. *International Journal of Eating Disorders*, 49, pp. 407–12.

Steinhausen, H. C. (2002) 'The outcome of anorexia nervosa in the 20th century'. *American Journal of Psychiatry*, 159, pp. 1284–93.

Trachsel, M., Irwin, S. A., Biller-Andorno, N., Hoff, P. and Riese, F. (2016) 'Palliative psychiatry for severe persistent mental illness as a new approach to psychiatry? Definition, scope, benefits, and risks'. *BMC Psychiatry*, 16, p. 260.

Westmoreland, P. and Mehler, P. S. (2016) 'Caring for patients with Severe and Enduring Eating Disorders (SEED): certification, harm reduction, palliative care, and the question of futility'. *Journal of Psychiatric Practice*, 22, pp. 313–20.

Williams, C. J., Pieri, L. and Sims, A. (1998) 'Does palliative care have a role in treatment of anorexia nervosa? We should strive to keep patients alive'. *British Medical Journal*, 317, pp. 195–6.

Yager, J. (2015) 'The futility of arguing about medical futility in anorexia nervosa: the question is how would you handle highly specific circumstances'? *American Journal of Bioethics*, 15, 47–50.

To Learn More

Touyz, S., Le Grange, D., Lacey, H. and Hay P. (2016) *Managing Severe and Enduring Eating Disorders: A Clinicians Guide.* 1st edition. New York, NY: Routledge.

Trachsel, M., Irwin, S. A., Biller-Andorno, N., Hoff, P. and Riese, F. (2016) 'Palliative psychiatry for severe persistent mental illness as a new approach to psychiatry? Definition, scope, benefits, and risks'. *BMC Psychiatry*, 16, p. 260.

Westmoreland, P. and Mehler, P. S. (2016) 'Caring for patients with Severe and Enduring Eating Disorders (SEED): certification, harm reduction, palliative care, and the question of futility'. *Journal of Psychiatric Practice*, 22, pp. 313–20.

CHAPTER 19

Suicide Awareness and Prevention

Annessa Rebair

INTRODUCTION

In nursing, we may relate to spirituality, belonging and hope in our exploration and attempt to gauge and understand wellbeing. It is of course central to our practice to notice and respond to spiritual despair and disconnectedness manifesting itself as loss of hope and a desire to end one's life. To respond with compassion when this is uttered is arguably the duty of every nurse. However, the stigma associated with suicide can be disabling, preventing those in need from seeking help and preventing those able to help from engaging in a meaningful conversation about suicide.

Themes from the literature tell us that those who are suicidal would like engagement, time to tell their story, to be met with a genuine human response to their despair and to be asked about suicide (Cutcliffe et al. 2006; Lees, Procter & Fassett 2014). One can assume from this that nurses would be equipped to listen, ask, connect human-to-human and be genuine in their response to an expression of distress. This transaction is far more complex than initially perceived notwithstanding the supposition that the nurse has the emotional capacity, ability and willingness to go there. If the implicit assumption is that nurses are concerned with what it means to be human, in strength and in despair, all nurses must be equipped and motivated to intervene and explore the edges of humanity.

Breathing life into national strategies and workforce training not only requires a fuzzy degree of alignment from the macro to the micro level but it also requires social thrust, the creation of new movement to change the stigma and myths surrounding suicide as is currently told.

KEY POINT 19.1

It is still considered difficult to talk about suicide. To hold out one's hand, to feel confident to explore and ask outright about suicide requires courage as it is not an easy conversation to have and, as Barker (2004) comments, 'it is not for the faint-hearted'.

That said, 'what do nurses need to engage in conversations about suicide'? Educational needs, kindness, the focus of the meeting place, issues with dissonance and preparation will be discussed in the following pages. This chapter is by no means an exhaustive account of all of the variables, rather it echoes important rhetoric of the past combined with political drivers of the present, and serves to contribute to the discussion of how best to address nurses needs in order to meet the needs of those in distress.

THE CASE FOR EDUCATION AND TRAINING

The body of evidence is growing regarding nurses' responses and care of suicidal people. Positive outcomes are reported from participants in receipt of suicide training programmes and include increased understanding about suicide, changes in attitude, skills acquisition and increased confidence (Isaac et al. 2009; Talseth & Gilje 2011; Heyman, Webster & Tee 2015; Pullen, Gilje & Tesar 2016; Ramberg, Di Lucca & Hadlaczky 2016). The need for training in suicide awareness and prevention for nurses and health professionals is consistent across the health literature. Surprisingly, this is not a feature in pre-registration nurse education. None of the fields of nursing in the UK (apart from mental health) are currently required to complete competencies concerning suicide before registering (Nursing and Midwifery Council – NMC – 2009; 2010). This has recently been addressed and the draft publication of the revised pre-registration nursing proficiencies identify nurses of all fields to: 'use best evidence to take a history, observe and accurately assess signs of mental and emotional distress including suicidal ideation' (Nursing and Midwifery Council – NMC 2017, p. 27). Not only does this ossify the tenets implicit in The Code of Conduct (Nursing and Midwifery Council – NMC 2015) but it also supports the vision for workforce development plans, recommendations for emergency and primary care set out by the Department of Health (DoH 2017) and Public Health England (PHE 2015) and aligns with plans for suicide risk training in medical education (General Medical Council (GMC 2017). The pending challenge for delivery in nurse education will be deciding what form the training will take and how compatible it is with the language of care.

Although training approaches are generally positively received and reported in the literature, key findings conclude that more research is needed to evaluate the efficacy of suicide prevention programmes (Heyman, Webster & Tee 2015; Zalsman et al. 2016). The lasting impact of receiving training is unknown, suggesting the need for mandatory refresher training to be built into delivery plans. In addition, little is understood regarding individuals' experience and the subsequent impact on therapeutic engagement and quality experiences after training is received as viewed by the individual and family in receipt of care. Those who have been in receipt of intervention when suicidal, relay the need for human-to-human meaningful contact. Soul-less information gathering serves as a barrier to connecting with the person, therefore just as interactions need to be based in meaning to be effective, one could argue so does the framework in which training is delivered.

Careful consideration to training delivery is necessary to avoid the tick box application that we strive to avoid in practice. There is a need for appreciation of the complexity that sits behind attending and delivering programmes. There is no one agreed structure to delivery or content and there appears to be little evidence underpinning the actual methods of delivery (Heyman, Webster & Tee 2015). These features may be key in the preparation and subsequent construction of meaning for nurses embarking on such a programme as they may have no previous experience to refer to. Suicide can be an imperceptible construct for some people. Identification of smaller groups for supportive peer learning, psychological safety and considerations of personal and cultural sensitivities (*See* Chapter 6) are considered core to initiating a deeper personal experience of suicide prevention (Heyman, Webster & Tee 2015). Here, Heyman and colleagues refer specifically to ASIST (Acquired Suicide Intervention Skills Training). This is the perceivable difference of delivering skills training as opposed to awareness training to clinical staff. The latter raises awareness to participants, whereas the former dedicates substantial time to helping participants connect with and understand personal attitudes and beliefs towards suicide in the context of an open and safe forum. A degree of personal exposure and anxiety is part of the course, activated in subsequent role play and emotional exchange, and with this the hope of an emergent renewed understanding of self and the world of the suicidal person. The framework of delivery is carefully constructed to emphasise the power of intervention and equip participants with skills and confidence to ask about suicide. Unfortunately, not all courses follow such a considered approach; some confuse awareness with intervention without due exploration and preparation of participants. Potentially, participants leave more 'suicide aware' but not necessarily possessing confidence or skills to intervene. Delivering training in pre-registration nursing contexts can afford a scaffolded approach but adequate thought is needed to address content to ensure that nurses are being prepared adequately. In post registration contexts, accessibility of training, regular updates and duration of delivery is advised along with a variation of mediums to receive the information (Heyman, Webster & Tee 2015; Rebair and Hullatt 2016).

In the likelihood of expressed trepidation of attending said courses, nurses would do well to self-affirm and recall the plethora of transferable skills they already possess, which are woven into the fabric of their daily work.

The need for nurses to experience kindness from colleagues is a healthy starting point. Maybe there is a need to relinquish the boundaries that define us as different (as colleague, peer, manager, patient, nurse) and embrace that which celebrates our similarities. Ballat and Campling (2011, p. 37) suggest that 'kind staff have a sense of shared humanity and see in the patient someone who is part of the flow of life and essentially the same as themselves' (2011, p. 37). They extend this concept to the importance of kindness in and throughout organisations, acknowledging that little assessment is done to understand the impact of caring throughout organisations and connections throughout whole systems. This is particularly poignant when considering support after suicide; nurses go on caring and are likely to experience mental distress after inpatient suicide as well as shock and blame and fear of consequences (Takahashi et al. 2011). In the aftermath of suicide, support systems such as counselling and availability of support for health care professionals are required to minimise the impact on personal and professional lives (Draper et al. 2014). Authors of the same study identified that females are more vulnerable to the experience impacting upon them and the latest Office of National Statistics (ONS), Suicide by Occupation Report (2017) states female nurses in England are at higher risk than the general population for suicide. Affording kindness, support and an open-hearted response to others is therefore, essential when considering this information.

The importance of kindness and compassion is the basis of Cole-King et al. (2013) suicide mitigation quest, where all claims of suicide are met with compassion and taken seriously, and steps taken to engage positively with the person using strengths based intervention. Extending compassion is, according to the author, the only way to engage with a suicidal person. Cole-King and Gilbert (2011) describe the relationship between compassion and motivation with motivation being attributed to caring about wellbeing. By the same principal and shared sense of humanity, nurses who possess motivation and compassion may well extend their care of wellbeing to team colleagues, as unbeknown to them someone close by may be struggling with suicide. In a Royal College of Nursing survey (Rebair & Hullatt 2016) nurses remarked upon the presence of stigma about suicide in clinical teams. This unduly impacted upon nurses' ability to openly share feelings and thoughts about suicide in the clinical realm. In some cases, attitudes of colleagues compounded feelings of isolation for nurses struggling with attempted suicide of loved ones, bereavement by suicide and or personal thoughts of suicide.

REFLECTIVE PRACTICE EXERCISE 19.1

> **Time: 15 minutes**
> Take a step back and refocus on the starting point; ourselves, and how we meet each other.

ESTABLISHING THE MEETING PLACE

'All real living is meeting'

(Martin Buber 1958)

Each nurse reading this text will be reacting in their own way, accepting, rejecting, contemplating, ruminating on what they have read. Not everyone will agree. Some will feel frustrated; others may want more guidance, a formula of what to say and do. Some have already traversed the existential limits of themselves and have their own relationship with suicide. Just as the factors that lead a person to have thoughts of suicide are complex and multifaceted, so are the factors influencing the nurses' responses and ability to 'meet' a suicidal other.

There are many theories in nursing to which one can turn to help gain an understanding of how people interact and how self emerges relating. However, it is the philosophical anthropologist Martin Buber who offers an explanation of a meeting place. Buber explains that there are two main orientations of addressing relationships; I-Thou and I-It. Buber believed that human existence was about relationships and the continued desire to meet and be met hence 'all real living is meeting' (Buber 1958, pp. 24–25). Importantly, it is the nature of the relationship that defines I-Thou and I-It rather than the object of what they relate to (*See* Chapter 7). According to Buber (1970), the I-Thou relationship has openness, directness, mutuality and presence and establishing I-Thou meets the object in its entirety. The meeting of the object creates a whole experience and is termed the site of relation.

Conversely, the I-It refers to the subject – object relationship. The I in me and the I in Thou have distance where there is no connection; we do not share a whole experience; we do not relate. This is of interest to nursing and conversations about suicide because the co-creation of the I -Thou' is reached through what Buber (1970) terms 'will and grace'. Here, participants work to create I-Thou, I-Thou is co-created, it is what happens between participants and it requires a continual desire for mutuality. This focus is crucial when working with suicidal people and requires the nurse to be open and present to the unfolding situation and willing to engage, willing to see the whole person. Long and colleagues (Long, Long & Smyth 1998) discuss the dilemmas in caring for suicidal people, when referring to Buber's philosophy noting initial contact phases and the paradox of construing meaning in a shared space. They comment: 'as an I-it, the individual is considered to contain information or data that are wanted by the nurse, but there is no need to engage with the presence of the patient in any meaningful way. When the gathering of information becomes more important than making a connection with the presence of the patient, as nurses, we are diminished in our humanity' (Long, Long & Smyth 1998, p. 6). The universal tool is the nurse themselves, capable of creating or disabling opportunities to connect. Distancing and maintaining the I-it relationship is less emotionally demanding in stressful clinical situations and nurses may knowingly or unknowingly hide behind the mechanics of the assessment to protect themselves for a variety of reasons. Friedman (2002, p. xiii) explains, 'I can prevent such a relationship from coming into being if I am not ready to respond or if I attempt to respond with anything less than my whole being insofar as my resources in this particular situation allows' (2002, p. xiii).

In a call for theory-based interventions about nursing suicidal people, Cutcliffe et al. (2006), theorised 'reconnecting the person with humanity' as the first stage in a process of engaging with suicidal people. The nurse's input reflects the need for 'warm, care-based, human to human contact' understanding and being with the person without judgement. Experiencing wholeness in the continual quest to co-create I-Thou as offered by Buber (1958). It is described as a place of stillness, co-presence, the focus is on accepting and being with the person. This nurtured connectivity to the nurse, creating a site where the person could share feelings. It is only when the connectivity is established that sharing of stories occurred. Stage 1 is a critical encounter and the site of genuine kindness and concern for the person. This is echoed in the author's current research along with an unfolding emphasis on the fear and vulnerability of the nurse as the protagonist of willingness to engage.

KEY POINT 19.2

Nurses have a professional responsibility to notice their limitations, care for their wellbeing and notice if they may be compromised in affecting care. The need for self-compassion and care must be a priority.

KEY POINT 19.3

Nurses are key in crafting a meeting place through which humanity is enacted though this can be impeded by fear and uncertainty, despite adorning the moral code of offering care.

EXPLORING DISSONANCE

One such area of fear and uncertainty arises when there is discord between what a nurse believes and what is expected of them as governed by The Code of Conduct for Nursing and Midwifery (2015) and the Mental Health Act Code of Practice (MHA 1983, updated 2015). Thus, dissonance arises through conflicting values and beliefs implicit in the caring role. In a two-part article (Cutcliffe & Links 2008a; Cutcliffe and Links 2008b) provide a compelling presentation of the moral distress that may occur in nurses who believe that suicide is a personal right whilst operating in a system expected to prevent people from taking their own life. Rich and Butts (2004) term this 'uncertain moral ground' presenting the tensions and paradoxes in greater detail than this section can do justice. Legal and professional positions are highlighted through exploring the Mental Health Act Code of Practice presenting an understandable portrayal of why nurses become conflicted. While there is an emphasis on preserving safety, and preventing harm the nurse must also consider capacity bearing in mind what appears to be an unwise decision may not denote the person as lacking capacity. Herein lies the tension: the nurse is accountable and responsible for actions and omissions. He or she is bound by the code of conduct and law and the nurse must consider and assess capacity of the individual in the context of a meaningful conversation whilst espousing the person's view of human rights and confidentiality. All of this is done whilst potentially struggling with their own moral perspective and the counter argument of 'rational' suicide.

The Consensus Statement for Information Sharing and Suicide Prevention was developed by several professional organisations to help support professionals make decisions about sharing information about a suicidal person, an excerpt from the document reads:

> The Mental Capacity Act makes it clear that a person must be assumed to have capacity unless it is established that they lack capacity, and that a person is not to be treated as unable to make a decision merely because they make an unwise decision. However, if a person is at imminent risk of suicide there may well be sufficient doubts about their mental capacity at that time.
>
> (DoH, Office of Public Guardian 2014, p. 5)

The extract above gives permission to doubt mental capacity that subverts arguments regarding rational suicide (Werth 1996) because it suggests that imminence of suicide and mental capacity are not mutually exclusive. Assessing if the person is at imminent risk is also a challenge and suggests that non-imminent responses are less concerning, what timing differentiates them? Moreover, is establishing the imminence of suicide a sole reason to share information? Changing and unfolding circumstances render the person in need of support either way. The National Confidential Enquiry (2010) report that predicting suicide is thwart with difficulty and levels of prediction is low and for these reasons NICE CG133 (National Institute for Health and Care Excellence 2011) do not recommend the use of risk assessment tools and scales to predict future suicide. This then presents yet more conflict regarding what to do for the greater good of the person whilst demonstrating adherence to professional codes.

There is an identified need for nurses to be afforded time and space to explore dissonance as fear of reprisal, professional accountability and the desire to practice none maleficence have been cited as key reasons for avoiding conversations about suicide (Rebair & Hullatt 2016).

It might be helpful to shift focus to another site of discussion, that of the ethic of caring. Rich and Butts (2004, p. 276) refer to the obligation of nurses to promote caring through:

respectful, compassionate exploration of the patient's feelings; anything less and a caregiver would be remiss in fulfilling the role of caring . . . the caring relationship facilitates exploration of feelings, including the caregiver's feelings, meaningful communication and thoughtful decision making that facilitates the autonomous patient's best interests as the patient views it.

(2004, p. 276)

The emphasis here is in the interaction, the meeting and the shared understanding and decision making. The nurse is duty-bound to think about how they are expressing care in the context and are upholding the code with sincerity and expressing humanity. Suicide prevention takes place in the context of a caring relationship with a shared understanding of where each person is and so in the advent of disagreement regarding safety the person has had an experience of being cared for and understands the nurse's genuine concern. Barker (2004) upholds that in all accounts 'it is better to be safe than sorry' offering the person an opportunity to explore the edges of their distress and the cause of 'psychache' can allow a turning point to emerge as the story between nurse and person unfolds. It is this that is the primary goal.

PREPARATION

May we go to the places that scare us, may we lead the life of a warrior.

(Chodron 2003)

Information is limited regarding the preparation of nurses to discuss, explore and be with the subject of suicide. Hem and Heggen (2003), offer that vulnerability is important and that this is the site to which professional nursing development can emerge. Similarly, sensitive and considered approaches to suicide in the oncology nursing literature refer to nurses' professional responsibility of first understanding and addressing their own feelings of suicide. This would appear to be the starting point, being with the places that scare us. As with a home, the foundations need to be constructed to withstand the impending structure. It is acknowledged that readers will be in various stages of their own building, some may be at planning stage, others may have built the house and are attending to repair work as the nature of our interactions bear weathering, rebuilds and construction of extensions over time. The house is never finished.

Nurses openly refer to the fear of starting a conversation about suicide, fear of what they might say and hear, fear of making the situation worse, fear of opening the proverbial 'can of worms'. Facing the fear requires considering the sacred space inside ourselves, the inevitability of acknowledging mortality and that of the ones we love. Thinking about untimely loss can be enough to initiate tears and great sadness; therefore, willingly engaging with our vulnerabilities seems counterintuitive. Yet, nurses are faced with this in the context of practice every day. The difference is that preparation in safe spaces heeds warning and care can be initiated.

In her book about facing fear, Pema Chodron (2003), refers to the Buddhist practice of Bodhicitta. Bodhicitta exists on two levels, the first being unconditional Bodhicitta, practicing an open, free and un-opinionated response. The second level is relative Bodhicitta, working to stay open hearted through pain and suffering. The practice of Bodhicitta acknowledges that humans look for safety and security, the need to stay safe and not venture out of the safety. The focus is how we relate to discomfort as opposed to avoiding uncertainty and fear. Through the practice of Bodhicitta the subject of suicide and associated fear is not to be avoided but instead one is asked to look at how one relates to the discomfort that arises.

One would suggest that this requires a degree of curiosity of self and of the other, knowing that discomfort and fear are unavoidable conditions of the human spirit. It encompasses the term feel the fear and do it anyway but enter with kindness and care of where one is treading for self and other.

CONCLUSION

The needs of nurses in delivering meaningful care with a suicidal person is as multifaceted and complex as the reasons one may present with suicidal feelings. The current evidence base surrounding suicide prevention training is reported to be helpful by those attending, but due to the various applications, content and methods of presenting, there is little understating of what actual elements are helpful and the medium to longer term impact is unknown. Fear and stigma underlie difficulties in conversations about suicide, therefore, preparation of self and the reality of facing acute end-of-life conversation should be addressed to create confidence within the nurse. Being open to uncertainty and discomfort encourages willingness. Willingly entering the space of another with kindness creates a connection and a meeting place where a story can be shared, and the power of meaningful and efficacious dialogue can occur. This is the key to co-creating potential lifesaving interventions.

Nurses need support to explore and unravel the paradox in which they operate to create self-awareness. Moreover, there needs to be a way to incorporate this as a fundamental aspect of teaching and development. Nurses would benefit from what they personally understand as being professional. By traversing the I-It and I-Thou, nurses can be both without diminishing themselves of humanity, the essence of what suicidal persons need.

The power of simply asking if someone is OK is often overlooked. The story of Kevin Hines and the Golden Gate Bridge is testament to this. Up until the point that he let go of the bridge, Kevin was prepared to talk to someone. He was desperate for someone to acknowledge his distress and ask the question, "Are you OK?", "Are you thinking about ending your life?" (Hines, Cole-King & Blaustein 2013). Let us have faith in those that have survived their distress and lived to tell their story. We are told not to be afraid. We are invited to ask about suicide. Throughout the literature and collective voices of the other, nurses are given permission to ask about suicide, permission to be human and to care.

REFERENCES

Ballatt, J. and Campling, P. (2011) *Intelligent Kindness; Reforming the Culture of Healthcare.* London: Royal College of Psychiatry Publications.

Barker, P. J. (2004) *Assessment in Psychiatric and Mental Health Nursing; In Search of the Whole Person* (2nd edition). Andover, Hampshire: Cengage Learning EMEA.

Buber, M. (1958) *I and Thou.* 2nd edition. Edinburgh. T and T Clark. Translated by R. Gregory Smith, pp. 24–5.

Buber, M. (1970) *I and Thou.* New York: Charles Scribner's Sons. Translated by W. Kaufmann.

Buber, M. (2002) *Between Man and Man.* London/New York: Routledge. Translated from German by R. Gregor-Smith.

Cole-King, A., Parker, V., Williams, H. and Platt, S. (2013) 'Suicide prevention: are we doing enough'? *Advances in Psychiatric Treatment*, 19, pp. 284–91.

Cole-King, A. and Gilbert, P. (2011) 'Compassionate care: the theory and the reality'. *Journal of Holistic Healthcare*, 8, pp. 29–36.

Cutcliffe, J. R., Stevenson, C., Jackson, S. and Smith, P. (2006) 'A modified grounded theory study of how psychiatric nurses work with suicidal people'. *International Journal of Nursing Studies*, 43, pp. 791–802.

Cutcliffe, J. R. and Links, P. S. (2008a) 'Whose life is it anyway? An exploration of five contemporary ethical issues that pertain to the psychiatric nursing care of the person who is suicidal. Part one'. *International Journal of Mental Health Nursing*, 17, pp. 236–45.

Cutcliffe, J. R. and Links, P. S. (2008b) 'Whose life is it anyway? An exploration of five contemporary ethical issues that pertain to the psychiatric nursing care of the person who is suicidal. Part two'. *International Journal of Mental Health Nursing*, 17, pp. 246–54.

Chodron, P. (2003) *The Places that Scare You, a Guide to Fearlessness.* London: Element.

Department of Health. Mental Health, Equality and Disability Division (2014) *Information Sharing and Suicide Prevention. Consensus Statement.* London: Her Majesty's Government.

Department of Health. (2017) *Preventing Suicide Ion England; Third Progress Report of the Cross-Government Outcome Strategy to Save Lives.* London: Her Majesty's Government. London.

Draper, B., Kolves, K., De Leo, D. and Snowdon, J. (2014) 'The impact of patient suicide and sudden death on health care professionals'. *General Hospital Psychiatry*, 36, pp. 721–5.

Friedman, M. (2002) 'Introduction' in Buber, M. (2002) '*Between Man and Man*'. Translated from by R. Gregor-Smith. London/New York: Routledge.

General Medical Council. (2017) *Generic Professional Capabilities Framework. Working with Doctors Working with People.* Available at: www.gmc-uk.org/education/postgraduate/GPC.asp (Accessed: 22 October 2017)

Hem, M. H. and Heggen, K. (2003) 'Being professional and being human: one nurse's relationship with a psychiatric patient'. *Journal of Advanced Nursing*, 43, pp. 101–8.

Heyman, I., Webster, B. J. and Tee, S. (2015) 'Curriculum development through understanding the student nurse experience of suicide intervention education- a phenomenographic study'. *Nurse Education in Practice*, 15, pp. 498–506.

Hines, K., Cole-King, A. and Blaustein, M. (2013) 'Hey kid, are you OK? A story of suicide survived'. *Advances in Psychiatric Treatment*, 19, pp. 292–4.

Isaac, M., Elias, B., Katz, Y. L., Belik, S. L. Deane, F. P. et al. (2009) 'Gatekeeper training as a preventative intervention for suicide. A systematic review'. *The Canadian Journal of Psychiatry*, 54, pp. 260–8.

Lees, D., Procer, N. and Fassett, D. (2014) 'Therapeutic engagement between consumers in suicidal crisis and mental health nurses'. *International Journal of Mental Health Nursing*, 23, pp. 306–15.

Long, A. and Smyth, A. (1998) 'Suicide: a statement of suffering'. *Nursing Ethics*, 5, pp. 3–15.

Mental Capacity Act (2014) London: Office of Public Guardian. Available at: www.gov.uk/government/collections/mental-capacity-act-making-decisions (Accessed: 22 October 2017)

Mental Health Act. (1983, updated 2015) London: Department of Health. Available at: www.gov.uk/government/publications/code-of-practice-mental-health-act-1983 (Accessed: 22 October 2017)

National Confidential Inquiry into Suicide and Homicide by People with a Mental Illness (2010) Annual report. England and Wales. July 2010. Manchester: University of Manchester. Available at: http://research.bmh.manchester.ac.uk/cmhs/research/centreforsuicideprevention/nci/reports/2016-report.pdf (Accessed 22 October 2017)

National Institute for Health and Care Excellence -NICE CG133 (2011) *Self harm in over 8's. Long term management.* Available at: www.nice.org.uk/guidance/cg133 (Accessed: 22 October 2017)

Nursing and Midwifery Council – NMC. (2009) *Standards for Pre-registration midwifery education.* London: Nursing and Midwifery Council. Available at: www.nmc.org.uk/globalassets/sitedocuments/standards/nmc-standards-for-preregistration-midwifery-education.pdf (Accessed: 22 October 2017)

Nursing and Midwifery Council – NMC. (2010) *Standards for Pre-registration nurse education.* London: Nursing and Midwifery Council. Available at: www.nmc.org.uk/globalassets/sitedocuments/standards/nmc-standards-for-pre-registration-nursing-education.pdf (Accessed: 22 October 2017)

Nursing and Midwifery Council – NMC (2015) *The Code. Professional Standard for Practice and Behaviour for Nurses and Midwives.* London: Nursing and Midwifery Council.

Nursing and Midwifery Council – NMC (2017) *Standards of proficiency for registered nurses.* London: Nursing and Midwifery Council. Available at: www.nmc.org.uk/globalassets/sitedocuments/edcons/ec7-draft-standards-of-proficiency-for-registered-nurses.pdf (Accessed 22 October 2017)

Office for National Statistics – ONS. (2017) *Suicide by occupation. England 2011–2015.* Available at: www.ons.gov.uk/peoplepopulationandcommunity/birthsdeathsandmarriages/deaths/articles/suicidebyoccupation/england2011to2015 (Accessed 22 October 2017)

Public Health England – PHE. (2015) *Public mental health leadership and workforce development framework. Competence, confidence, commitment.* London: Public Health England. Available at: www.gov.uk/government/uploads/system/uploads/attachment_data/file/410356/Public_Mental_Health_Leadership_and_Workforce_Development_Framework.pdf (Accessed: 22 October 2017).

Pullen, M. J., Gilje, F. and Tesar, E. (2016) 'A descriptive study of baccalaureate nursing students' responses to suicide prevention education'. *Nurse Education in Practice,* 16, pp. 104–10.

Ramberg, I., Di Lucca, M. A. and Hadlaczky, G. (2016) 'The impact of knowledge of suicide prevention and work experience among clinical staff on attitudes towards working with suicidal patients and suicide prevention'. *International Journal of Environmental Research and Public Health,* 13, p. 195.

Rebair, A. and Hullatt, I. (2016) 'Identifying nurses needs in relation to suicide awareness and prevention'. *Nursing Standard,* 31, pp. 4–51.

Rich, K. L. and Butts, J. B. (2004) 'Rational suicide: uncertain moral ground'. *Philosophical and Ethical Issues,* 46, pp. 270–83.

Talseth, A. G and Gilje, F. L. (2011) 'Nurses' responses to suicide and suicidal patients: a critical interpretive synthesis'. *Journal of Clinical Nursing,* 20, pp. 1651–67.

Takahashi, C., Chida, F., Nakamura, H., Akasaka, H., Yagi, J. et al. (2011) 'The impact of in-patient suicide on psychiatric nurses and their need for support'. *BioMed Central Psychiatry.* Available at: https://bmcpsychiatry.biomedcentral.com/articles/10.1186/1471-244X-11-38 (Accessed: 22 October 2017).

Werth, J. L. (1996) *Rational Suicide? Implications for Mental Health Professionals.* Washington: Taylor and Francis International.

Zalsman, G. Hawton, K. Wasserman, D. Heeringen, K. Arensman, E. et al. (2016) 'Suicide prevention strategies revisited: 10-year systematic review'. *The Lancet Psychiatry,* 3, pp. 646–59.

To Learn More

Barker, P. J. and Buchanan Barker, P. (eds) (2003) *Spirituality and Mental Health. Breakthrough.* Wiley and Sons Ltd: UK.

Chodron, P. (2012) *Living Beautifully with Uncertainty and Change.* Shambhala: Boston and London.

National Suicide Prevention Alliance (NSPA) www.nspa.org.uk/

Plath, S. (2005) *The Bell Jar.* Harper Collins: US.

Prevention of Young Suicide (PAYRUS) www.papyrus-uk.org

Support After Suicide Partnership supportaftersuicide.org.uk/

CHAPTER 20

Supportive Decision Making

Geralyn Hynes and Agnes Higgins

INTRODUCTION

The term supportive care was introduced in the 1990s to describe: 'the provision of the necessary services for those living with or affected by cancer to meet their informational, emotional, spiritual, social, or physical need during their diagnostic treatment or follow up phases encompassing issues of health promotion, and prevention, survivorship, palliation and bereavement' (Altilio & Otis-Green 2006, p. 1994). Since then there is a notable lack of consistency in how the term is defined.

More recently, a systematic review of the literature to identify concepts and definitions for palliative, hospice and supportive care provided a preliminary conceptual framework unifying these terms along the continuum of care (Hui et al. 2013). This framework positions supportive care throughout the cancer disease trajectory from diagnosis and includes survivorship and bereavement with palliative care viewed as coming in under the umbrella of supportive care. Supportive care is broadly understood as 'helping the patient and family get through the illness in the best possible condition' (Bruera & Hui 2016, p. 98).

For our purposes, we understand supportive decision making as beginning with all those involved in care of the individual experiencing ill-health and their family, acknowledging and engaging with the concept of total pain which is fundamental to understanding palliative care.

KEY POINT 20.1

Of note, supportive care applies to any life-limiting condition including cancer.

In this chapter we will discuss the implications of our understanding of supportive decision making in palliative care within a mental health context. In particular, we refer to the everyday challenges associated with different and potentially conflicting philosophies of care that are represented by different disciplines and specialist teams working in acute care, mental health and palliative care. From there, we will present a case study that illustrates the challenges and then, begin to unpack how supportive decision making might be addressed. We do this using reflective questions and follow-up points in the case study presentation.

KEY POINT 20.2

Core to palliative care are two moral attitudes. First, an unconditional respect for human life and second, dignity and acceptance of human finitude and death. These moral attitudes are accompanied by truthfulness, prudence and compassion.

(Taboada 2016)

CONCEPTS FOR SUPPORTIVE DECISION MAKING

Disease Versus Ill-Health

In keeping with the distinction drawn by medical anthropologists between disease and ill-health (Helman 1981), we understand disease as referring to patho-physiological abnormalities that can be identified and described as distinct entities in terms of structure and function/disfunction. In contrast, ill-health refers to the individual's perspective of their disease, including its significance for all aspects of living and the meaning that the person attributes to this experience. From this distinction, terms such as ill-health oriented and disease oriented care have become established short hand for reflecting care approaches with the former often used interchangeably with person-centred care. The concept of disease-oriented care is often used in a way that goes well beyond the patho-physiological, to reflect the reductionism of health service management and policy implementation. Here, guidelines and protocols are standardised in a way that privileges certain kinds of evidence over the subjective experience, and the person is viewed as a passive recipient of the 'wisdom' of the 'expert professional'.

Total Pain

Since palliative care is fundamentally concerned with the individual's subjective experience of pain and suffering, we will adopt the term ill-health oriented care accordingly. Total pain recognises pain as multi-dimensional. These dimensions include physical symptoms, mental and existential distress and social problems, all or any combination of which can be inter-related and interdependent. Addressing total pain implies an emphasis on whole-person care (Hutchinson 2011). In laying the foundations for what we understand as palliative care today, Cecily Saunders conceptualised total pain in a now famous quote from one of her patients who described her pain thus: 'It began in my back, but now it seems that all of me is wrong' (Saunders 1964, p. viii). The woman went on to explain her physical pain, its emotional and social impact and her need for security or safety. Saunders (2006, p. 280) held that total pain is 'the complex of physical, mental, social and spiritual elements that make up the patient's whole experience' and that crucially, neither the individual nor the doctor can separate these elements. Thus, to deny any one dimension of a person's whole experience is to deny their whole experience, in other words, their personhood. Engaging with and acknowledging the concept of total pain presents immediate challenges for those involved in care of individuals who are under different teams (e.g. oncology, medical, mental health and palliative care). Each team or specialty brings its own language, history and underlying values that influence how knowledge of a person's needs are understood and addressed. It is against this background that the person must navigate their understanding and participation in decisions about treatment and care. Supportive decision making might therefore, be understood as enabling the individual and family to understand and process information about ill-health, and its symptoms and to actively participate in decisions about treatment options from different perspectives in what is likely to be a dynamic situation as the disease evolves. For this to happen, the individual with an advanced chronic ill-health, and their family, should be aware of the distinct specialism and contribution of each team (medical, mental health and palliative care for example) but should equally experience a seamlessness in how care is delivered, and problems are managed.

Supportive Decision-making in Context

Supportive decision making rests on how the individual's suffering is acknowledged and understood by health care teams, and these teams' capacity to enable individuals both to articulate their suffering, and actively pursue goals that are important to them at a given point in time. Supportive decision making requires a recognition that the individual's goals will shift and evolve over the course of the ill-health trajectory. Figure 20.1 illustrates a basis for framing supportive decision making from two intersecting perspectives.

The vertical line (A) reflects a continuum depicting how suffering is understood in health care from unidimensional perspective at one extreme to the concept of total pain at the other end. The horizontal line (B) reflects another continuum from, at one end, a disciplinary view of symptom management with disciplines working independently,

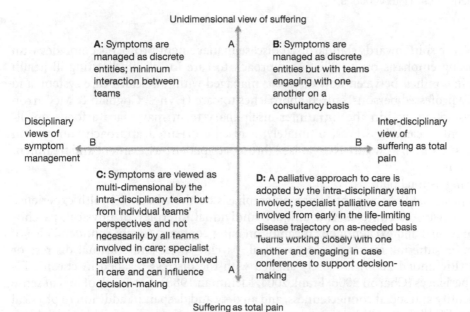

Figure 20.1 Perspectives on and context for supportive decision making

bringing their own particular perspectives. At the other end of this continuum lies an inter-disciplinary view of suffering as total pain and brings an integrated approach to care.

(A) Vertical line

(1) A unidimensional perspective on suffering

At one end of the vertical line, the concept of total pain is rejected though perhaps, unintentionally. Instead, a unidimensional approach to disease and symptom management dominates whereby, for example, a disease is diagnosed and managed from a patho-physiological perspective (Figure 20.1). In the case of multiple morbidities where a person may experience life-limiting ill-health such as cancer, heart failure, renal failure or chronic obstructive pulmonary disease (COPD), in addition to a mental health diagnosis such as depression, these are treated as separate disease entities with their respective discrete sets of signs and symptoms. This places the health care professional in the mode of expert with little focus on what the combined ill-health experience as a whole means to the person. Standardised protocols associated with treatments for common life-limiting diseases such as cancers, COPD, and mental health problems such as, depression, place an emphasis on bio-medicine or what some might refer to as disease oriented rather than ill-health oriented care; the former representing a bio-medical view and the latter reflecting a whole experience oriented view.

KEY POINT 20.3

Disease or bio-medically focused care that denies ill-health experiences increases suffering and ultimately iatrogenesis that is to say, inadvertent and preventable suffering arising from treatment of care interventions.

Ironically, the shift towards standardised disease management protocols coincides with an increasing emphasis on a palliative approach to care for all life-limiting ill-health resulting in conflicts between how disease is managed within a health care system, and disciplines professed person-centred approaches to care (Hynes, Coghlan & McCarron 2014). Disciplines within the intra/inter-disciplinary team may place a focus on ill-health oriented care. However, ultimately, a disease-oriented approach can remain dominant such as, in how care is organised through to patient-assessment and treatment interventions.

(2) Suffering as total pain

At the opposite end of the continuum, an emphasis on the whole ill-health experience is dominant with its complex and uniquely individual interplay of physical, psycho-social, emotional and existential or meaning-making contexts. Cicely Saunders' idea of total pain as suffering encompassing physical, psycho-social and spiritual distress or struggles (Richmond 2005) is closely aligned with the distress recalled in chronic ill-health experiences (Charon 2006; Frank 2004; Kleinman 1988) that speak of loss of sense of self, identity and social connectedness, and anxiety and despair in addition to physical symptoms. Multiple morbidity experiences are greater than the sum of their individual diseases both in terms of how symptoms are experienced and the degree of integrated care required by specialist oncology, medical, mental health and palliative care teams. Much of the palliative care and wider health care literature draws on Eric Cassell's definition of suffering as: 'the specific distress that occurs when persons feel their intactness or integrity as persons threatened or disintegrating, and it continues until the threat is gone or intactness or integrity is restored' (Cassell 2011, p. 10). Suffering in this sense includes pain but is not bounded by it; they are phenomenologically distinct from one another. Central to Cassell's definition for suffering is his understanding of the person. For Cassell (2011, p. 12) the person is an 'embodied, purposeful, thinking, feeling, emotional, reflective, relational very complex human individual of a certain personality and temperament, existing through time in a narrative sense, whose life in all spheres points both outward and inward and who does things'. Individuals need to be able to pursue goals that are important to them and are unique to each person.

Cassell (1991) describes a person as having a past with memories, built-up truths, life experiences, family, relationships, cultural background (*See* Chapter 6), roles with social and political influences, and a relationship with self. The person is aware of and can assign meaning to a past and future. Cassell's concept of personhood stands against mind-body dualism. He argues that the person is 'of a piece' and that all aspects of personhood are susceptible to damage and loss. Thus, for Cassell, it is incorrect to refer to suffering as existential or psychological or physical. Rather existential, physical or psychological issues may be the cause of my suffering but the suffering impacts on all of me. In other words, if I am suffering mentally then that will manifest in every other part: my social, political, physical self and so on. This is because suffering threatens the wholeness of me (Cassell 2013). Supportive decision-making therefore, requires all those involved to recognise suffering as intensely personal and an embodied experience.

Not surprisingly, palliative care specialists such as Byock (2004) have placed an emphasis on the importance of recognising the unique needs of an individual at the end-of-life. For this to happen, active total care of the individual is paramount, including control of pain and other symptoms, and acknowledging and addressing psycho-social and existential problems. Such total care depends on in-depth knowledge of the individual's ill-health, aetiologies and patho-physiologies, expression of symptoms including global suffering, factors influencing suffering such as family and significant life events, and the meaning the person attaches to each experience. Therein lies the paradox for modern health care whereby the use of terms such as physical, psycho-social, existential and so on to reflect an understanding of pain in all its multi-dimensionality can also serve to set these up as discrete entities and so infer a more disease oriented or reductionist view.

(B) Horizontal line: Disciplinary engagement and approaches to symptom management and decision making

Persons receiving care from specialist palliative care (SPC) teams typically remain under the care of their primary health care teams. In the case of co-existing ill health, a person will remain under the care of several teams and services such as oncology, medical and mental health with each team needing to support complex treatment decisions and symptom management (inter-disciplinary team).

(1) Uni-dimensional perspective on disease and symptom management
At one end of the continuum, each team brings its own specialist knowledge, ways of working, language and values that may reflect the reductionism of a dominant

patho-physiological focus on disease and symptom management. Here, an intra- inter-disciplinary team may follow its own standardised ways of working and consult with other teams on an as needed basis. Each team has its own culture in terms of the nature of decision making, the degree to which this reflects the participation of different professional groups within the team, and the nature and quality of engagement. Engagement with other teams and the individual reflects a consultative process at the level of technical support. There is limited if any engagement with another team's ways of working, language and values, questioning of one's own assumptions and values or acknowledging the uniqueness of an individual's suffering and personhood.

The degree to which each team can recognise a person's whole ill-health experience can vary not least because of the system's structures and processes within which the team works. A medical team must, for example, follow protocols for the management of an acute exacerbation of COPD, which include criteria for admission, lengths of stay in hospital, treatments and so on. These privilege the reductionism and techno-rationality of bio-medicine and quantifiable measures for assessment with less emphasis on suffering as total pain and its irreducibility (Hynes et al. 2014; Hynes et al. 2015). Palliative care and psychiatry, on the other hand, may, at first glance, have a closer relationship since both place an emphasis on a person's life experience, emotions and suffering. However, any such comparison can be brought into question with psychiatry's focus on bio-medicine and reductionism (Billings & Block 2009). Though emerging recovery-oriented approaches to care within mental health reflect a greater emphasis on the whole-person experience and alignment with palliative care principles, embedding such practices within the service has proven to be challenging (Storm & Edwards 2013). This is in part, because traditional care models are wedded to a bio-medical view of mental distress and approaches to care.

KEY POINT 20.4

Features that render palliative care significantly different from other specialist areas such as oncology, internal medicine and psychiatry include palliative care's focus on quality of life, and view of the individual and family as the unit of care.

Palliative care recognises the individual and family as the unit of care thus recognising the importance of family caregiver experiences. Where the specialist palliative care (SPC) team is involved in care of an individual and the family, this may counter the dominant disease and symptom management focus of other teams, that tend to marginalise the role of family and significant others (*See* Chapter 16). The degree to which the SPC team can influence a more whole-person and family-focused care approach across the different teams will help determine the degree of supportive decision making that can be introduced.

(2) An interdisciplinary view of suffering

Against a background of different ways of working, team cultures and so on, enabling supportive decision making with the person and family requires attention to how teams understand one another and are able to question their own assumptions and values.

At the other end of the continuum of disciplinary approaches to care and decision making, an intra- inter-disciplinary view of suffering begins with active engagement with the principles of palliative care and embedding a palliative approach to care in everyday practice. Intra- inter-disciplinary teams that can interrogate their understanding of person-centeredness and family-focused care are well placed to adopt a palliative approach to care within their everyday practice. This ensures three important facets of supportive decision making. First, the intra-disciplinary team introduces and practises non-specialist palliative care early in the trajectory of a life-limiting ill-health with its focus on the whole-person experience and personhood. Second, the intra/inter-disciplinary team can ensure that the person is fully informed from an early stage and can set the pace for information and decision making. Third, the intra- inter-disciplinary team is well placed to recognise and respond to the shifting dynamics of a person's whole ill-health experience and to bring in the specialist palliative care team for help with symptom management on an as-needed basis. This also ensures that the person is not faced with a new team late in the ill-health trajectory and at a point when advanced care planning is more difficult to introduce. Since palliative care views the individual and family as the unit of care, the intra- inter-disciplinary team moves away from the dyadic person/professional relationship that characterises modern health care and towards shared decision making. Shared decision making in this context can be understood as a continuum moving from person-driven decision making, through to partnership with care providers, and eventually to physician-driven decision making (Kon 2010, 2012). This process of decision making should be shaped and guided by the wishes of the individual or the surrogate decision maker.

IMPLICATIONS OF PERSPECTIVES ON, AND CONTEXT FOR, SUPPORTIVE DECISION MAKING

Psychological problems such as depression and anxiety are common among individual cohorts with a life-limiting ill-health but may remain undiagnosed (Mitchell et al. 2011; Garrido et al. 2017). Over the past decade there has been a significant body of research on various advanced chronic ill-health pointing to poor health status, and all-encompassing loss experienced by the individual, including loss of sense of self, of identity, roles and purpose, and of social interaction. These findings stem from health status measurement and qualitative research and all resonate with the concept of total pain and Cassell's (1991) concept of suffering. As people live longer they are more likely to experience multiple-morbidity that may or may not arise from treatment side effects. This is likely to result in an increased need for a greater number of intra/inter-disciplinary teams involved in the care of a person experiencing increasingly complex decision making about treatment. For instance, for those people experiencing a pre-existing mental health problem, poorly integrated systems of medical and psychiatric care may inhibit or delay access to services (Foti 2009). This increases the likelihood of poorly integrated care with the person's experience thought of as a collection of conditions and symptoms that are treated as separate entities (Figure 20.1, quadrant A). Tragically, the lack of integrated care means these individuals are less likely to be supported in advanced care planning or making advanced care directives for their medical conditions. There appears to be some evidence that people experiencing pre-existing mental ill-health have difficulties in accessing palliative care services though the scale and nature of the problem is woefully under-researched (Lloyd-Williams, Abba & Crowther 2014). In mental health services where recovery-oriented models of care are established and embedded, one might anticipate that a more whole-person approach to care is practised and with accompanying recognition of suffering reflecting quadrant B in Figure 20.1. Palliative and supportive care is limited by the lack or late engagement of the SPC (specialist palliative care) team and few examples of good practice that would reflect quadrant D in Figure 20.1 and the basis for supportive decision making.

Case Study 20.1.1

Amyotrophic lateral sclerosis (ALS) including motor neurone disease (MND) is typically a rapidly progressive, degenerative life-limiting condition involving degeneration of motor nerves (known as neurons) with an average life expectancy of between two and five years from the onset of symptoms though there is considerable variation and some people live much longer. Neurones control the muscles that enable movement, speech, breathing and swallowing. With neurone degeneration muscles weaken and waste. The person experiences symptoms such as muscle weakness and paralysis, and impaired speech, swallowing and breathing.

Supportive Care Issues for Kate and Her Family

Kate is 54 years old with a long history of anxiety and substance use (*See* Chapter 17). She was married and is now divorced and lives alone. She has two adult children who live some distance away and who keep in touch but do not visit regularly. She has been attending the mental health services off and on over many years. She has a number of friends whose company she enjoys but with whom she is not very close.

Kate received a diagnosis of motor neuron disease (MND) a month ago. Kate is now depressed and talking of wanting to end her life. While she can still engage in her normal social activities including shopping and socialising with friends, she is already aware of increased fatigue, of friends straining to understand her and of staggering at times.

Kate is shocked that this is happening to her and is struggling to accept her diagnosis and prognosis. She is experiencing feelings of guilt and fears that her previous substance use and associated lifestyle have contributed to her ill-health. She wonders if life is somehow punishing her. She is terrified of the future and of the pace at which symptoms are worsening, and fears the rapid progression of her condition.

REFLECTIVE PRACTICE EXERCISE 20.1

Time: 15 minutes

What are your immediate concerns upon receiving information about Kate's diagnosis from the neurology team and from Kate herself?

Case Study 20.1.2

At the time of diagnosis, Kate will likely be aware of muscle weakness and may or may not be anticipating a potentially serious diagnosis. Irrespective, the diagnosis of ALS is traumatic and can lead to the development or exacerbation of mental health problems such as depression or anxiety. A recent study found that people experiencing ALS are at a higher risk of a depression diagnosis and use of antidepressant drugs, before and after diagnosis (Roos et al. 2016). In addition, people with a history of clinically significant depression or anxiety are at high risk of relapse. A Swedish study also found that people experiencing ALS are at higher risk of suicide than the population in general (Fang et al. 2008). Even though depression and anxiety are prevalent among people experiencing life-limiting ill-health and may co-exist when nearing end-of-life, they frequently go unrecognised, underdiagnosed and undertreated in palliative care (Breitbart & Alici 2014). For those experiencing pre-existing depression or anxiety, they are likely to get worse following diagnosis. People experiencing ALS are also faced with malnutrition related to dysphagia, and compounded by problems with using utensils including cutlery. Such problems, in turn, can further exacerbate a sense of powerlessness with the knock-on effect of increasing depression and anxiety levels in a vicious cycle. In addition, individuals are at high risk of respiratory problems, and increased anxiety is often associated with fear of the future not least, of choking to death. Combined, these problems and fears bring Saunders' concept of total pain as 'all of me is wrong' very much to the fore. Resolution comes not from treating anxiety or malnutrition as separate symptoms. Rather, resolution of such problems demands a total care approach.

With Kate's mental health and substance use history, there is a high risk that Kate may return to substance use. Someone who is predisposed to anxiety will already be experiencing high levels of anxiety. In the mistaken belief that Kate's symptoms were associated with her anxiety (diagnostic overshadowing) or, in an effort to minimise her 'anxiety' she may have received misleading reassurances that 'there is nothing to worry about' from members of the mental health team before being diagnosed by the neurologist. While MND is not an uncommon condition, it is likely that Kate's formal carers from her mental health service will not be familiar with the condition at least initially, and will have difficulty in supporting Kate appropriately. They may struggle with her fears about the future and how her final months will be. At the same time, both the neurology and palliative care teams may be unsure of how best to treat Kate considering her mental health history and increased risk of suicide (*See* Chapter 19). Her current state of hopelessness needs to be addressed urgently. This might lead to the neurology team seeking an urgent consultation with the psychiatrist.

REFLECTION PRACTICE EXERCISE 20.2

Time: 30 minutes
What actions need to be taken considering Kate's depressed state and suicidal thoughts?

There can be considerable variations in how MND presents and the degree to which upper and/or lower groups of motor neurons are affected. As a consequence, people experiencing MND can experience symptoms differently. There are no known curative treatments for MND and therefore care is palliative from the time of diagnosis. Neurology teams need to adopt a palliative approach to care from the outset and ensure early referral to the specialist palliative care team.

Motor Neurone Disease (MND) requires significant input from a large intra/inter-disciplinary team including neurologists, nurses, occupational therapists, physiotherapists, speech and language therapists, and social workers. The specialist palliative care team may be involved in care from an early stage and can assist in alleviating the pain, psychological distress and terror of worsening symptoms such as choking. Although there may be a well-established neurology intra- inter-disciplinary team that has a culture of supportive decision making within it, collaborating with the mental health team may prove more challenging given the differences in how each team works, the language and values that reflect different care philosophies, histories and expertise.

REFLECTIVE PRACTICE EXERCISE 20.3

Time: 30 minutes

Thinking about disciplinary engagement and approaches to symptom management and decision making (horizontal line in Figure 20.1) what are the implications for Kate's care outcomes for Kate depending on how the mental health, neurology and SPC teams collaborate?

Case Study 20.1.3

There is a risk that the mental health team who have known Kate for years may view Kate's MND management as being solely the remit of the neurology team. The mental health team may also have expectations that the MND team will seek advice on the treatment of Kate's anxiety and suicidal feelings. This possible response from the mental health team could set the scene for a more fragmented approach to caring for Kate (quadrant A in Figure 20.1). There is some evidence that people experiencing motor neuron disease may not be referred to the specialist palliative care team until the second year of their ill-health trajectory and that, until then, concerns associated with anxiety, depression and loss are dealt with by the mental health team while muscle weakness, dysarthria, dysphasia, saliva management, nutrition and respiratory insufficiency are managed by the medical team (Harris 2016). By not referring to specialist palliative care teams earlier and by not addressing existential concerns, anxieties and hopelessness, important conversations about future care options and advanced care planning are delayed. This is significant in MND because the person may no longer be able to speak clearly and may experience cognitive changes that are associated with the condition by the second year following diagnosis.

Commitment to supportive decision making will require the teams to move beyond the consultation type relationship that typifies communication between medical teams. Each team needs to share their experiences of working alongside Kate and then engage in joint

continued . . .

problem solving in terms of treatment options and communication with Kate. Discussions between teams are key to this. A palliative approach needs to be adopted by both the neurology and mental health teams so that palliative care principles are applied with the adoption of a whole-person approach (Cassell 2011; Hutchinson 2011, Cruess & Cruess 2011) in all interactions with Kate. For the teams to engage fully in supportive decision making they need to comprehend the uniqueness of Kate's ill-health experience, and her fears and expectations for the future.

Though Kate attends the neurology clinic regularly and has the support of the social worker, speech and language therapist, physiotherapist, occupational health therapist and specialist nurse, she finds it easier to speak with the two members of the mental health team who have supported her for some years. Kate seeks confirmation of information from them that she has already received from the neurology team. She wants to remain at home but will become increasingly dependent in the near future. She is terrifed of choking but does not want to 'end up on a ventilator'. She wants to die before 'things get that bad'.

She believes that she pushed her two daughters away and that they have their own lives to lead but has informed them of her diagnosis. She feels guilty about their childhood experiences and does not know how they will react upon seeing her. She is conscious that her speech is becoming affected but she is understood at present. However, the last few times a member of the mental health team saw her and offered her a coffee, she refused. This is something she would not have done in the past.

REFLECTION PRACTICE EXERCISE 20.4

Time: 20 minutes
- How might you prioritise Kate's immediate needs and your concerns for her?
- What actions might you take to support Kate in the short, medium and long term?

Case Study 20.1.4

An initial conference meeting involving the neurology, palliative and mental health teams is important to ensure that the teams work towards integrating their respective specialist knowledge into a comprehensive and individualised care plan. Given the progressive nature of ALS, close communication between the teams and disciplines and commitment to follow up conference meetings are needed despite the considerable demands this places on teams. Creating this environment of team collaboration will not only assist the teams to share expertise, it will generate a space for Kate to process information and participate in her advanced care planning. This will allow the teams to ensure that discussions on end-of-life and advanced care planning are paced and timed according to her receptivity. She needs to be fully aware that she can review any decisions regularly and to be confident that in the continuum of shared decision making her wishes will be respected and will guide decisions when she is no longer able to fully engage in her care planning (Kon 2010, 2012).

continued . . .

Individual and Family as the Unit of Care

Specialist palliative care (SPC) teams view the individual with the ill-health and family as the unit of care. Family means those who are closest to and who are most significant for the individual. Accordingly, the family is who the individual says it is (*See* Chapter 16). Nevertheless, there is some evidence that families' experiential knowledge gained from caring for people experiencing motor neuron disease is not always acknowledged (Hubbard et al. 2012). Interventions to support caregivers are under-developed (Aoun et al. 2015). Apart from alleviating practical and emotional concerns, such interventions may also play an important role in enabling families to talk about the ill-health and resolve historical tensions. Given Kate's history with alcohol there may be pain and grief within the family, about which, her children may wish to speak. Equally Kate may feel distressed as she reviews her life and relationships with her children and remembers opportunities missed and hurts experienced.

Having a family member with high dependency care needs, who is increasingly unable to communicate and who wishes to remain at home brings its own particular stressors to families. They need guidance on what to expect. Family meetings remain a key element of palliative care (Lichtenthal & Kissane 2008). Assisting the individual and family to set goals for current and future treatment should ensure the ground is set for fully comprehending and working alongside the person's preferences and values so that they have control in decision making over interventions such as non-invasive ventilation or gastrostomy (Creutzfeldt, Robinson & Holloway 2016; Martin et al. 2016).

Advanced care planning should take place over a period of time and involve many discussions so that Kate can obtain and process what information she wants and to ensure the decision making is shared (Sykes 2014). In this way, even after Kate has lost the ability to communicate, decision making is more likely to be aligned with her preferences and values. All advanced care planning discussions need to be recorded so that all those involved in the person's care (health care professionals and family members) are fully informed. Engagement with the family early on following diagnosis will help the individual and family on several fronts. First, the family will have greater confidence in knowing the individual's wishes. Second, the family are more informed about the ill-health and what to expect over its course. Third, the effects of caregiving such as exhaustion, anxiety and so on, can be identified early and interventions put in place to minimise these. Advanced care planning may relieve the caregiver burden by reducing the burden of decision making and subsequent feelings of regret (Murray et al. 2016).

Adult children frequently live some distance from their parents rendering distant caregiving prevalent in the form of instrumental and or emotional support. Unresolved issues and conflicts can impede the development of shared goals and decisions for end-of-life. Byock (2004, 2012) claims that resolving such issues are integral to pain management, and end-of-life including bereavement care (*See* Chapters 21–23). Thus, it is important to support individual Kate in dealing with her concerns should she wish it.

CONCLUSION

At its heart, supportive decision making is a whole-person approach to care that recognises all dimensions of suffering. As is the case for most life-limiting ill-health, barriers to palliative care provision for people experiencing ALS include failure to recognise the need for palliative care from diagnosis and the significance of progressive loss and disability for the person (Oliver 2014). This includes the recognition of the importance, regardless of discipline and speciality background, of the application of palliative care principles by all those involved in the care of such individuals. Supportive decision making rests on this application of palliative care principles within and across disciplinary teams. This means a move away from consultation and towards close collaboration in all aspects of care delivery. Individual team cultures are an important mediator of supportive decision making.

KEY POINT 20.5

Supportive decision making is an organisational concern since it is influenced by how different teams can work together and how the system can facilitate this.

REFERENCES

Altilio, T. and Otis-Green, S. (2006) ' "Res Ipsa Loquitur" . . . it speaks for itself . . . social work—values, pain, and palliative care', *Journal of Social Work in End-of-Life and Palliative Care*, 1, pp. 3–6. Available at: DOI: 10.1300/J457v01n04_02 (Accessed: 29 October 2017)

Aoun, S., Toye, C., Deas, K., Howting, D.,Ewing, G., Grande, G. and Stajduhar, K. (2015) 'Enabling a family caregiver-led assessment of support needs in home-based palliative care: Potential translation into practice'. *Palliative Medicine*, 29, pp. 929–38. Available at: DOI: 10.1177/02692163 15583436 (Accessed: 20 October 2017).

Billings, J. A. and Block, S. (2009) 'Integrating psychiatry and palliative medicine: the challenges and opportunities', in Chochinov H. M. and Breitbart W. (eds.) *Handbook of Psychiatry in Palliative Medicine*. 2nd edition. New York: Oxford University Press, pp. 13–19.

Breitbart, W. S. and Alici, Y. (2014) *Psychosocial Palliative Care*. New York: Oxford University Press.

Bruera, E. and Hui, D. (2016) 'Palliative and supportive care', in Bruera, E., Higginson, I., von Gunten, C. F. and Morita T. (eds.) *Textbook of Palliative Medicine And Supportive Care*. 2nd edition. Boca Raton: CRC Press, pp. 97–102.

Byock, I. (2004) *The Four Things That Matter Most: A Book About Living*. New York: Free Press Simon and Schuster, Inc.

Byock, I. (2012) *The Best Care Possible*. London: Penguin.

Cassell, E. J. (2013) *The Nature of Healing: The Modern Practice of Medicine*. New York: Oxford University Press.

Cassell, E. J. (1991) *The Nature of Suffering and the Goals of Medicine*. New York: Oxford University Press.

Cassell, E. J. (2011) 'Suffering, whole-person care, and the goals of medicine', in Hutchinson, T. A. (ed.) *Whole-person Care*. New York: Springer, pp. 9–22.

Charon, R. (2006) *Narrative Medicine: Honoring the Stories of Illness*. New York: Oxford University Press.

Cruess, R. L. and Cruess, S. R. (2011) 'Whole person care, professionalism, and the medical mandate', in Hutchinson T. (ed.) *Whole Person Care*. New York: Springer, pp. 201–7.

Creutzfeldt, C. J., Robinson, M. T. and Holloway, R. G. (2016) 'Neurologists as primary palliative care providers: communication and practice approach', *Neurology Clinical Practice*, 6, 6–40.

Fang, F., Valdimarsdóttir, U., Fürst, C. J., Hultman, C., Fall, K., Sparén, P. and Ye, W. (2008) 'Suicide among patients with amyotrophic lateral sclerosis'. *Brain*, 13, pp. 2729–33.

Foti, M. E. (2009) 'Palliative care for patients with serious mental illness', in Chochinov, H. M. and Breitbart W. (eds) *Handbook of Psychiatry in Palliative Medicine* (2nd editon). New York: Oxford University Press, pp. 113–21.

Frank, A. W. (2004) *The Renewal of Generosity: Illness, Medicine, and How to Live*. London: University of Chicago Press.

Garrido, M. M., Prigerson, H. G., Neupane, S., Penrod, J. D., Johnson, C. E. and Boockvar, K. S. (2017) 'Mental illness and mental healthcare receipt among hospitalized veterans with serious physical illnesses', *Journal of Palliative Medicine*, 20, pp. 247–52.

Harris, D. A. (2016) 'Existential concerns for people with motor neurone disease: Who is listening to their needs, priorities and preferences'? *British Journal of Occupational Therapy*, 79, pp. 391–3.

Helman, C. G. (1981) 'Disease versus illness in general practice'. *Journal of the Royal College of General Practitioner*, 31, pp. 548–52.

Hubbard, G., McLachlan, K., Forbat, L. and Munday, D. (2012) 'Recognition by family members that relatives with neurodegenerative disease are likely to die within a year: A meta-ethnography'. *Palliative Medicine*, 26, pp. 108–22.

Hui, D., De La Cruz, M., Mori, M., Parsons, H. A., Kwon, J. H. et al. (2013) 'Concepts and definitions for "supportive care," "best supportive care," "palliative care," and "hospice care" in the published literature, dictionaries, and textbooks'. *Supportive Care in Cancer*, 21, pp. 659–85.

Hutchinson, T. A. (2011) *Whole-person Care*. New York: Springer.

Hynes, G., Coghlan, D. and McCarron, M. (2014) 'Giving voice in a multi-voiced environment: the challenges of palliative care policy implementation in acute care', in Keating, M. A., Montgomery, K. and McDermott A (eds) *Patient-centred Healthcare: Achieving Co-ordination, Communication and Innovation*. Basingstoke: Palgrave Macmillan, pp. 133–44.

Hynes, G., Kavanagh, F., Hogan, C., Ryan, K.,Rogers, L., Brosnan, J. and Coghlan, D. (2015) 'Understanding the challenges of palliative care in everyday clinical practice: an example from a COPD action research project'. *Nursing Inquiry*, 22, 249–60.

Kleinman, A. (1988) *The Illness Narratives: Suffering, Healing and the Human Condition*. New York: Basic Books.

Kon, A. A. (2010) 'The shared decision-making continuum'. *Journal of the American Medical Association*, 304, pp. 903–4.

Kon, A. A. (2012) 'Difficulties in judging patient preferences for shared decision-making'. *Journal of Medical Ethics*, 38, pp 719–20.

Lichtenthal, W. G. and Kissane, D. W. (2008) 'The management of family conflict in palliative care'. *Progress in Palliative Care*, 16, pp. 39–45.

Lloyd-Williams, M., Abba, K. and Crowther, J. (2014) 'Supportive and palliative care for patients with chronic mental illness including dementia'. *Current Opinion in Supportive and Palliative Care*, 8, pp. 303–7.

Martin, N. H., Lawrence, V., Murray, J., Janssen, A., Higginson, I. et al. (2016) 'Decision making about gastrostomy and noninvasive ventilation in amyotrophic lateral sclerosis'. *Qualitative Health Research*, 26, pp. 1366–81.

Mitchell, A., Chan, M., Bhatti, H., Halton, M., Grassi, L. et al. (2011) 'Prevalence of depression, anxiety, and adjustment disorder in oncological, haematological, and palliative-care settings: a meta-analysis of 94 interview-based studies'. *The Lancet Oncology*, 12, pp. 160–74.

Murray, L., Butow, P. N., White, K., Kiernan, M. C., D'Abrew, N. and Herz, H. (2016) 'Advance care planning in motor neuron disease: A qualitative study of caregiver perspectives'. *Palliative Medicine*, 30, pp. 471–8.

Oliver, D. (2014) 'Palliative are', in Oliver, D., Borasio, G. D. and Johnston W. (eds) *Palliative Care in Amyotrophic Lateral Sclerosis: From Diagnosis to Bereavement* (3rd edition.) Oxford: Oxford University Press.

Page, B. (1994) 'What is supportive care'. *Canadian Oncolology Nursing Journal*, 4, pp. 62–3.

Richmond, C. (2005) 'Dame Cicely Saunders'. *British Medical Journal*, 331, p. 238.

Roos, E., Mariosa, D., Ingre, C., Lundholm, C. Wirdefeldt, K. et al. (2016) 'Depression in amyotrophic lateral sclerosis'. *Neurology*, 86, pp. 2271–7.

Saunders, C. M. (2006) 'Introduction (management of advanced disease)', in Saunders, C. M. (with an introduction by David Clark) (ed.) *Cicely Saunders Selected Writings 1958–2004*, New York: Oxford University Press, pp. 279–84.

Saunders, C. M. (1964) 'Care of patients suffering from terminal illness at St Joseph's Hospice, Hackney, London'. *Nursing Mirror*, 14 February, pp. vii-x.

Storm, M. and Edwards, A. (2013) 'Models of user involvement in the mental health context: intentions and implementation challenges'. *Psychiatric Quarterly*, 84, pp. 313–27.

Sykes, N. (2014) 'End of life care in ALS', in D. Oliver, G. D. Borasio and W. Johnston (eds), *Palliative Care in Amyotrophic Lateral Sclerosis*. New York: Oxford University Press, pp. 277–92.

Taboada, P. (2016) 'Bioethical principles in palliative care', in Bruera, E., Higginson, I., von Gunten, C. and Morita, T. (eds), *Textbook of Palliative Medicine and Supportive Care*. Boca Raton, FL: CRC Press, pp. 105–18.

To Learn More

American Academy of Hospice and Palliative Medice http://aahpm.org

Breitbart, W., Rosenfeld, B., Pessin, H., Applebaum, A., Kulikowski, J. and Lichtenthal, W. G. (2015) 'Meaning-centered group psychotherapy: an effective intervention for improving psychological well-being in patients with advanced cancer'. *Journal of Clinical Oncology*, 33, pp. 749–54.

Hayes, A., Henry, C., Holloway, M., Lindsey, K., Sherwen, E. and Smith, T. (2013) *Pathways through Care at the End of Life: A Guide to Person-Centred Care*. Jessica Kingsley Publishers: London.

The Irish Hospice Foundation http://hospicefoundation.ie/programmes/public-awareness/think-ahead/

McPhee, S. J., Winker, M. A., Rabow, M. W., Pantilat, S. Z. and Markowtiz, A. J. (eds). (2011) *Care at the Close of Life: Evidence and Experience*. New York: McGraw-Hill Press.

National Council for Palliative Care www.ncpc.org.uk

NHS Choices: End-of-life care www.nhs.uk/planners/end-of-life-care/Pages/End-of-life-care.aspx

Palliative Care Wales http://wales.pallcare.info

Speck, P. W. (2006) *Teamwork in Palliative Care: Fulfilling or Frustrating?* New York: Oxford University Press.

Worldwide Hospice Palliative Care Alliance www.thewhpca.org

CHAPTER 21

End-of-Life Care

Alcohol and Other Drugs

Sarah Galvani and Gemma Anne Yarwood

INTRODUCTION

This chapter bases its discussion of ethics around an innovative research project exploring end-of-life care for people with a history of problematic alcohol or other drug use (hereafter, substance use). The project was led by researchers at Manchester Metropolitan University in partnership with professionals from three hospices, three substance use agencies and one community-based organisation in England. The research set out to explore whether people experiencing problematic substance use, and their family members, friends and carers (FMFC), faced health inequalities in accessing end-of-life care or substance use support, in part through documenting their experience of services. Further, it sought the experiences of the professionals involved in delivering services to this group of people including key professionals from different disciplinary areas around the UK, for example, social workers, hepatologists, community nurses and general practitioners (GPs).

During the development of the project, the design of the research tools, and the collection and analysis of data, there were a number of important and highly sensitive ethical issues to address. Most of these had been identified by the research team ahead of time but others, as in practice, emerged as the project progressed. Throughout the project, practice partners and members of the research team debated and discussed ethical questions as they emerged. This was vital to ensuring our research practice was informed and as sensitive as possible to the needs of the people receiving services and the professionals delivering them.

This chapter will present six ethical questions organised in a chronological order and broadly located around the following core questions:
- should we do the research if there is the potential for causing distress?
- how do we do it ethically – with sensitivity towards people who experience problematic substance use and end-of-life care needs, and their family members, friends and carers?
- what are some of the key ethical dilemmas professionals face when working with these combined issues?

In social and health care practice, there is a parallel process of questioning and reflection about ethical practice, sensitive and non-judgemental intervention, and concern for the impact on people who use services.

Of the six ethical challenges presented – four were raised by the research process, and two were raised by participants. In starting out, we thought these challenges would split into two clear camps: research- or practice-based. In most cases, we found that the reality of research that is practice focused means the two are inextricably linked. Challenges in one have clear parallels in the other. In addition, we found ourselves debating the blurred margins between what was a practice or research challenge and what was an ethical challenge. In navigating these margins, we asked ourselves 'what would be unethical research or practice in this situation'? Where relevant we have illustrated the discussion with pseudonymised quotations of the people we spoke to.

We begin by summarising the key concepts used throughout the chapter before offering some background evidence to contextualise the research and chapter. A summative policy context is then provided before moving on to discuss the selected ethical challenges, our reflections on them and the implications for practice. The chapter concludes with a summary of key points and resources for further learning.

BOX 21.1 Learning the language

> Problematic substance use – this refers to the use of substances that has become problematic in some way for the person using them. This could be problems relating to physical or mental health, finances, relationships, crime and employment. This terminology is preferred to alternatives that have become increasingly stigmatising and labelling, such as addiction or addict. Moreover, substance 'abuse' or 'misuse' are often little understood and taken to mean any use – problematic or not – of any type of illicit drug use, often excluding alcohol. 'Problematic substance use' terminology stems more from a social and non-judgemental model and lends itself to asking, 'what problems is it causing' as a practical next step in the conversation.
>
> End-of-life – the end of someone's life can be sudden or spread out over many years depending on a range of factors including diagnosis, lifestyle factors, treatment access and availability. This makes clear definitions difficult. The National Institute for Care and Clinical Excellence (NICE) define it as: 'people who are likely to die within 12 months, people with advanced, progressive, incurable conditions and people with life-threatening acute conditions' (NICE 2017, online). However, the end of life could mean years, months, weeks or days of remaining life.

WHAT IS THE PROBLEM?

Life limiting conditions including liver cirrhosis, chronic obstructive pulmonary disease, various forms of cancer, heart disease and dementia are linked to the problematic use of substances and alcohol (Institute of Alcohol Studies 2013). There are no figures on how many people are living with chronic or terminal ill-health and using substances problematically; nor is their demographic profile known. For some people, their problematic substance use can lead directly to their chronic or terminal ill-health, while for others their substance use may co-exist with their ill-health.

While problematic substance use can seriously damage the health of younger people (Effiong et al. 2012), older people are disproportionately affected given the increased likelihood of other pre-existing health conditions (Department of Health 2008; Rao 2013). Evidence shows an increase in the rate of alcohol-related hospital admissions among older people (Wadd & Popadopoulos 2014) and an increase in illicit drug use among older age groups (Beynon, Stimson & Lawson 2010). This is predicted to grow further, placing significant demand on end-of-life and palliative care services (Dixon et al. 2015).

While some people may change their substance use behaviour as they age or become ill, not everyone does (Holdsworth et al. 2014). While there is much written about the importance of palliative and end-of-life care services being ready to meet the needs of our ageing population, little is known about how these services support people experiencing substance problems and if, or how, they do so at present. At the core of service provision sit the professionals who deliver it. It is their attitudes and engagement with these co-existing issues that are likely to be key to the engagement and care of individuals and their family members. It is vital not to forget the needs of family members in this context (*See* Chapter 16). There can be considerable negative impact on family members, friends and carers from an individual's problematic substance use alone (Orford et al. 2010). This is likely to be exacerbated as their relative nears the end-of-life (Valentine & Templeton 2013).

To summarise, the number of people with problematic substance use histories is likely to increase among our ageing population. This is in addition to the increasing complexity of health conditions that longevity and older age bring. Specialist services need to be prepared to address the ethical and practice challenges posed by a substance using population at the end-of-life and policy initiatives need to be ready for the challenge.

POLICY ENVIRONMENT

From an ecological theoretical standpoint, understanding the impact of wider socio-political environment in which we exist as individuals, organisations, communities and society is paramount (Bronfenbrenner 1977, 1986). Among the influences that affect change in this environment are changes in government. The impact of such changes is felt at national and local policy levels and ultimately by front line services and the people who use them. At the time of this research project there were four key policy considerations that are important to understand in contextualising the research, its ethical challenges, and its practice implications:

1. A focus on health inequalities including in end-of-life care.

    In England, the government set out clear goals to reduce the health inequalities resulting from 'social, geographical, biological or other factors' (NICE 2012a online). [It states there is a need to address health inequalities] 'to reduce the difference in mortality and morbidity rates between rich and poor and to increase the quality of life and sense of wellbeing of the whole local community' (NICE 2012a online). Pre-existing government policy on palliative and end-of-life care seeks to offer all people approaching end-of-life a needs assessment and high-quality care (Department of Health 2008), but it is unclear to what extent this applies to people experiencing problematic substance use who are often marginalised in health and social care services (Room 2004; Schiffer & Shatz 2008).

2. Austerity measures and their impact on service commissioning.
   The British government's economic policy under its coalition government pledged to reduce the UK's deficit bill (Her Majesties (HM) Treasury and Osborne 2013). The pledge continued with successive annual budgets (HM Treasury and Osborne 2015; HM Treasury 2017) in which the government announced further austerity measures or funding cuts. As a result, there were direct consequences to regional government budgets and, in turn, to health and social care commissioning. In the substance use field there was a rapid recommissioning of services, which saw the closure and reduction of a number of services, or transitions to new providers (Public Health England 2014). This context of austerity, job losses, system change and shrinking resources was the operational context in which this project was conducted.
3. Concern about an ageing demographic and its impact on service provision.
   By 2036, the percentage of the population over 65 years old will have increased from its current 18 per cent to 23.9 per cent (Office for National Statistics (ONS) 2017). Simultaneously, in the four nations of the UK, people in the age group, 65–74 years, are either increasing their alcohol intake compared to other age groups or drinking above daily guidelines (Wadd et al. 2017). Thus, the emerging picture is one of an increasing number of older people requiring health and social care services, a lack of funding to support those services (Age UK 2017) and a trend of increasing alcohol and other drug use among older age groups.
4. A 'recovery' focused substance use commissioning landscape.
   The 2017 Drug Strategy adopted the language of 'recovery', promoting an emphasis on full recovery from 'dependence' on substances, with peer-led, community and family support (HM Government 2017). For people experiencing problematic substance use and end-of-life care needs, such notions of, and mechanisms to, recovery are not appropriate. This raises professional challenges for those delivering such care and support as they need to step out of the dominant policy discourse within which their wider service provision is framed and find a way to defend and promote their work while providing complex level of care. Moreover, it potentially alienates a group of people for whom full recovery is not an option because of their health status.

Thus, the current policy context highlights the importance of identifying and addressing health inequalities while at the same time expects solutions to be delivered within existing or shrinking resources. At times of economic recession and budgetary restraint it is often the services or the needs of people in minority or marginalised groups that are lost in order to deliver to the majority or mainstream. This political context raised the first ethical consideration:

Ethical Challenge 21.1

Question
Is it ethical to conduct research if there is doubt about whether or not the findings and recommendations will be operationalised?

Reflections
Our reflections and discussions with our practice partners provided the solution. The co-existing issues of substance use and end-of-life care were presenting concerns and

problems operationally and the partner organisations were keen to have some research to underpin service development. However, whatever the funding and other resource limitations in relation to implementing larger scale change, professional attitudes and genuine engagement with people remain the key to good service delivery. Testimony from individuals, families, friends and carers who use end-of-life and substance use services was needed to evidence their experiences, identify their support needs, and inform future policy and practice models that were responsive to their needs. This research set out to collect such testimony and to disseminate it as widely as possible to try to positively influence operational issues for the benefit of people using services and those delivering them. While operational change at service level is beyond the control of the research team, the commitment to translating project findings to operational practice and disseminating that guidance widely is not.

Implications for Practice

The parallel for practice would be conducting an assessment of the individual's needs knowing that nothing could be provided. Arguably, it is unethical practice if an individual in a position of power asks for information that is personal and sensitive, knowing that the information will be recorded but not actioned in any way. Operational change can take place at individual and organisational levels and professionals can control the former while advocating for the latter if required. What is important is having clarity from the start about what the information requested is for, who will see it, and what will be done with it. The decision of whether, what and how much to disclose is then with the individual concerned.

Having resolved the first challenge in collaboration with our practice and community partners, there was another ethical question right at the heart of the research project:

Ethical Challenge 21.2

Question

To what extent is it ethical to discuss sensitive issues relating to people's current or previous problematic substance use with a person who is at (or near) the end-of-life?

Reflections

Underpinning this question are two ethical concerns. The first relates to the general concern about invading people's privacy, and the limited time they have left, when they are so near to the end-of-life; the second, relates specifically to the discussion of problematic substance use, and the stigma and sensitivities that accompany substance use. There were concerns that in asking people about it they may be embarrassed or uncomfortable or defensive. In other words, as a team of researchers and practitioners, we questioned whether it was ethical to engage in discussions with individuals which we anticipated would likely prompt a range of negative emotions – something they could do without in the final period of their lives. However, one of the main aims of the project was to explore whether people experiencing problematic substance use received the best possible care at the end-of-life. Without talking to people about their experience this was not going to be possible. To omit people with experience from the project because of:

- the potential sensitivities of the subject matter and
- their health status

. . . without providing them with a choice felt assumptive and patronising.

The primary consideration here was about people's choice to participate and whether or not they had capacity to do so. If they agreed to participate, it was the researchers' responsibility to ensure it was done in a way that was sensitive to their social and health care needs, for example, not taking too much time.

To give people a voice about their experiences and care is not just about informing future service development, it would also allow people to be heard in a way they may not have been heard before. Quite often people reported being dismissed or overlooked in health and social care settings because of their substance use. One of the people we spoke to about her experience was Barbara, (57). Her experience involved a range of health professionals who had failed to ask her questions relevant to her treatment.

Barbara 21.1

[The gastroenterologist] treated me as another person who just drank. He didn't know my background, he didn't know I was abused mentally and physically, he didn't know anything, but he just, he just saw a six-stone alcoholic and that is all he could see. There was no, no delving into my past. And his words were in 2010, when I left, He said "we'll discharge you now" he said, "but no doubt we'll see you again in the future". Now how un-motivational is that?

In this scenario Barbara wanted to be asked about her substance use and reasons for it, and to have conversations about her health. She was not aware of what the diagnosis meant nor what she had to do to improve her chances:

Barbara 21.2

. . . I'd been told I'd got cirrhosis,[1] I didn't really know much about cirrhosis. The doctors told me "you've got ascites."[2] I thought, "what the hell is ascites?" I couldn't spell it never mind know it at the time. And I was discharged from the hospital after two weeks of being drained . . . And within four weeks I was back in again because I was given no knowledge of diet, such as low salt, you can't do this, you can't do that, I didn't pick up a drink but my stomach grew and grew and I thought "hang on a minute what's going on here?" So I was back in again for another four weeks, where I had another two drains and I said to them "Look, I'm not leaving this hospital until somebody tells me what is going on".

People experiencing alcohol and other drug problems, and those who support them or work with them, have long reported stigmatising and dismissive attitudes towards them in relation to their health care needs. Throughout this project we heard many more examples of poor care than good care, often at primary and acute care facilities.

Implications for Practice

Understanding the importance of having conversations with people about their health and substance use, without passing judgement, is fundamental to delivering care effectively.

Indeed, it is arguably unethical not to ask about such co-existing issues when it could have such a bearing on their treatment, comfort and care. These conversations may need repeating, particularly if there is cognitive impairment related to the person's substance use or health condition, but people need the information if they are to make informed choices. Professionals need to develop an awareness of the impact of their language. Medical terminology like that used with Barbara (above) may need clear explanation accompanied by checking the person's understanding of their condition, diagnosis or prognosis. However, this is not just about providing information, rather it is about being prepared to have a conversation about substance use and end-of-life care of which that information is part. Even if the person's choice is to continue their problematic substance use, a caring, non-judgemental discussion needs to be had about what the implications are for their health, well-being and death, and how they would like to be supported in the time they have remaining.

Having decided that it was ethical to conduct the research, the next related ethical challenge was how to go about it:

Ethical challenge 21.3

Question

What would be the most ethical and sensitive way of collecting data from people experiencing problematic substance use who may only have weeks to live and whose health and capacity to participate might change daily?

Reflections

First, qualitative data collection was felt to be the most appropriate way to collect data on people's experience, but the type of data collection, for example, semi-structured interviews, focus groups, digital stories, was open for discussion. Through our consultation with the hospice, substance use and community partners, it became clear that there was no single approach to data collection that would suit everyone due to the varying needs and preferences of the people who experience it. We had to consider that people at the end-of-life had limited time and their ill-health probably meant limited energy and attention. Therefore, we needed to be flexible about how we collected the data while staying focused in order not to waste, or take up, too much of the person's time. We were aware that going back to people for further information or to verify our findings was not going to be an option for some people, so a clear focus for data collection while giving people a voice was needed. This was resolved through offering a menu of data collection options from which the person could choose, or circumstances might dictate. This became known as P.E.M. or Person-centred Evolving Method, a process that began with initial tentative conversations about the research and possible participation and moved towards options of data collection combined with flexibility about when to do them, for how long and who could be present.

   Second, the language we used to explain what the research was about also required careful consideration. Being transparent about 'end-of-life' research would be more appropriate with people accessed through the hospice services, but they may be resistant to discussing their substance use, particularly if their previous experience of discussing it with care services had been negative and judgemental. Similarly, people in substance use services may be able to talk freely about their alcohol or other drug consumption but not consider themselves at the end-of-life, even though they may be very unwell. It was not our place to inform or remind someone, however inadvertently, that they were at the end-of-life. To avoid this, we drew on the expertise of our practice partners and members of the research team who helped us understand the language we should use.

Implications for Practice

There are clear parallels between collection of data in a research context and the collection of information for ongoing health and social care assessments in end-of-life or substance use services. Both are often driven by procedural models of questioning (Smale, Tuson & Statham 2000) with professionals required to complete at least one form as part of the process. Such models often drive the order and type of questions posed and the type of language used. Further, there is usually a set timeframe within which the information needs to be gathered and reported. As with the research data collection, there is often a range of ways to collect information from people about their needs, which avoid a question and answer model and are far more person-centred. People experiencing problematic substance use often have fluctuating capacity depending on levels of intoxication and people with life limiting ill-health will also have peaks and troughs in their health status and ability to function. A combination of the two therefore, can result in uncertain behaviour and capacity. Therefore, professionals need to adopt a flexible approach to assessment and care grounded in an understanding of the potential impact of substance use on the person's capacity to participate, in addition to their other health needs.

In addition to the needs of individuals with problematic substance use who were receiving end-of-life care, an important strand of the project was talking to family members, friends and carers (FMFC) about their experiences of, and perspectives on, services. In preparing for collecting new data from FMFCs, the research used an approach called Secondary Analysis of Qualitative Data (Yarwood and Galvani, forthcoming). By conducting secondary analysis of an existing dataset of family members bereaved through substance use (Templeton et al. 2016), the team was able to ensure that it avoided ethical pitfalls, for example, asking questions that had already been addressed in other research. Moreover, it facilitated some understanding of the issues FMFCs faced, enabling the researchers to prepare both emotionally and practically for the new data collection. This included an awareness that some FMFCs would have their own current or historical substance problems. This raised the next ethical challenge:

Ethical Challenge 21.4

Question

Family members, friends and carers (FMFC) can also have problems with substance use. How can we capture their experiences of end-of-life care as a FMFC without their substance use stories diverting the focus?

Reflections

Throughout interviews with some FMFCs, they shared their own experiences of being stigmatised due to problematic substance use. They were keen to share their wider experiences of stigma, that is, beyond the end-of-life and substance use services that were the focus of this study. The challenge for the researchers was to ensure research objectives were met in the time available but also avoid 'closing down' the voices of FMFCs in a quest to do so. Research time had to be used to meet the aims of the research; collecting data that would not be used is unethical. However, we needed to give the FMFCs space to voice their experiences of being stigmatised, not only to engage them in the research but also to respect their starting point for their experiences of being a FMFC for someone with problematic substance use receiving end-of-life care.

Cheryl (62), an ex-partner and friend of someone at the end-of-life, wanted to share her own history of substance use and her response to people who had a problem with it. She described feeling stigmatised by professionals and society throughout her life as a result of problematic substance use from the age of 14 years old. By referring to her own life experiences of feeling 'instantly judged' by health and social care professionals, she explained why she felt angry and 'in conflict' with professionals:

Cheryl 21.1

> ... the main thing for me, obviously there's nothing that can be done to change what happened, but all I really want is to know, even if just one person feels "I've been listened to" and "when I needed help, it was there, and I wasn't being judged".

Cheryl felt the interview was an opportunity to share her own life experiences of being stigmatised and the ways in which she had 'shored up' feelings of anger towards professionals in practice who she felt had stigmatised her because of her past substance use. This was reinforced further by the health and social care professionals she came into contact with when she adopted the caring role for her ex-partner at the end of his life.

Ultimately, the researchers had to use their sensitivity and skills to listen and give time to the person's story as well as be tentatively directive in moving the focus towards their experiences of end-of-life care for their relative and their own needs as a family member, friend or carer. Researchers and professionals should aim to capture the particularities of an individual's situation such as Cheryl's to reflect on the implications for practice. This can feel challenging for the researcher if the respondent is deemed un-obliging in their interview performativity because they may have been under the influence of substances or they may 'hijack' the interview by discussing their own agenda (Alldred & Gillies 2012).

Implications for Practice

It is good research and practice to reflect on feelings of discomfort raised by an interview as it enriches knowledge about the nuances of people's experiences of problematic substance use, stigma and end-of-life care. Interactions are sites of performativity where identity (re)construction takes place. It was important that the researcher facilitated FMFCs opportunities to voice their, often unheard, experiences of being stigmatised themselves through their own or their friend/relatives' substance use. Research around end-of-life care and problematic substance use involves capturing information about the private lives of others in a similar way to social and health care practice (Hillman 2017). The stigma associated with problematic substance use is immense and can result in defensiveness. In research and practice, understanding our own attitudes towards substance use and dying, and ensuring we apply our learned principles of anti-discriminatory practice, should be at the heart of an empathic and non-judgemental practice. Giving people the time to tell their story prior to meeting the professional's agenda is far more likely to engage people in conversation and access relevant information than rushing in with a list of questions. Professionals can improve practice by developing an awareness of the ways in which uncomfortable interactions with the FMFCs of those receiving end-of-life care can enrich their knowledge and enhance their understanding about experiences of stigma and problematic substance use.

The following ethical considerations stem from the experiences of the professionals who participated in the research.

Ethical Challenge 21.5

Question

How do we work with an individual who continues their problematic substance use in spite of their end-of-life prognosis?

Reflections

While both the hospice and substance use professionals were non-judgemental of people who chose to continue their use, it nevertheless provided ethical challenges in their day-to-day work and in their personal and professional responses to people who made that choice. For hospice professionals, there was an acceptance of people's substance use although only alcohol was allowed in the hospices. It was also common practice to offer an alcoholic drink to people on the day unit or ward at meal times. One nursing professional recalled giving an agitated man in the hospice a drink of Bourbon, the brand of which he kept repeating in his limited communication. The professional subsequently struggled with how contrary this course of action was to their training as a medical professional:

Hospice professional 21.1

It's important you know, if he hadn't had been able to say [Bourbon] and he was agitated as hell and everybody is trying to give him some water and some [medication] and actually he's been a drinker all his life, [I said] to his wife, "what is his favourite tipple"? . . . This sort of thought process and advice goes against everything, when you go and do your nurse training . . . if you wrote that in your nursing exam, you'd fail wouldn't you?! Talking about how to address psychological needs and things, "give them some alcohol", you'd fail wouldn't you?

For some of the substance use professionals, the concern was 'missing' offering people the support they needed, or lacking the knowledge of how to do so:

Substance use professional 21.1

> . . . some clients we know will never stop drinking and so it's actually how we
> . . . work with those because if we don't, it costs a lot of money bouncing back
> through treatment services, they don't really want to stop drinking, they're not
> going to, so I suppose that's where we're missing it and those people die at
> home on their own.

In these examples, both sets of professionals expressed concern about actions they took, or failed to take, that provided ethical challenges. Providing alcohol to someone in distress felt unethical for the hospice professional concerned; failing to provide an adequate, or any service to the person who is drinking and dying in the community was a heavy burden for the substance use professional. Clearly, there are no single solutions. The hospice professional in this example used their initiative and was totally person-centred in doing so. Their creativity and flexibility to step outside their normal practice led to a solution for the person in their care. They were able to affect the support required even though it felt uncomfortable in doing so. For the substance use professional, they were aware of missing people but unclear about how to intervene.

Implications for Practice

The fluctuating capacity and needs of people experiencing problematic substance use at the end-of-life requires a flexible and creative approach to practice. Sitting comfortably with professional discomfort may be part of that process providing practice is ethical and value based. Further, the impact on the professionals of these frustrating and challenging situations needs recognition. An important part of supporting people experiencing problematic substance use at the end-of-life is self-care of the professional. Being emotionally and psychologically able to do the work needs considered attention. Thus, making good use of internal or external supervision to process the frustrations, emotions and sadness of some situations is equally as important as the knowledge or training on the topic. Supporting someone through a process of self-harm using substances is difficult when it is exacerbating their condition and hastening their end. Further, reflecting on how the behaviour supports or challenges our values is vital in order to prepare adequately for practice and to understand that we may have to work and live with some element of discomfort if care is to be as person-centred and needs led as possible.

Ethical Challenge 21.6

Question

How do we manage pain medication for people with current or previous histories of problematic substance use?

Reflections

Concerns about under- or over-prescribing pain medication were probably the key concern raised by professionals in the hospice settings. For people with current or previous opiate use, the professionals spoke of difficulties in knowing how much opiate-based painkillers to prescribe and whether the prescribed amount would be sufficient or too much. The risk of under prescribing was leaving someone in pain potentially; prescribing too much risked overdosing them. The practice of medicating strong opioids for pain relief (NICE 2012b) must consider the individual's levels of tolerance to painkillers and the interaction with other prescribed or illicit medication or drugs.

Hospice professional 21.2

Poly-prescribing is a big issue, poly-pharmacy is a big issue so when you've got lots of different people prescribing, you can't keep track of what they're getting and when they get it, or from whom.

Hospice professional 21.3

And people start taking . . . cumin, turmeric and mushrooms and cannabis oil, a lot of these things . . . but it made it very difficult because we're prescribing drugs that we know interact to a degree that you can't predict because there's no trials but they know from the pharmacy that there's an interaction, and I think more and more, there are people taking particularly cannabis in various forms, oils, smoke, whatever it is and it's those unknown interactions that also add a new layer of complexity that you don't really know what these herbal homeopathic remedies are doing.

Implications for practice

The challenges for prescribing practice do not have easy solutions. The variations in who has taken what and its impact on prescribed medication interactions will be many and varied. Getting a more honest and open answer about other substances used is, however, far more likely when the professional has proven their trust in their approach, genuine manner and care for the person concerned. If the person feels judged by the tone or manner of the questions then, understandably, they are more likely to be deceptive. If their honesty is met with condemnation and criticism, why would they be honest? Setting out the professional's concerns in a non-judgemental manner and encouraging a dialogue rather than a one-way lecture about drug interactions is more likely to achieve the desired result. The use of various substances can then remain a topic for reconsideration each time medication, treatment and wider care is reviewed.

KEY POINTS 21.1

➤ Listening to people's experiences of services is an important part of research and practice. It is crucial to ensure that something is done with the information gathered. Operational change can take place at individual and organisational levels and professionals need to be clear on their agency and remit to act on information supplied.

➤ Having conversations with people about their health, substance use, death and dying are important components of providing effective health and social care, including appropriate medical treatment and social support.

➤ Flexibility with 'normal' procedures of assessment and the time taken to collect information may be required. Professionals working alongside people with current problematic substance use and end-of-life care needs must be prepared to respond with patience to a person's fluctuating capacity.

➤ Being honest about our attitudes towards problematic substance use, and our personal and professional experiences of it, will help to ready professionals for meeting it in practice and responding appropriately.

➤ Sitting comfortably with discomfort is likely to be part of the role of health and social care professionals working alongside people who are at the end of their lives who choose to continue to use substances. Seeking support appropriately is an important part of professional self-care.

SELF-ASSESSMENT EXERCISES 21.1 – OPENING A BOX FULL OF EMOTIONS

> **Time: 30 minutes**
>
> Drawing on what you have read here, identify a situation or interaction where you avoided discussing your feelings and emotions.
> - What was the situation and why did you avoid discussing your feelings?
> - What strategies did you use to avoid talking about feelings and emotions?
> - In what ways, did your avoidance behaviour impact on the interaction and those involved in it?

It is not uncommon for people to avoid talking about emotions. Talking about our emotions can make us feel exposed. For people experiencing problematic substance use who are receiving end-of-life care, talking about their emotions can add to their feelings of vulnerability. These feelings may include fear, frustration, distress, shame and denial. Past unhelpful experiences of interactions with health and social care professionals can compound a person's unwillingness to openly discuss their feelings for fear of further stigmatisation whilst needing end-of-life care. Our role as current or aspiring professionals is to use skills, experience and knowledge to support a person at end-of-life in ways which minimise any distress or difficulties they may be experiencing whatever their choice of lifestyle.

SELF-ASSESSMENT EXERCISE 21.2 – TALKING TO PEOPLE ABOUT SUBSTANCE USE AT THE END OF THEIR LIVES

> **Time: 20 minutes**
>
> Talking to a person about their substance use initially does not require an assessment tool or set of questions. First and foremost, it is a conversation with compassion.
> - Devise two questions about substance use and two questions about death and dying that would help begin a conversation and be appropriate for your practice context.

The questions of what substances people are using, when, how and why, do not need asking at this early stage. The questions can be open and broad, for example, "How does your drinking/drug use help you"? "Would you like to change your drinking/drug use in any way"? Your tone of voice and the way the questions are asked are hugely important. Further resources to help conversations about substance use can be found below.

Questions about death and dying also need to be approached with warmth and care, for example, "Have you ever thought about the end of your life and how you would like that to be?" or "I understand that you would like to continue drinking (or using substances). Can we have a conversation about the implications of that for your care and treatment from this point on, so we can meet your needs?"

Asking people about their substance use or serious health conditions can be uncomfortable for professionals if they do not feel knowledgeable or confident enough. The key to asking people about their substance use is to remember they, not us, are the expert. We are there to learn from them.

CONCLUSION

This chapter has identified ethical challenges in research and practice with people whose use of substances is problematic and who are receiving end-of-life care. It illustrates how this combination of conditions can challenge received practice and research wisdom. Many health and social care professionals are well equipped to respond to complexity within set structures and systems. We argue that overcoming this particular set of challenges requires a commitment to a truly needs-led and person-centred approach that may involve breaking with traditional ways of working. Further, it requires the professional to reflect on their knowledge and skills base and to seek support to improve in any areas as needed. People experiencing substance problems are often marginalised and stigmatised within service provision. The voices of the people who took part in the study reflect this sense of exclusion. As this chapter has illustrated, their needs are often not heard, or they are overlooked by professionals who perceive them as somehow undeserving. While their use of substances can present psychological, behavioural, and physiological challenges to those who seek to support them, people do not start out using substances with the intention of developing a problem or being viewed as untrustworthy, troublesome, and unreliable. As separate issues, both substance use and end-of-life care pose professional and personal challenges. Combined, these challenges are magnified, but people experiencing substance problems, at the end of their lives, still deserve choice, respect, care and compassion, regardless of their lifestyle choices.

NOTES

1 Cirrhosis is 'scarring of the liver caused by long-term liver damage. . . . Cirrhosis can eventually lead to liver failure . . . which can be fatal' (NHS 2017, online)
2 Ascites is a 'build up of fluid in [the] abdomen (tummy) and around the intestines' (NHS 2017, online)
3 Contact the authors for resources currently in progress.

REFERENCES

Age UK (2017) *Briefing: Health and Care of Older People in England 2017*. Available at: www.ageuk. org.uk/Documents/EN-GB/For-professionals/Research/The_Health_and_Care_of_Older_People_ in_England_2016.pdf?dtrk=true (Accessed: 2 January 2018)

Alldred, P. and Gillies, V. (2012) 'Eliciting research accounts: reproducing modern subjects'? in Mauthner, M., Birch, M., Jessop, J. and Miller, T (eds.), *Ethics in Qualitative Research*. London: Sage, pp. 146–66.

Beynon, C., Stimson, G. and Lawson, E. (2010) 'Illegal drug use in the age of ageing'. *British Journal of General Practice*, 60, pp. 481–2.

Bronfenbrenner, U. (1977) 'Toward an experimental ecology of human development'. *American Psychologist*, 32, pp. 513–31. Available at: doi: 10.1037/0003-066X.32.7.513. (Accessed: 2 January 2018)

Bronfenbrenner, U. (1986) 'Ecology of the family as a context for human development: research perspectives'. *Developmental Psychology*, 22, pp. 723–42. Available at: www.scirp.org/(S(351jmbntv nsjt1aadkposzje))/reference/ReferencesPapers.aspx?ReferenceID=1808979 (Accessed: 2 January 2018)

Department of Health (2008) *End of Life Care Strategy. Promoting High Quality Care for All Adults at the End of Life.* London: Department of Health.

Dixon, J., King, D., Matosevic, T., Clark, M. and Knapp, M. (2015) *Equity in the Provision of Palliative Care in the UK: Review of Evidence. PSSRU*, London: London School of Economics and Political Science. Available at: www.pssru.ac.uk/publication-details.php?id=4962 (Accessed: 2 January 2018)

Effiong, K., Osinowo, A., Pring, A. and Verne, J. (2012) *Deaths from Liver Disease. Implications for End of Life Care in England.* Bristol: National End of Life Care Intelligence Network.

Her Majesties Government (2017) *2017 Drug Strategy.* Available at: www.gov.uk/government/publications/drug-strategy-2017 (Accessed: 2 January 2018)

Her Majesties Treasury and Osborne, G. (2015) *2010 to 2015 Government Policy: Deficit Reduction.* Available at: www.gov.uk/government/publications/2010-to-2015-government-policy-deficit-reduction/2010-to-2015-government-policy-deficit-reduction (Accessed: 2 January 2018)

Her Majesties Treasury (2017) '*Autumn Budget 2017*'. Available at: www.gov.uk/government/publications/autumn-budget-2017-documents/autumn-budget-2017 (Accessed: 2 January 2018).

Her Majesties Treasury and Osborne, G. (2013) *Spending Round 2013: next stage in government's plan to move from rescue to recovery.* Available at: www.gov.uk/government/news/spending-round-2013-next-stage-in-governments-plan-to-move-from-rescue-to-recovery (Accessed: 2 January 2018).

Hillman, A. (2017) 'Diagnosing dementia: ethnography, interactional ethics and everyday moral reasoning'. *Social Theory & Health*, 15, pp. 44–65.

Holdsworth, C., Frisher, M., Mendonça, M., de Oliveira, C., Pikhart, H. and Shelton, N. (2014) *Life course transitions, gender and drinking in later life. Summary of Findings.* Available at: www.ncbi.nlm.nih.gov/pmc/articles/PMC5426316/ (Accessed: 2 January 2018).

Institute of Alcohol Studies (2013) *Health impacts.* Available at: www.ias.org.uk/Alcohol-knowledge-centre/Health-impacts.aspx (Accessed: 2 January 2018).

National Health Service Choices (2017) 'Cirrhosis'. Available at: https://www.nhs.uk/conditions/cirrhosis/ (Accessed: 2 January 2018)

National Health Service Choices (2017) 'Alcohol-related liver disease: ascites'. Available at: https://www.nhs.uk/conditions/alcohol-related-liver-disease-arld/complications/ (Accessed: 2 January 2018)

National Institute for Care and Clinical Excellence. (2012a) *Health Inequalities and Population Health.* Available at: www.nice.org.uk/advice/lgb4/chapter/Introduction (Accessed: 2 January 2018)

National Institute for Care and Clinical Excellence. (2012b) *Palliative Care for Adults: Strong Opioids for Pain Relief.* Available at: www.nice.org.uk/guidance/cg140/chapter/introduction (Accessed: 2 January 2018)

National Institute for Care and Clinical Excellence. (2017) *End of Life Care for Adults.* Available at: www.nice.org.uk/guidance/qs13 (Accessed: 2 January 2018)

Office for National Statistics (2017) *Overview of the UK Population 2017.* Available at: https://www.ons.gov.uk/peoplepopulationandcommunity/populationandmigration/populationestimates/articles/overviewoftheukpopulation/july2017 (Accessed: 2 January 2018)

Orford, J., Velleman, R., Copello, A., Templeton, L. and Ibanga, A. (2010) 'The experiences of affected family members: a summary of two decades of qualitative research'. *Drugs: Education, Prevention and Policy*, 17, pp. 44–62.

Public Health England. (2014) *Review of Drug and Alcohol Commissioning. A joint review conducted by Public Health England and the Association of Directors of Public Health.* Available at: https://www.basw.co.uk/resource/?id=4077 (Accessed: 2 January 2018).

Rao, T. (2013) 'Trends in alcohol related admissions for older people with mental health problems: 2002 to 2012'. *Alcohol Concern Briefing.* London: Alcohol Concern. Available at: www.ias.org.uk/uploads/pdf/Older%20people/Alcohol%20Concern%20Briefing%20-%20alcohol%20and%20older%20people.pdf (Accessed: 2 January 2018).

Room, R. (2004) 'Thinking about how social inequalities relate to alcohol and drug use and problems'. Presentation at the 1st International Summer School on Inequalities and Addictions, at the National Centre for Education and Training in Addictions, 25–27 February, 2004, Adelaide, South Australia.

Schiffer, K. and Schatz, E. (2008) *Marginalisation, Social Inclusion and Health. Experiences based on the work of Correlation – European Network Social Inclusion and Health.* Amsterdam, Netherlands: Foundation Regenboog AMOC.

Smale, G., Tuson, G. and Statham, D. (2000) *Social Work And Social Problems: Working Towards Social Inclusion and Social Change.* Basingstoke: Macmillan.

Templeton, L., Ford, A., McKell, J., Valentine, C. and Walter, T. (2016) 'Bereavement through substance use: findings from an interview study with adults in England and Scotland'. *Addiction Research & Theory*, 24, pp. 341–54.

Valentine, C. A. and Templeton, L. (2013) 'When drink kills: Biographical construction by those left behind'. *Paper presented at British Sociological Association Alcohol Study Group; Drinking Dilemmas Conference, 12 December, Cardiff, Wales.* Available at: http://opus.bath.ac.uk/38931/6/BSA_Drinking_Dilemmas_presentation_final091213_2_4_.pdf (Accessed: 2 January 2018).

Wadd, S. and Papadopoulos, C. (2014) 'Drinking behaviour and alcohol-related harm amongst older adults: analysis of existing UK datasets'. *BMC Research Notes*, 7, p. 741.

Wadd, S., Holley-Moore, G., Riaz, A. and Jones, R. (2017) *Calling Time. Addressing ageism and age discrimination in alcohol policy, practice and research.* Available at: www.drinkwiseagewell.org.uk/wp-content/uploads/2017/11/DWAW_Yr3_Report-FOR-WEB4.pdf (Accessed: 2 January 2018).

Yarwood, G. and Galvani, S. (forthcoming =) 'Secondary analysis of qualitative data in social work research and practice: a case study exploring end of life care for family members of people with substance problems'. *European Journal of Social Work* (submitted)

To Learn More

This is a new area of research and practice development and therefore current resources are scarce. There is some literature focusing on aspects of care, for example, on pain management for people with histories of substance use, or on particular groups of people with co-existing substance use and end-of-life care needs, for example, homeless people. We have included a sample of this literature below. Until more targeted resources are available,[3] we have also provided a number of resource links to broadly relevant areas including research reports, websites and journal articles.

Articles

Carmichael, A. N., Morgan, L. and Del Fabbro, E. (2016) 'Identifying and assessing the risk of opioid abuse in patients with cancer: an integrative review'. *Substance Abuse and Rehabilitation*, 7, pp. 71–9.

Collier, R. R. (2011) 'Bringing palliative care to the homeless'. *Canadian Medical Association Journal*, 183, pp. E317–E318.

Hudson, B. F. (2016) 'Challenges to access and provision of palliative care for people who are homeless: a systematic review of qualitative research'. *BMC Palliative Care*, 15, p. 96.

Kirsh, K. and Passik, S. (2006) 'Palliative care of the terminally ill drug addict'. *Cancer Investigation*, 24, pp. 425–31.

Mundt-Leach, R. (2016) 'End of life and palliative care of patients with drug and alcohol addiction'. *Mental Health Practice*, 20, pp. 17–21.

Reports and Guidance

British Association of Social Workers series of pocket guides for working with alcohol and other drugs (2012): www.basw.co.uk/pocket-guides/

Care Quality Commission (2016) *A different ending. Addressing inequalities in end of life care. Good practice case studies.* www.cqc.org.uk/publications/themed-work/different-ending-end-life-care-review

Centre for Death and Society, University of Bath (2015) *Understanding and responding to those bereaved through their family members substance misuse.* www.bath.ac.uk/cdas/research/understanding-those-bereaved-through-substance-misuse/

Homelessness and end of life care report and information pack. www.mariecurie.org.uk/globalassets/media/documents/commissioning-our-services/current-partnerships/homeless_report.pdf

Websites

Alcohol Concern – national alcohol charity in England and Wales www.alcoholconcern.org.uk

BEAD Project (Bereaved through alcohol or drugs) – www.beadproject.org.uk/

Marie Curie – webpage on addiction at end of life for healthcare professionals www.mariecurie.org.uk/professionals/palliative-care-knowledge-zone/symptom- control/addiction-at-end-of-life

Working with substance use – Open Educational Resource from Health Education North West – https://workingwithsubstanceuse.wordpress.com

CHAPTER 22

Last Few Days of Life and Bereavement

Sue Read, Sotirios Santatzoglou and Anthony Wrigley

INTRODUCTION

One of the author's recalls when they first seriously thought of death:

> I was about six years of age when I realised that my mother was not immortal.
> We were watching a programme on the television, when it suddenly occurred to
> me that someday I would have to watch such programmes on my own – that
> mum would not always be there because she would die. I remember this moment
> vividly. I was inconsolable, and my mother couldn't understand my distress; she
> tried to placate me with empty platitudes. When my mother eventually died
> many years later from cancer that moment when I faced death all those years
> previously came flooding back without conscious thought. Death really is an
> important part of life, yet we rarely treat it as such unless it is happening to us
> or those around us.

Most people will have similar stories around their first conscious thoughts of mortality.
Everyone will come to a dying part in their lives, whether it be a sudden or protracted
death borne out over months or years. Whilst dying and death are recognised as the only
certainty within life itself, they remain fundamentally important topics that are not
always talked about as much as they should be. This often leaves many issues around
death and dying that may be important to an individual unspoken or unconsidered, with
little chance for developing a detailed understanding of such a significant aspect of
everyone's lives.

Read (2011) describes death as having a number of different roles or characters: as
a regular or constant companion; as a sudden and unexpected visitor, when it arrives
without warning or time to prepare, and is perceived as untimely. Death can be a
welcomed friend, after times of enduring pain and no expectation of release; death can
also be a stranger, when, for example, death and loss are shrouded in secrecy and
individuals are not allowed to know about death and loss until absolutely necessary, for
example, when the person involved has an intellectual disability or mental health issues
(Read 2011). However, whilst 'death is inevitable, the experience of death and dying may

not be universal' (Todd 2009, p. 245). This is particularly likely to be the case if you are part of a recognised marginalised group and have, for example, an intellectual disability or a mental health diagnosis.

Loss, dying and death experiences remain unique experiences to each individual, as people all grieve in different ways (Worden 2008), and any responses are dependent on a range of factors: 'If we understand the different ways people react to loss, we understand something about what it means to be human . . . something about the way we experience life and death, love and meaning, sadness and joy.' (Bonanno 2009, p. 3).

Death and dying never occurs in a vacuum but within a social context and the nature of that context can influence greatly how the person faces the end of their life and how others accommodate the death of their friend/family member (Read 2008). That social context can have a huge impact on:

➤ how the experience is lived
➤ where people receive their care and support
➤ when they can expect care and support
➤ who they receive this care and support from.

Whilst death is a tangible loss, and for the most part, the most difficult of losses to accommodate, people experience many other losses throughout their lives that can feel equally painful, but may be less tangible or visible, and subsequently not be as easily acknowledged or constructively and consistently supported.

For the person experiencing a mental health condition, general ethical issues are often seen to centre on concerns over coercion (both subtle and overt – *See* Chapter 8) and the attributional assumption of irrationality and unreasonableness, which usually suggest a lack of capacity to self-govern (Barker 2011a). If we add the dimension of palliative or end-of-life care to the person experiencing a mental health condition, then these ethical issues are likely to be compounded. This, in turn, can lead to concerns that genuinely held beliefs and wishes may not be respected in the dying process or that other aspects of end-of-life care that may contribute to a good death for that individual are not always fully realised. However, to appreciate these potential complexities we have to first understand palliative and end-of-life care.

APPROACHING THE END-OF-LIFE

Approaching one's own death can be one of the most difficult tasks that anyone has to face; whilst simultaneously supporting someone as they near the end-of-life remains one of the humblest but is also challenging too. For anyone diagnosed with a palliative, terminal condition, they know that they are living with a condition that cannot be cured that will ultimately and eventually kill them. Palliative care is therefore described as an approach that: 'improves the quality of life of patients and their families facing the problem associated with life-threatening illness, through the prevention and relief of suffering by means of early identification and impeccable assessment and treatment of pain and other problems, physical, psychosocial and spiritual' (World Health Organisation 2017). Underlying this, the concept of palliative care is strongly morally motivated (Have & Clarke 2002). Whilst palliative care can last for many months and sometimes years, end-of-life care is recognised as a specific stage of that care which: 'End of life care is simply acknowledged to be the provision of supportive and palliative care in response to the assessed needs of patient and family during the last phase of life'

(National Council for Palliative Care 2006, p.7). End-of-life care is usually seen to be only the last 24–48 hours of life.

There are a range of different professionals involved in the palliative care journey, some of whom have contributed to this book, and such carers are pivotal in ensuring that individuals receive the holistic care and support they need, at the time they need it most. To care for another is, according to Mayeroff, to help the other grow and entails encouraging and assisting them to care for something or someone other than themselves, as well as for themselves (Mayeroff 1971). The caring relationship is mutual and is primarily a process, not simply a series of goal-orientated services. According to Mayeroff, caring has a number of characteristics, as indicated in Box 22.1.

Box 22.1 Characteristics of Caring (Mayeroff 1971)

- Knowledge
- Patience
- Honesty
- Trust
- Humility
- Hope
- Courage

Caring involves trusting the individual to grow in his or her own time and way. There may be a lack of trust when guarantees are required regarding the outcome of caring, or when one 'cares too much' (Mayeroff 1971). More recently, following the Department of Health (DoH's) strategy, Compassion in Practice (2012), the 6C's campaign was launched, where the values essential to compassionate care were highlighted and recognised as underpinning care in England. These underpinning values are:
1. care
2. compassion
3. confidence
4. communication
5. courage
6. commitment.

The 6Cs are adopted as being fundamental to care practice, wherever that care is delivered or received. Carers in the palliative care field are crucial in supporting palliative and end-of-life care for those with a life limiting diagnosis, regardless of multi morbidity or co-conditions.

The therapeutic relationship is fundamentally important to both the individual and the carers/family at the end-of-life. Based on the core values of the 6 Cs, the therapeutic relationship can be fruitful if it adopts two-way, reciprocal communications with the individual and the family; and is based on honesty and openness. This is crucial when a person discovers that they have a life limiting condition.

FINDING OUT AND SUPPORTING SENSITIVE CONVERSATIONS

Finding out that you have a life limiting condition, or that the end-of-life is fast approaching, can obviously be very difficult to hear and comprehend, particularly if you have a mental health condition. Even before any sensitive conversations can be held, it is likely that some discussions between health professionals, and even perhaps with associated family members, may have already taken place to explore whether the person is able to hear and understand about his or her condition. Finding out what the person knows and needs, and identifying how such needs can be met, are the first steps in the healing, helping and caring process. Professionals should actively listen to the person (including using body language, eye contact, facial expressions, etc.) to look for common responses distress and perceived difficulties in grieving. It should be noted that in R. (Tracey) [2014], the Court of Appeal recognised the significant and also critical nature of the management of the end-of-life phase, the '. . . closing days and moments of one's life', [wherein difficult and sensitive care decisions, which affect] 'personal autonomy, integrity, dignity and quality of life', [have to be made and communicated] (R. (Tracey) [2014] at paras 32, 85 and 95).

Sometimes, starting a conversation around a difficult topic area is the hardest part for any professional. Some people have indicated that saying nothing at all, and ignoring the loss and pain, is worse than any clumsy language used. Therefore, it is not necessary to have accurate answers to all the complex questions raised; just being there, available, and eager to listen is what matters most. Doing this is to offer that most precious commodity: a time to talk. Many professionals call this 'providing an invitation to talk'. One can tell an awful lot from the professional's body language; that they have found 10 minutes in a busy calendar to come and find the person and offer them this time. So, it is never the case that a professional has nothing to offer – you have yourself, and a wealth of personal and professional experience.

Breaking news that is difficult and sensitive in nature, and which is likely to be perceived as 'bad news' by the recipient, can be challenging for any professional. Buckman describes bad news as any news that drastically and negatively alters someone's perceptions of their future (Buckman 1991), and he offers a useful six-step protocol or framework that professionals have often found useful (*See* To Learn More web-link).

People experiencing a mental health diagnosis need to be reassured that whatever choices they make they will be given the necessary help and support to carry out their decisions (such as ensuring their preferred place of death), wherever feasible and possible. This is also important for minimising the amount of potential distress that might accompany such choices. For example, for a bereaved person, one choice they may have to make is whether they wish to see the body. For those people who wish to view the body at the Chapel of Rest or elsewhere, and have permission to do so, further preparation is important. The person needs to know that the body will not look the same, that it may smell distinctly different. That a dead body will feel cold to the touch, will not be breathing, and will normally be in a box called a coffin. Such preparation is crucial in helping the person experiencing a mental health diagnosis to make an informed decision and in helping them to anticipate what they might see, hear and smell when viewing a dead body, to minimise excessive distress. Although difficult to support, viewing the body and saying goodbye to a loved one can be an important part of the bereavement healing process.

Conversations around these topic areas may be difficult for any professional, the key is to offer an invitation to talk, and not being afraid to admit you do not know the answer to all of their questions. If you do need to find out certain information, you should try and do so in a timely manner. Many of these issues carry ethical dimensions, particularly around truth telling, and particularly if you have a mental health issue. Professionals may have important discussions with fellow professionals, and without the person themselves, and make decisions that they feel are the most appropriate under a particular set of circumstances. This has the potential to disempower the individual at the time they really need to feel a sense of control around what is happening to them. An example of these issues is found in the following Case Study 22.1.

Case Study 22.1 – Sue's story

Sue was 28, had an intellectual disability and associated mental health issues. Sue lived at home with her elderly mother, for whom she was the primary carer. With support from Meals on Wheels and a regular Social Worker, Sue and her mother lived in a ground floor flat on the outskirts of a busy town.

Following a series of investigations, Sue was diagnosed with an advanced primary brain tumour, with the recommendation of no active treatment. She was referred to the local hospice initially for day care and eventually was admitted to the inpatient unit where she died a year later.

Supporting Sue was difficult throughout, not least because of her role as the major carer for an aging mother with dementia. To support Sue accessing appropriate support at the hospice also meant accessing support for her mother in her absence, and there were many 'Best interest discussion groups' regarding this issue and how to appropriately manage it with Sue's family members.

A further ethical dilemma was that Sue refused to acknowledge her condition, and despite numerous opportunities to explore this, she always closed down and would not engage with the conversation. However, the day before she died, when a professional entered her room at the hospice, she became very distressed, claiming that she had a brain tumour and that she was going to die and didn't know how her mother would cope. Whether Sue had deliberately ignored the severity of her ill-health until she absolutely had no choice as death was becoming imminent, or whether she simply refused to engage with her condition and the fact that she would die, because it was too big to contemplate, one will never know for sure. However, Sue was supported throughout until the time she needed to know and felt she could engage with what was inevitably happening to her. The counsellor supporting her provided frequent invitations to learn more about her condition, and to explore the future for her mum, but had to wait until Sue was ready to talk for these conversations to happen.

KEY POINT 22.1

Remember:
➤ Finding out what the person knows, and needs, and identifying how such needs can be met are the first steps in the healing and helping process
➤ Don't feel that you need to have all the answers to complex questions raised
➤ You are offering that most precious commodity: time to talk

➤ Never feel that you have nothing to offer – you have yourself
➤ Providing an invitation to talk is an opportunity for the person to talk about their sadness
➤ Communication involves what you say, what you don't say and what you do – body language is a very powerful tool
➤ People need time to think about difficult topics and cannot be hurried.

FACING THE END-OF-LIFE

Kubler-Ross's seminal text (*On Death and Dying* 1969) has guided many people through their dying phase of life. She identified a number of tasks that dying people usually experience at some stage of the end-of-life phase, which are listed in Box 22.2.

BOX 22.2 On dying (Kubler-Ross 1969) Denial

- Anger
- Bargaining
- Depression
- Acceptance

These phases may not be experienced in this linear order and may be revisited many times by different people; but at least help professionals to appreciate and anticipate the challenges faced by each individual. Anyone experiencing existing mental health conditions might find these are compounded as they near the end-of-life. Anyone facing the end of their life goes through a plethora of emotions, one of which is fear. Whilst 'fear often aggravates itself' (Parkes 1998) it also involves a number of different features or elements, as indicated in Box 22.3.

BOX 22.3 Fear of dying (Parkes 1998)

- Fear of separation from loved people, homes, jobs, etc
- Fear of becoming a burden to others
- Fear of losing control
- Fear for dependents
- Fear of pain or other worsening symptoms
- Fear of being unable to complete life tasks or responsibilities
- Fear of dying
- Fear of being dead
- Fear of the fears of others (reflected fear).

Whilst there may be many physical symptoms associated with fear, ranging from the physiological effects of disturbance of the autonomic nervous system to the secondary effects of over breathing, when they occur in people who are already physically (or mentally) ill the resulting tangle of physical and psychosomatic symptoms is not always easy to unravel (Parkes 1998) or to treat.

Despite knowing that a particular diagnosis of, for example, cancer is likely to end fatally, professionals can never give an accurate prognosis, and living with this uncertainty and unpredictability can have a huge impact on the person and their family, particularly if the person already has a mental health condition.

Parkes reminds us that there is always something that can be done to help people through the long periods of waiting, be it a regular chat with a trusted doctor with whom the individual can air their fears or the prescription of additional medication that may break the vicious circle of fear and symptoms (Parkes 1998). Whilst there may be additional issues to consider regarding the habitual use of certain medications for those experiencing a mental health diagnosis, one needs to think about the shorter-term benefits against the probability of no longer term usage because of impending death.

DISENFRANCHISED DYING AND DEATH

'No soul remembered is ever really gone' (Albom 2013).

Disenfranchised grief can be described as the grief that people experience when they incur a loss that cannot be openly acknowledged, publicly mourned, or socially supported (Doka 2002). Disenfranchisement is seen amongst populations '. . . who are not recognised as having the status of persons who experience grief' (Corr 2002, p. 44) or where people are deemed not to have the right to grieve (Doka 2002). Particular populations likely to experience disenfranchised grief include: people experiencing mental health issues; children and young people; older people; prisoners; and people with intellectual disabilities (PWID) (Doka 2002). With respect to prisoners (*See* Read & Santatzoglou 2018), these populations become doubly disadvantaged as some of these characteristics are combined. For example, PWID living in secure environments; or prisoners experiencing mental health and mental well-being problems (*See* Warrilow 2018); or children and young people who are dealt with by the criminal justice system (*See* Vaswani 2018). In these cases, the disenfranchising effects will be more so, as evidenced in Chapters 12–15. The typology of disenfranchised grief is identified in Box 22.4.

BOX 22.4 Typology of disenfranchised grief (Doka 2002, pp.10–14)

- The relationship is not recognised
- The loss is not acknowledged
- The griever is excluded
- The ways that individuals grieve
- The circumstances surrounding the death.

Whilst Doka ably articulated the challenges of disenfranchised grief for certain marginalised populations (Doka 2002), Read (2006) highlighted the plight of marginalised groups being exposed to disenfranchised dying, and coined the phrase 'disenfranchised death', particularly in relation to people with intellectual disabilities. Read defined disenfranchised death as the death that cannot be openly acknowledged with the dying person, where the dying person is socially excluded from the process of dying and deliberately excluded from the decision-making processes surrounding the terminal condition (2006, p. 96). Common features of disenfranchised death include a lack of autonomy with the dying person; where the pending death of the person is not recognised or legitimised with the dying person themselves; the person's rights to know are overlooked; and the recognition of specific circumstance surrounding the death which may preclude appropriate communication (Read 2006, p. 97).

Clearly it is entirely plausible that the concept of disenfranchised death may also be a feature with those individuals experiencing a mental health condition, for a whole host of reasons.

IMPACT ON PROFESSIONALS

Whilst supporting people with dying and death can be difficult but also extremely rewarding and often humbling, the impact on professionals working in difficult, sensitive and complex situations can itself be multifaceted and complex. Jeffreys (2011) describes such people as 'exquisite witnesses', symbolising anyone who steps in to help a grieving or dying person. Worden (2008) identifies that working with loss and bereavement can impact on helpers in three distinct ways.
1. it can remind us of our own previous losses
2. it makes us aware of our potential future losses
3. it reminds us of our own pending mortality.

Clearly this indicates the need for support for the helpers too, whether in the form of regular peer support, professional supervision, or counselling. A healthy helper means healthy support, so this aspect should not be overlooked or neglected by managers or service providers.

The concept of compassion fatigue has been around since the early 1990s and refers to healers, helpers or rescuers who are tending to those suffering in a range of contexts (Figley 2002). Kottler (1992) recognised the importance of compassion in relation to supporting difficult and resistant people, and Sacco et al. indicated that 'population of patients cared for' is influencing the levels of compassion fatigue which is experienced by critical care nurses (2015, p. 41). More recently the term compassion fatigue has been adopted to describe 'secondary traumatic stress' (Figley 2002, p. 2) and recognised as the 'cost of caring' for empathic pain (Figley 1982). Supporting people experiencing mental health conditions as they approach the end-of-life can be challenging, and the impact on professional carers should not be underestimated.

ETHICAL DIMENSIONS TO END-OF-LIFE CARE

End-of-life care is, as we have already indicated, a sensitive area that brings with it an array of challenges. These challenges create a range of important ethical considerations for anyone involved in the end-of-life care or treatment of an individual. The complexity of these ethical concerns is magnified when dealing with people experiencing mental health problems, both when they are the ones who are dying or when they are experiencing bereavement. Now that the nature of palliative and end-of-life care and also of bereavement has been outlined, we are in a position to consider some of the more salient ethical issues that can directly arise in this area.

The general ethical considerations surrounding end-of-life care mirror many of the ethical considerations that are present when caring for any individual but with some important additional considerations that are a consequence of the end-of-life setting or context. Therefore, although we remain concerned with many of the ethical issues we are generally familiar with surrounding preventing harms, improving the well-being, and respecting the autonomy of each individual, these can all take on important new dimensions and interpretations at the end-of-life, particularly when caring for those experiencing mental health conditions. As we have seen, dealing with feelings of loss and grief, fear or other negative psychological states surrounding death and dying, and effectively communicating with individuals at end-of-life are all major considerations; each of which fall within the scope of our major ethical duties of care and treatment. What surrounds many of the ethical challenges is the central aim of palliative and end-of-life care . . . to help an individual have a good death. It is this goal that impacts on how we may interpret and act upon our ethical concerns.

What constitutes a good death can vary considerably depending upon the individual in question and establishing this will help give us answers as to what it is to help prevent or reduce harm, to improve well-being, to respect autonomy, and so on. The importance of establishing, as far as is reasonably possible, what a good death might be for a given individual entering or encountering end-of-life will therefore have significant ethical implications. For example, how someone envisages what their good death might be may result in changes to their care or treatment, depending upon what they value most (freedom from pain, lucidity, symptom relief, etc.). Working towards that goal can also fulfil other important aspects of care, such as helping to address some of the individuals' fears about dying, or by showing that her or his wishes and values are being followed, so alleviating any concerns about their treatment.

When dealing with any mental health condition, one of the most fundamentally important ethical concerns is the consideration as to whether the person with the condition is fully autonomous. The answer to this question has some significant implications, although it is by no means the only ethical concern that is at stake. The reason we are so interested in autonomy is that it grounds our duty to respect the wishes, consent, or refusal of an individual when it comes to their various care and treatment options. End-of-life care, in this regard, is no different from any other area of care. However, the very fact that it is end-of-life; that we have one chance to get the care of the individual right and to assist them in having as good a death as possible, is reason why we need to ensure we are maintaining the highest ethical standards towards every person in this stage of care.

There are aspects of certain mental health conditions that may mean that a person is no longer an autonomous agent. In order to understand the implications of this and why respect for autonomy is such an important ethical consideration, we first need to be clear as to what it is for someone to be autonomous. Although there are several different conceptions of personal autonomy available (Feinberg 1989), there are enough common features amongst them to mean there is broad agreement that autonomy, in this sense, can be understood as a form of self-governance or self-rule that allows a person to freely choose her own actions and make decisions about herself, provided certain conditions are met (Beauchamp & Childress 2001). These conditions surround both capacities that the individual may possess and the circumstances under which a decision is made, usually taken to involve the voluntariness or freedom from controlling influence under which a deliberation was made: the level of understanding with which the decision was made, and capacity to rule oneself (Dworkin 1988).

Often, personal autonomy is conflated with competence, but competence may not always capture all the aspects relevant to determining autonomy, depending upon what account of competence is being applied. Competence is generally used as an ethical and legal standard to determine whether a person's decisions should be accepted, whereas autonomy may also consider wider factors, such as emotional maturity, voluntariness, authenticity, and quality of deliberation. Furthermore, competence itself is not quite the same thing as capacity, which is often what is assessed in a medical setting and tends to concern whether someone has an ability within a given context. It may be, for example, that an individual with locked-in syndrome may have the rational capacity to make judgements about all sorts of matters but lacks competence to make decisions because they are unable to communicate. Despite the nuances surrounding different interpretations of all of these important concepts within debates surrounding autonomy, the connection between all these elements is very strong and usually it will be the case that a person who lacks decision-making capacity would also be considered incompetent and, accordingly, also considered to lack autonomy. (Buchanan & Brock 1990).

Mental health conditions can affect competency, and therefore, the autonomy of an individual. The importance of determining whether an individual is autonomous is that it is respect for autonomy that grounds our ethical obligation to respect the decisions made by an individual, regardless as to our own views or attitudes as to whether those decisions are in that person's interests or not. Even seemingly irrational decisions are not, by themselves, grounds to reject an individual's competence or autonomy. This is because autonomy is not merely an ability or capacity, it is to possess a right to self-govern (albeit a right that may be forfeited in certain situations, such as criminal conviction). It is therefore, what grounds our requirement to obtain consent before intervening in the care or treatment of another person. It also guarantees individuals the freedom to be able to make decisions that they value that others might not, something established both in the ethical literature and in legal cases (Mill 1859; re C [1994]). Accordingly, it is of the utmost importance that we do not lightly dismiss an individual as lacking autonomy, for such rights and freedoms can be lost in favour of paternalistic, best interest considerations for non-autonomous individuals, albeit with some exceptions as will be discussed below. This places a significant burden upon the quality of assessment of anyone experiencing a mental health condition to determine whether they lack autonomy. This is a task made all the more demanding because of the complexities surrounding different types of condition but also because of the additional demands that arise when a person is at the end of their life.

Terminal ill-health, particularly in the last few days or hours of life, can render an individual particularly vulnerable in a number of ways that have significant ethical implications. Even those who have no mental health conditions may be experiencing significant psychological distress at the prospect of their impending death, which may impact on their ability to make clear and rational choices, their understanding of information or options given to them, or their ability to communicate. There may also be a desperate desire based on false views of hope for unwarranted or excessive interventions at end-of-life stages. In all cases, this means that in order to respect autonomy or to promote autonomy in situations where this may be impaired, extra attention needs to be paid to addressing these issues.

Yet the requirement for extra care and effort to be taken addressing issues of understanding can be something of a double-edged sword. Although good palliative care encourages individuals to come to terms with and subsequently accept their terminal condition, excessive presentations or reminders of facts of one's impending death can be extremely distressing to an individual. Whilst promotion and enhancement of autonomous choice is often presented within discussions of ethics as being of primary concern, this does not mean it should override other considerations. Sensitivity, judgement and balance when discussing end-of-life issues with an individual must therefore take precedence over a slavish devotion to attempting to capture constant autonomous decisions from the terminally ill person. Of course, this also doesn't mean simply reverting to paternalistic judgement on the part of the health care professional. In particular, it is important to look out for signs of refusal or dissent from any intervention, particularly if this is consistent with previously established wishes or views about the dying process that the individual has made known. Again, insight and judgement will be needed to distinguish such refusals from simply aversions to discomfort, etc. that are inevitable side-effects of certain kinds of intervention. However, refusal and dissent, even from those lacking autonomy, is extremely important to consider, as it is often easier for a person to indicate their refusal of an intervention – implicitly or explicitly – than to enter into a clear discourse with their carers about their needs, wants and values.

In raising the issue of previously established wishes, some additional distinctions and considerations need to be made about who it is that decisions surrounding end-of-life care are being made for, and the way in which those decisions are made. In considering those who are unable to make autonomous decisions, we might further distinguish between previously autonomous adults who have made future provisions for their wishes to be known for their end-of-life care, previously autonomous adults who have not made such provision, adults who have never been considered fully autonomous, and adults with fluctuating capacities who may be considered at certain times to be autonomous and at other times not to be so. For the purposes of this chapter, the authors will not discuss the other significant distinction that covers the case of children, as this brings with it its own set of significant issues.

Where previously autonomous adults have made future provision for their wishes to be known, this raises the question as to the means by which they have done this. The way in which such provision is made will require different approaches to decision-making. In some cases, the individual is seen to have provided consent in advance for certain decisions through a legally authoritative advance directive. In other cases, interpretation as to the exact nature of their wishes or consent is required from an appointed 'proxy' third party, which can now have recognised legal status in the UK through the Lasting Power of Attorney provision under The Mental Capacity Act (2005). Although the nature and quality of these methods of decision-making has been open to a great deal of debate as to their use due to such concerns as lack of information provision, understanding, and lack of experience about living with certain conditions (Buchanan 1988; Buchanan & Brock 1990; Davis 2004 and 2009; Dworkin 1988; Wrigley 2007a, 2007b and 2015), they can still prove useful indicators as to what sorts of treatment options an individual wishes to receive at the end-of-life when they are no longer able to make decisions for themselves. Understanding and interpreting decisions made in these ways can have a significant impact on what that individual might consider to be the best way to achieve a good death.

With previous autonomous adults who have not made any future provision, additional challenges are raised surrounding decisions for their care and treatment. It may not be clear what their values and wishes were regarding their end-of-life care but, even if they are known, these can only be taken into account rather than be definitively binding. Instead, decisions will need to be based on a best interests' standard and that may mean that certain decisions that may shorten or prolong life might need additional approval. The same holds for adults who have never been competent and been considered autonomous, except that there may be even less information about values and wishes to consider. However, in both cases, although an individual might be considered to have fallen below the threshold standard for autonomy, they may still be able to communicate assent and dissent in certain cases. Although this lacks the ethical and legal force of consent or refusal, they can still play a role in determining the most appropriate decision for that person's treatment. The final group, those adults with fluctuating capacities that might be a result of mental ill-health or disorder, form an interesting and challenging concern surrounding end-of-life decision-making. Episodic loss of competence might raise concerns about express refusals issued by the individual during those phases that seem to override or contradict previously formed instructions as to treatment choice. Wherever possible, it is therefore preferable to attempt to gain a clear account of a person's wishes during a lucid phase that covers periodic lapses. These are often known as 'Ulysses contracts' (Walker 2012) and function in a similar manner to advance directives, albeit without the same legal authority.

Use of various means of extending autonomous decision-making, such as advance directives or proxies, is not a perfect solution to treatment decision-making at end-of-life. For example, there may be circumstances or areas that are not covered by the advance directive or the proxy may not be available at a crucial time. Family members are often involved in decision-making. However, although they are often seen as an important source of information and a useful means of enhancing communication with the individual, there is neither an ethical nor a legal requirement to consider family decisions binding if they have not been formally appointed as a proxy. Indeed, certain safeguarding issues may arise in the case of family involvement, particularly if their involvement seems unwarranted, in conflict with the perceived best interests, or seeks to impose views that may not be in accord with those of the individual. It is important to make sure that the individual is in no way being coerced or otherwise unduly influenced by family members to decide to undergo or forfeit treatments that they might not wish to have otherwise perform.

The demands of making treatment decisions leave many decisions in the hands of medical teams. Although there are many advantages to medical treatment decisions being made by a team with specialist knowledge and understanding who are able to make immediate decisions when needed, this can be burdensome and outside their field of expertise when it comes to decisions requiring some moral judgement. Even in the context of making best interests judgements, some of the most demanding decisions at end-of-life, such as withdrawal of life-prolonging treatments, require a wider knowledge and understanding of the person's values and interests than they may possess.

This brings us on to another major area of ethical concern in end-of-life settings to do with how we address and understand the nature of harms and benefits. With decisions that are genuinely matters of life and death and with only one chance to effectively deliver a good death, the demands surrounding the choices to be made can be demanding and stringent. Although there is a widely held view that continued life is a good thing, we are also faced with situations where either the person has made clear provision that they do not want continued life-sustaining interventions or where continued intervention will be either futile or bring about significant suffering. It is certainly the case that loss of competence does not necessarily mean the loss of enjoyment of life and therefore those experiencing mental health conditions should not be seen as having life bereft of quality experience or even of the desire to have a good death. Yet questions surrounding whether continued life is bearable or not are particularly difficult to answer where communication and information provision is difficult or challenging. It is not just decisions about withdrawing and withholding life-sustaining treatments that are at stake. Decisions to prolong life at all costs have to be considered on balance as well.

It is not simply questions of physical pain and suffering that need to be assessed in these cases. Psychological and existential suffering can be significant factors at the end-of-life. For example, someone might value prolonging life at all costs and so may be willing to undergo greater amounts of physical pain and suffering than someone else. However, the conscious anticipation of their impending death can lead to states of fear and despair, which themselves need to be addressed. States of fear and hopelessness can be even greater for those who have limited capacities. It is therefore, vital that end-of-life care must engage with all these areas. Although this makes the scope of considerations potentially much wider than in other areas of care, it is attention to such areas that help to fulfil the central tenant of palliative care in helping people live until they die.

CONCLUSION

> 'To be ethical is to be human. If we shirk the challenge of ethics, we risk sacrificing our right to be called human'.
>
> (Barker 2011b, p. 26)

This chapter has considered some of the main ethical issues associated primarily with palliative care, end-of-life care and people with a diagnosis of a mental health condition. These elements, together, raise some significant challenges for providing good quality end-of-life care. However, they are not insurmountable in themselves. It is possible to provide excellent care, even for those with considerable limitations on their understanding or ability to comprehend and express the difficult feelings and concerns that arise in this setting. Working towards understanding what a good death might be for any individual is at the heart of many of these concerns and recognising the many ways that this can manifest itself and what is needed to achieve this will be at the heart of good, ethical care for some of the most vulnerable people and one of the most vulnerable stages of their life.

KEY POINT 22.2 – FOR DISCUSSION WITHIN A SMALL GROUP AND MAY PRODUCE SOME INTERESTING AND VALUABLE MATERIAL

➤ Explore what the person's needs and wants might be
➤ Think about when the right time and place might be to have difficult conversations
➤ Consider what the person might need to support them at this time, and who would be best placed to support them
➤ Think about what communication skills are going to be important when inviting the person experiencing a mental health diagnosis to talk

➤ Think about how disenfranchised death and dying may be a factor to the person experiencing a mental health condition who is dying

➤ Think about treatment options from a holistic perspective.

REFERENCES

Albom, M. (2013) *The First Phone Call From Heaven*. Great Britain: Sphere.

Barker, P. (2011a) 'The keystone of psychiatric ethics', in Barker, P. (ed.). *Mental Health Ethics: The Human Context*. London: Routledge.

Barker, P. (2011b) 'Ethics: in search of the good life', in Barker, P. (ed.). *Mental Health Ethics: The Human Context*. London: Routledge.

Beauchamp, T. L. and Childress, J. F. (2001) *Principles of Biomedical Ethics*, 5th edition, Oxford: Oxford University Press.

Bonanno, G. A. (2009) *The Other Side of Sadness: What the New Science of Bereavement Tells Us About Life After Loss*. New York: Basic Books.

Buchanan, A. (1988) 'Advance directives and the personal identity problem'. *Philosophy and Public Affairs*, 17, pp. 277–302.

Buchanan, A. E. and Brock, D. W. (1990) *Deciding for Others: The Ethics of Surrogate Decision Making*. Cambridge: Cambridge University Press.

Buckman, R. (1991) *How to break bad news: A guide for healthcare professionals*. London: Papermac. Available at: www.med.unc.edu/aging/fellowship/current/curriculum/palliative-care/Communi cating_Bad_News_Reading_Module.pdf (Accessed: 16 January 2018).

Corr, C. (2002) 'Revisiting the concepts of disenfranchised grief', in Doka, K. (ed.). *Disenfranchised Grief: New Directions, Challenges and Strategies for Practice*. Champaign, IL: Research Press.

Davis, J. K. (2004) 'Precedent autonomy and subsequent consent'. *Ethical Theory and Moral Practice*, 7, pp. 267–91.

Davis, J. K. (2009) 'Precedent autonomy, advance directives, and end-of-life care', in Steinbock, B. (ed.) *The Oxford Handbook of Bioethics*. New York: Oxford University Press, pp. 349–74.

Department of Health. (2012) *Compassion in Practice*. London: Department of Health. Available at: www.england.nhs.uk/wp-content/uploads/2012/12/compassion-in-practice.pdf (Accessed: 17 January 2018).

Doka, K. J. (ed.) (2002) *Disenfranchised Grief: New Directions, Challenges and Strategies for Practice*. Champaign, IL: Research Press.

Dworkin, G. (1988) *The Theory and Practice of Autonomy*. Cambridge: Cambridge University Press.

Figley, C. R. (ed.) (2002) *Treating Compassion Fatigue*. London: Routledge.

Figley, C. R. (1982) *Traumatization and Comfort: Close Relationships May Be Hazardous to Your Health*. Keynote Presentation at the Conference on Families and Close Relationships: Individuals in Social Interaction. Texas Tech University: Lubbock, TX.

Feinberg, J. (1989) 'Autonomy', in J. Christman, (ed.), *The Inner Citadel: Essays on Individual Autonomy*. New York: Oxford University Press, pp. 27–53.

Have, H. and Clarke, D. (2002) 'Introduction: the work of the Pallium project', in ten Have, H. and Clarke, D. (2002) *The Ethics of Palliative Care: European Perspectives*. Buckingham: Open University Press.

Jeffreys, J. S. (2011) *Helping Grieving People -Hen Tears Are Not Enough*. New York: Routledge.

Kottler, J. A. (1992) *Compassionate Therapy: Working With Difficult Clients*. San Francisco: Jossey Bass.

Kubler-Ross, E. (1969) *On Death and Dying*. New York: Touchstone.

Mayeroff, M. (1971) *On Caring*. New York: Harper & Row.

Mill, J. S. (1859) *On Liberty*. London: Penguin Classics, reproduced. 1985.

National Council for Palliative Care. (2006) End of Life Care Strategy. London: National Council for Palliative Care. Available at: www.ncpc.org.uk/sites/default/files/NCPC_EoLC_Submission.pdf (Accessed: 17 January 2018).

Parkes, C. M. (1998) 'The dying adult'. *British Medical Journal*, 316, pp. 1313–15.

re C (Adult: Refusal of Treatment), [1994] 1 WLR 290.

R. (Tracey) v Cambridge University Hospitals NHS Foundation Trust and another (Equality and Human Rights Commission and another intervening) [2014] EWCA Civ 822.

Read, S. (2006) 'Communication in the dying context', in Read, S. (ed.). *Palliative Care for People with Learning Disabilities.* London: Quay Books.

Read, S. (2008) 'Loss, bereavement, counselling and support: An intellectual disability perspective'. *Grief Matters*, 11, 54–59.

Read, S. (2011) 'End of life', in Atheron, H. and Crickmore, D. (eds). *Learning Disabilities: Towards Social Inclusion* (6th edition). London: Churchill Livingstone Elsevier.

Read, S. and Santatzoglou, S. (2018) 'Death, social losses and the continuum of disenfranchised grief for prisoners', in Read, S., Santatzoglou, S. and Wrigley, A. (eds). *Loss, Dying and Bereavement in the Criminal Justice System.* London: Routledge.

Sacco, T. L., Ciurzynski, S. M., Harvey, M. E. and Ingersoll, G. L. (2015) 'Compassion satisfaction and compassion fatigue among critical care nurses'. *Critical Care Nurse*, 35, pp. 32–43.

The Mental Capacity Act. (2005) UK. Available at: http://www.legislation.gov.uk/ukpga/2005/9/contents (Accessed: 17 January 2018).

Todd, S. (2009) 'The absence of death and dying in intellectual disability research', in Earle, S., Komaromy, C. and Bartholomew, C. (eds) *Death and Dying: A Reader.* Milton Keynes: Open University Press, p. 245.

Vaswani, N. (2018) 'Beyond loss of liberty: how loss, bereavement and grief can affect young men's prison journeys', in Read, S., Santatzoglou, S. and Wrigley, A. (eds). *Loss, Dying and Bereavement in the Criminal Justice System.* London: Routledge.

Walker, T. (2012) 'Ulysses contracts in medicine'. *Law and Philosophy*, 31, pp. 77–98.

Warrilow, A. (2018) 'The impact of loss on mental health: implications for practice', in Read, S., Santatzoglou, S. and Wrigley, A. (eds). *Loss, Dying and Bereavement in the Criminal Justice System.* London: Routledge.

Worden, J. W. (2008) *Grief Counselling and Grief Therapy: A Handbook for the Mental Health Practitioner* (4th edition). London: Routledge.

World Health Organisation. (WHO) (2017) *WHO Definition of Palliative Care.* Available at: www.who.int/cancer/palliative/definition/en/ (Accessed: 17 January 2018).

Wrigley, A. (2007a) 'Personal identity, autonomy and advance statements'. *Journal of Applied Philosophy*, 24, pp. 381–96.

Wrigley, A. (2007b) 'Proxy consent: moral authority misconceived'. *Journal of Medical Ethics*, 33, pp. 527–31.

Wrigley, A. (2015) 'Moral authority and proxy decision-making'. *Ethical Theory and Moral Practice*, 18, pp. 631–47.

To Learn More

Buckman, R. (1991) *How to break bad news: A guide for healthcare professionals.* London: Papermac. Available at: www.med.unc.edu/aging/fellowship/current/curriculum/palliative-care/Communicating_Bad_News_Reading_Module.pdf (Accessed: 16 January 2018).

Figley, C. R. (ed.) (2002) *Treating Compassion Fatigue.* London: Routledge. An informative text that addresses issues of the human spirit in a fundamental but meaningful way. Primarily focuses on disaster experiences to illustrate the complexities but from a mental health perspective.

Worden, J. W. (2008) *Grief Counselling and Grief Therapy: A Handbook for the Mental Health Practitioner* (4th Edition). London: Routledge. An excellent, well established foundation text with a focus on bereavement and grief from the explicit perspective of the mental health professional.

CHAPTER 23

Making Sense
Death, Dying, and Mental Health

Dan Warrender and Scott Macpherson

INTRODUCTION

The causation of mental health problems remains burdened with an uncertainty that freely allows a variety of assertions to be made (Pilgrim 2014). It is therefore crucial, in this arena of confusion, that some sense be available. This chapter will bring together sociology, spirituality, and philosophy, and describe the human need to seek meaning, arguing the crucial role of spirituality in making sense of mental distress. The concepts of death and dying will be explored with a view to introducing spirituality, before arguments are applied specifically to mental health and the professional's role in spiritual care.

DEATH

> 'It always ends. That's what gives it value'
> (From: Death: The Deluxe Edition © 2012 DC Comics.
> Written by Neil Gaiman. Courtesy of DC Comics.)

Death. The concept is inescapably tied into systems of belief, which we the fragile and finite creatures of humanity use to make sense of the unknowable. Anyone reading this will only have had experience of death in the third person. We witness the death of others aware that the same inevitability waits for us all, able only to ponder the time we have left, and what if anything comes next. It is the final word and full stop to life, with a question mark on whether or not a new sentence follows.

Biologically speaking, death has been related to brain capacity and defined as the 'irreversible loss of the capacity for consciousness combined with the irreversible loss of the capacity to breathe' (Gardiner et al. 2012, p. i14). The impact of these functions on life is empirically verifiable, and this definition has gathered consensus. Whilst the reasons that our biological processes may cease can vary dramatically, there is no variation in the fact that regardless of our thoughts or feelings on the matter, we will die. How people deal with this knowledge is then a matter for each individual.

THE DENIAL OF DEATH

It has been suggested that by the age of nine children will have an understanding that everyone (including themselves) will die, and furthermore realise that death is final (Upton 2010). This can be a huge burden for one so young. Nonetheless, despite the inevitability of death, it has been argued to have become a much more unfamiliar concept, particularly to younger generations (Sidell 1993).

> **KEY POINT 23.1**
>
> Denial has been described as: 'cognitive acceptance of a painful event while the associated painful emotions are repudiated' (Bateman, Brown & Pedder 2010, p.32).

It could certainly be argued that whilst we are all aware that one day we will die, we 'choose to forget' as we live our lives. Ignorance is bliss.

This idea of a 'death denial' was championed by the French historian Aries (1976), who claimed that historical cultures were much more at ease with death, and modern progress in medical science has forced a shift. Medical science can now save people in ways that were not previously possible, prolonging life and contributing to the notion that death can be kept at bay by healthcare professionals (Beckett & Taylor 2016). Individuals in Western culture are not as in tune with mortality as was once the case.

SOCIAL DISENGAGEMENT

The theory of social disengagement (Cumming & Henry 1961) posits a potential contribution to this denial, suggesting that the ageing populous participate in a functional disengagement from society, thus allowing them to process the fact that they are nearing the end-of-life. It has however, been debated as to whether this is indeed a psychological need of the ageing individual, or a justification for marginalisation by society. Kearl (1989) argued that social disengagement was an intentional marginalisation to remove the dying from society so 'the living' would not be faced with a reminder of their mortality and the inevitability of death. This idea profoundly shifts the purpose of disengagement from one of psychological benefit to the individual, to one that ostracises the individual to the perceived 'greater good' of society.

Whether we agree or disagree with Kearl's view, the theory nonetheless retains its potential influence over a 'death denial' in society, as for whatever reason, society does keep the dying out of the way. Indeed, most people receiving end-of-life care in England will die in an acute hospital (National End-of-Life Care Intelligence Network 2010) rather than in their own homes and communities. Furthermore, there can be curious examination of the origin of the word 'palliative'. Whilst in modern language it is associated with end-of-life care, the word actually comes from the Medieval Latin 'pallitavus', the verb 'palliate' meaning 'to cloak' (Oxford University Press 2017). It could certainly be argued that care homes and hospitals serve as a cloak, under which we can hide death, and for a moment forget our mortality.

SELF-ASSESSMENT EXERCISE 23.1

Time: 20 minutes
Consider the statement
● What instantly comes to mind?
● Are we a society that hides or denies death?
● Write down your thoughts
● Do you perceive the word 'cloak' to refer 'to hide', or to offer protection?

SOCIAL DEATH

If disengagement is a prelude to biological death, then this process could perhaps be viewed as a form of social death. The treatment of people nearing death was originally presumed by Sudnow (1967) to be influenced by their perceived lessening social value. Once a human reaches a grand age, or receives a terminal diagnosis, they can be viewed to have more years behind them than in front, and society can effectively treat people as 'already dead'. Currently social death has been described as having three key components (Králová 2015 – *See* Box 23.1):

BOX 23.1 Social Death (Králová 2015)

● A loss of social identity
● A loss of social connectedness
● Losses associated with the disintegration of the body

Social disengagement of the ageing or dying population could be said to fit these criteria.

KEY POINT 23.2

Social identity can be lost through retirement from jobs and careers, which have given definition to an individual's life. An ageing individual is more likely to see friends and loved ones around them die, leading to a loss of social connectedness.

Finally, the disintegration of the body comes with the natural process of ageing, and is irreversible. Whilst it is not fair to generalise the ageing population as socially dead, we can speculate as to how, for some individuals, this could seem to be the case. Social death and the marginalisation of any group are consistent with the ideas of stigma, discrimination and prejudice, and these can come from external sources or be internalised.

Externally, social death is evident when an individual is viewed as less socially valuable, and therefore, is subject to behaviour from others which is prejudicial or discriminatory. An individual may receive less opportunities and even be viewed with less hope by healthcare professionals. Internally, social death is a form of self-stigma whereby an individual begins to adopt the beliefs of society. This could mean older people potentially believing that they are too old to change as a result of both internalising societal stereotypes of old age and their cohort beliefs (beliefs held by groups of people of similar ages that are indicative of collective life experiences). These beliefs can have huge influences on self-esteem, self-efficacy and locus of control, which impact on how people live. Further implications can be people not asking for help for distress, or if they do seek help then having diminished hope for the outcomes of any treatment.

Whereas biological death is the end-of-life as we understand it, the narrative provided by society can contribute to huge changes within life which could be described as a social death. Both deaths are huge milestones, and all individuals will attempt to make sense of not only their changing place in the world, but their place in the universe.

COMING TO TERMS WITH DYING

The need to make sense of death and dying belongs not only to the individual concerned, but also to their families, carers and responsible health and social care professionals. Based on work with terminally ill people, Kübler-Ross (1969) introduced one of the most influential and universally recognised models of grief through which an individual themselves or others around them may make sense of dying. Palliative care at the end-of-life will involve spending time with individuals working through these stages, in their own way, and at their own pace, which is different for each individual (*See* Box 23.2).

BOX 23.2 Five Stages of Grief Model (Kübler-Ross 1969)

1. Denial
2. Anger
3. Bargaining
4. Depression
5. Acceptance

This five-stage model suggests that a person begins their grief journey in denial, and being unwilling or unable to accept that what they have been told is true. There may be a rationalisation that views the news as a mistake, or seeks to avoid this offered truth. What follows is anger, whereby the news is realised as real yet not accepted as fair. During this phase the anger may be displaced, and without any objective 'death avatar' there may be a displaced channelling of anger towards professionals involved in care, or even anger at the spiritual concepts of gods or fate. Bargaining marks progress towards acceptance, however presents with a reluctance, which looks to make deals. These deals may again be with healthcare professionals, gods or fate, and involve an individual offering to do their part in extending life. This may mean offering to change lifestyle to 'appease' health and social care professionals, or offering prayer to gods.

The stage where professionals can have the greatest impact is during depression. This will involve discussion which may vary from the practical to the metaphysical, as an individual processes the knowledge of their dying. The model completes with acceptance, a person having made their own sense of their situation, and having become ready to face their biological end. However, for a minority, acceptance does not always arrive.

KEY POINT 23.3

It must be acknowledged that the reality of this model (and indeed any model describing human experience) may vary hugely from individual to individual.

Every human experience will be influenced by subjective traumas and varying degrees of stress vulnerability (Zubin & Spring 1977), and therefore, responses to life events and circumstances will filter through an individual and be uniquely processed. Whilst the five-stage model has been criticised for being too rigid, Kübler-Ross did acknowledge that these stages may not have a linear narrative, may present concurrently and have varying longevity (Torn & Greasley 2016). Furthermore, whilst a useful look at the emotional processes of grief or coming to terms with death and dying, the model cannot be viewed in isolation. The spiritual dimension is vital.

SPIRITUALITY

Spirituality and religion are familiar terms in day-to-day language, though these two concepts are often confused and require distinction and definition. Generally, well understood, religions are formal and organised belief systems, shared with others and focusing around one or more deities (Swinton 2001). Spirituality is inclusive of religious belief systems, although is altogether more subjective and unique to the individual. This breadth of scope has benefited spirituality in its distinction from religion, although it has nevertheless led to a plethora of definitions and left the term somewhat vague (Reinet & Koenig 2013). Beginning to unravel the concept, spirituality has been usefully categorised into five key attributes, which have presented in past definitions (Martsolf & Mickley 1998 – *See* Box 23.3).

BOX 23.3 Spirituality Key Components (Martsolf & Mickley 1998) Text Box

1. Meaning – finding purpose in existence and making sense of life situations
2. Value – beliefs and standards, which become principles and a way of living
3. Transcendence – experience and appreciation of a dimension beyond the self
4. Connecting – relationships with the self, others and higher powers
5. Becoming – the unfolding of a life and personal narrative.

These attributes provide an individual with a framework through which they can make sense of a complex world, and even more complex universe.

REFLECTIVE PRACTICE EXERCISE 23.1

Time: 40 minutes
- Consider your own spirituality in relation to these five attributes.
- How would you describe your experience of each of these attributes to another person?

Alongside Martsolf and Mickley's key components, two words that usefully refine the essence of spirituality are 'beyond' and 'between' (Kurtz & White 2015). The beyond relates to a vertical connection, which pulls upwards and outwards. This includes transcendence, whereby an individual can appreciate a dimension higher than the self. This dimension may be religious, in terms of a deity or god, but may even be an idea. The 'higher' aspect of beyond is not synonymous with some deity, heaven or god, but simply something experienced and appreciated as being higher than the self. This incorporates the concepts of meaning, value and transcendence, and may be defined as a goal, an ideology, a calling or a purpose.

KEY POINT 23.4

Considering what people may be driven to achieve and their reasons for doing so, we can highlight the spirituality in healthcare professionals which may potentially involve their higher dimension as the compassion and drive to help others, perhaps through a sense of moral duty or social justice, and a desire to change the world, even if only for one individual at a time.

The connecting to the higher dimension is realised through action that demonstrates the ideals.

'Between' posits the horizontal aspect of spirituality, with connections between an individual and other people expressed as mutual and collaborative relationships. Humans are social animals, and our basic needs to connect with others cannot be overstated.

KEY POINT 23.5

The value of social relationships and interactions with families, friends, carers and colleagues can provide the sense of belonging so crucial to human experience.

These interactions allow an expression of the self. Through others we see ourselves, and we can surely question how much we would know about ourselves and our place in the world without other people to act as our mirror. The concept of becoming can be realised as 'beyond' and 'between'. Each overlaps and complements the other, with a return to the example of health and social care professionals highlighting their inter-connectedness. The higher dimension and beyond may be evidenced as the values, ideology and moral duty, which inspires the dedication to the career, whilst the between is expressed through the connections, relationships and the day-to-day interactions with individuals. In this way, the beyond relies on the between as a vessel for its expression.

Taking the above ideas into account, this chapter defines spirituality as an individual's unique experience in applying meaning, value and purpose to existence, the self and life events, which develops into a personal narrative through which sense is made of their place in the world and beyond.

DEATH AND MENTAL HEALTH

The concepts of death and mental health may at first seem strange bedfellows. However, in terms of social theory, care and treatment, they do have common ground and can provide useful analogy. Whilst mental health care is not curative, it is not often referred to as 'palliative' given the association of this term with the end-of-life.

KEY POINT 23.6

There are arguments to not only suggest that palliation is appropriate as a definition and approach to mental health care, but that it relates to our entire understanding of it.

The rest of this chapter will apply the concepts of death, death denial and social death to the understanding of mental health diagnosis and distress, emphasise the importance of spirituality in making sense of mental health, as well as being a paramount aspect of care and treatment. There will be a reworking of the Kübler-Ross model to explore making sense of mental health, which includes key principles in the provision of spiritual care.

THE DENIAL OF MENTAL HEALTH

As discussed, there may be a denial of death in day-to-day living allowing people to enjoy life and contributing to the subject itself being somewhat taboo. This taboo status is shared with mental health, with this aspect of our holistic wellbeing often existing in the dim lit corners of society. Similarly, as people 'choose to forget' death and view it only as the business of the dying, mental health is in contention for the same denial, being viewed as an issue only for those in mental distress. Nonetheless, just as we value life as it always has an end, we so too should value good mental health, as it cannot be taken for granted.

It could be argued that the much trumpeted and widely recognised one in four statistics (that one in four people will experience a mental health condition throughout their lifetime) has brought mental health out from the shadows. Despite criticism of the validity of the evidence base, which has contributed to this statistic (Ginn & Horder 2012), it is used extensively with the aim of shifting the denial of mental health and making it relevant to all. However, despite the best of intentions, the statistic still carries the obvious implication that three in four of us will not be affected by mental health issues.

KEY POINT 23.7

It is difficult to describe human existence without mental health as a fluctuating state of wellbeing, which would be highly unlikely to remain 'perfect' throughout a lifetime.

Nonetheless the one in four statistic implies that some of us, in fact many more of us than not, will remain mentally healthy. While the statistic is well intended, it does not go far enough. A personal subjective idea of our own mental health is something we all have, and just as we will all die, we will all experience a fluctuation in the quality of our own mental health throughout our lifetimes. It could be debated that the idea of mental health being an issue only for a select group of people is actually counterproductive, allowing a socially visible mark of difference, and contributing to stigma, discrimination and prejudice.

SOCIAL DEATH AND MENTAL HEALTH

One probable reason for the denial of mental health by individuals may have its roots in how those in mental health distress have been treated by society. Historically treatment has ranged from the brutal to the misguided, often rooted in fear, apprehension and misunderstanding. From the fifteenth to the eighteenth century, estimates of up to 100,000 people were labelled and burned as witches, likely people in mental distress who became unfortunate victims of the social norms and superstitions of the era (Scull 2016). In Western society mental health is now better understood, and difference in behaviour or disclosure of difficulties thankfully no longer a life or death concern. Nonetheless, despite the progress, it can still be difficult for individuals to open up about their experiences of mental distress for fear of the social death associated with it. In addition to mental distress, the social death described by Králová (2015) alludes to a societal stigma and discrimination, which may be influenced by diagnosis or behaviour.

The validity of psychiatric diagnosis has been challenged for many years, with diagnosis criticised as unscientific and oppressive (Szasz 1961). The need for a shared language has potentially overshadowed the uniqueness of individuals, who may have the same clinical labels, but vastly different causal pathways and responses to treatment. Despite the questionable validity of diagnoses, what is evident is their potential sociological impact. A diagnosis is a tangible mark of difference in society, whereby an individual is labelled as different from others.

Even without a diagnosis however, when mental distress presents as behaviour outwith social and cultural norms, this itself can be enough to stigmatise. 'Normal' and 'stigmatised' are ultimately perspectives within a social script, with deviance not related to behaviour itself, but how behaviour relates to social norms (Curra 2014). The unfortunate cycle is that if diagnosis is a mark of difference, and deviance is different from social norms, then deviance can become diagnosis. As social norms can always shift, so too (and do) mental health diagnoses. Whether or not social death relies on diagnosis or behaviour, there is the chance that the two will always converge and present as a mark of difference, and legitimise social disengagement.

Stigma has been described as 'a mark or sign of disgrace usually eliciting negative attitudes to its bearer' (Thornicroft 2007, p.192), and though people may no longer be labelled as witches, challenges remain. Attitudes tend to have three key components: cognitive, affective and behavioural (Hogg & Vaughn 2008). Stigma towards people with mental health distress or diagnoses begins with a belief, not necessarily based on any evidence, with common misconceptions such as people being considered less socially valuable, less able to work, and likely to be violent and dangerous. These beliefs may lead to a negative evaluation of individuals, with feelings such as anger, fear or apprehension. The final element of a stigmatised attitude presents in behaviour, evidenced in discrimination and the consequential imposed social disengagement. This stigma has been described as having a 'double misfortune', as not only is there a societal misunderstanding of mental health and resulting discrimination, but individuals themselves may develop self-stigma, whereby they adopt negative attitudes about themselves and have lessened self-efficacy and self-esteem (Corrigan & Watson 2002, p. 35). Therefore, stigma in mental health can also fit Králová's (2015) definition of social death, with losses in social identity and social connectedness, and with society still largely favouring a medical model, mental ill-health being viewed as part of the body's disintegration.

Taking all of this into account, it is clear that when an individual comes to make sense of their mental distress, they also need to make sense of the sociological implications.

SPIRITUALITY FOR MENTAL HEALTH

Spirituality has been described as the fundamental dimension of peoples' overall health and well-being (Fisher 2011). One could argue that this is true especially and essentially for mental health where there remains so much debate around causation and effective treatment. The onset of mental distress and the receiving of a diagnosis can be difficult times for the individual, families and carers as well as professionals involved. One of the challenges is that similar to death and dying, mental distress does not have an established curative model of care.

KEY POINT 23.8

Care of the dying individual is palliative in nature as there is no reversing the dying process. It could be argued that there is no established method for the reversing of some forms of mental distress, although as with end-of-life care, this does not mean there is no appropriate and helpful role for professionals.

Death is commonly viewed as either an end or a transition. Either it is an end biologically with nothing remaining other than in the memories of others, or a transition to an afterlife or some other dimension. Socially, mental distress has been seen by some as an end, however with a growing focus on counter ideas such as recovery it can be viewed much more positively as a transition. Recovery in mental health, has been defined by the Scottish Recovery Network (2016) as an achievable, unique and personal experience, focused on a person's strengths and described individually as a journey or a destination. This entails an individual living a good life, as defined by them, in spite of any mental health difficulties they may experience. Mental distress may range from one short-lived episode with a return to relative 'normality' as defined by an individual, to a chronic and enduring condition, which has huge and lasting impacts on all aspects of a person's life. Either scenario still benefits from a recovery focus, and requires the spiritual dimension to facilitate understanding.

The ideas from recovery neatly match the notion of a transition, and relate well to spirituality and how spiritual care should be delivered. The spiritual transition model for mental health (see Box 23.2), influenced by the Kübler-Ross process of grief, collects the ideas and concepts discussed throughout this chapter, and hypothesises a process of making sense of mental distress. This model collates spiritual, philosophical and sociological ideas to posit a framework through which professionals may aid individuals in mental distress.

WARRENDER AND MACPHERSON'S 'SPIRITUAL TRANSITION MODEL'

This model proposes that beginning with the onset of mental health distress, an individual may move through five stages as they make a spiritual transition, adapt to their mental health distress and live a self-defined meaningful and satisfying life (*See* Box 23.4). Again, recognising the uniqueness and impossibly dynamic nature of human experience, this model is to be viewed as a framework to provoke discussion and aid understanding, not as universal truth.

BOX 23.4 Warrender and Macpherson's Spiritual Transition Model

1. Onset/Crisis
2. Confusion
3. Making sense
4. Acceptance
5. Adaption

Stage 1 – Onset/Crisis

The first stage of the model marks the onset or crisis point of mental distress. For some this may be an acute, sharp and sudden onset, and for others a slow deterioration in their experience of their own mental state. Regardless of the mental health issue, the onset stage is where mental distress is experienced at its most difficult for the individual. Self-efficacy may be impaired, and there may be the further challenge of whether the person has insight into their condition, as with a psychotic episode, for example. At this stage, a person may feel their own sense of crisis, and require urgent referral, acute care or other emergency intervention. Crisis has been usefully defined as 'a self-limiting moment outside of any person's normal manageable range' (Mental Health Foundation 2002) and it is self-limitation, which defines this stage. Whilst helping individuals in making sense should always be a key element of any professionals' care delivery, the gravity of mental health distress for some means that this may be difficult at this stage. Professionals should liaise with families and carers (*See* Chapter 16), communicate with empathy, carry out appropriate risk assessments and ensure safety.

It is recognised that for some people, crisis and distress may not be unique events, but a constant, chronic and enduring experience. In cases such as these, one could argue that the baseline has moved beyond onset, and an individual could then be in the process of making sense.

Stage 2 – Confusion

At the end of the onset and crisis and before making sense, we need to consider the array of issues that may need to be made sense of. People who had perhaps been in a 'mental health distress denial' could be faced with the devastating realisation of their own fragility. Many people regain insight to find themselves in hospital, and can have the uncomfortable process of learning their own story through the accounts of others, perhaps families, carers or professionals. People may carry shame or embarrassment on finding they have compromised their own values through unintended actions driven by their mental state. Furthermore, the experience of mental distress may challenge existing spiritual or religious beliefs, and open up many questions.

Confusion may be related to the social implications of mental distress or diagnosis. Individuals may wonder how their mental health will affect their relationships with others, their place in society and even question their place in the universe. This relates both to the beyond and the between, as connections with others may have been impacted by mental distress, and may cause anxiety regarding social death. People may come out of crisis to find very different landscapes in terms of their understanding of themselves, others, their place in society and the universe at large.

Stage 3 – Making sense

Spirituality should not be seen as the exclusive role of hospital chaplains and religious figures and should be a core consideration in the role of all professionals. It is important to first emphasise that a person's spiritual story is constructed by the individual and for them. Swinton (2005) describes the role of spirituality as the 'need to find satisfactory answers to the meaning of life, illness and death'.

The 'satisfactory' nature of these answers is to the individual, not the professional, and relates perfectly to the subjectivity of spirituality where people make their own sense in their own way. This does not mean however that professionals should avoid the issue. Whilst there should be no prescribed model of religious or spiritual belief and open acknowledgement that professionals will not have the answers, spirituality should be raised by asking at the very minimum, the question; "how do you make sense of what has happened"? Helping an individual find meaning and make sense of their mental health is not about providing the answers, rather it is evidencing the commitment to hear their story, and willingness to discuss the beyond, the between and related spiritual concepts.

The making sense stage may vary vastly in its longevity, it may be revisited, and it may take place across a lifetime. A key role of professionals should be to discuss this aspect of mental health by acting as a catalyst, beginning the conversations that set people on their own journeys of self-definition and spiritual growth. Then, upon finding their own sense in mental distress, a person may arrive at acceptance.

Stage 4 – Acceptance

Acceptance of mental distress as part of life is a hugely important step in spiritual growth. Whereas Kübler-Ross (1969) cites acceptance as the readiness to die, and an acceptance that the dying process cannot be reversed, this model posits acceptance as the recognition that mental health distress is a core aspect of the human experience, and that mental health care and treatment is not curative. A person need not be a passive recipient of standardised care (which should always be person centred), or accept clinical diagnoses or opinions, which have debatable validity and can change. People should however, aim to reach a point where they can make peace with their own fragility to mental distress, and recognise this as not being a stigmatising mark of being less than human, but as a defining feature of being human.

Stage 5 – Adaption

Acceptance is not the final stage as, unlike people who are dying, people in mental health distress have transitions, not ends. Therefore, in continuing to live, there must be a process of adaption. Acknowledging that there is no cure, people must adapt to circumstances that may include chronic mental health difficulties. A new self-paradigm will include a spiritual dimension of becoming, which includes mental health as part of a personal narrative as well as more tangible means of remaining in control of one's own mental state. This may include development of coping mechanisms, adjustment to living conditions and ensuring social connectedness. Adaption is in full harmony with the recovery movement, which has a strong presence in mental health policy.

CONCLUSION

Mental health, alongside death, is a human experience without cure, which we all share. Whilst care and treatment often have positive effects for people, there is no clear and established pathway for diagnosis and treatment that will be universally beneficial to all. Mental health care and treatment should, therefore, always include the spiritual dimension, where people are encouraged and given the space to discuss how they themselves make sense of their mental distress.

KEY POINT 23.9

Discussing spirituality will always be both palliative and person-centred and has a crucial role in finding subjective meaning in a life, which comes without reason or rule.

The experience of mental distress could be described as a spiritual transition, and professionals should be mindful of this process and recognise this as a key that may unlock a person's recovery.

SELF-ASSESSMENT EXERCISE 23.2

Time: 45 minutes

Case Study 23.1

Dean is a 23-year-old man who lives with his parents and younger sister. He has a job as a business support assistant for an information technology (IT) company that he has had for the past three years. Over a period of a year, Dean has experienced a series of psychotic episodes, having visual and auditory hallucinations and taking a significant amount of time away from work. For each episode he was admitted to an acute mental health ward where his psychosis was managed using medication and constant observations to assess risk. Dean is given a diagnosis of schizophrenia by his consultant psychiatrist, and informed that there is no cure for his condition but that it can be managed through medication and ongoing review by nursing and medical staff.

Points to Consider
- How may Dean and his family feel on hearing there is no cure for his condition?
- Considering the five components of spirituality, what are the spiritual implications of Dean's symptoms and diagnosis for him and his family?

- How might you feel when offering treatment to individuals that will not cure their symptoms or condition?
- Who should deliver spiritual care?
- How may spiritual care be delivered to Dean across a variety of mental health care contexts?

REFERENCES

Aries, P. (1976) *Western Attitudes Towards Death.* London: Marion Boyars.

Bateman, A., Brown, D. and Pedder, J. (2010) *Introduction to Psychotherapy: An Outline of Psychodynamic Principles and Practice.* 4th edition. Hove: Routledge.

Beckett, C. and Taylor, H. (2016) *Human Growth and Development.* London: Sage.

Corrigan, P. W. and Watson, A. C. (2002) 'The paradox of self-stigma and mental illness', *Clinical Psychology: Science and Practice,* 9, pp. 35–53.

Cumming, E. and Henry, W. E. (1961) *Growing Old: The Process of Disengagement.* New York: Basic Books.

Curra, J. (2014) *The Relativity of Deviance.* 3rd edition. London: Sage Publications.

Fisher, J. (2011) 'The four domains model: connecting spirituality, health and well-being', *Religions,* 2, pp.17–28.

Ginn, S. and Horder, J. (2012) '"One in four" with a mental health problem: the anatomy of a statistic', *British Medical Journal,* 344, pp. e1302.

Gardiner, D., Shemie, S., Manara, A. and Opdam, H. (2012) 'International perspective on the diagnosis of death', *British Journal of Anaesthesia,* 108, pp. i14–i28.

Hogg, M. A. and Vaughn, G. M. (2008) *Social Psychology.* 5th edition. Harlow: Pearson Education.

Kearl, M. (1989) *Endings: A Sociology of Death and Dying.* Oxford: Oxford University Press.

Králová, J. (2015) 'What is social death'? *Contemporary Social Science: Journal of the Academy of Social Sciences,* 10, pp. 235–48.

Kurtz, E. and White, W. L. (2015) 'Recovery spirituality'. *Religions,* 6, pp. 58–81.

Kübler-Ross, E. (1969) *On Death and Dying.* New York: Macmillan.

Martsolf, D. S. and Mickley, J. R. (1998) 'The concept of spirituality in nursing theories: differing world-views and extent of focus'. *Journal of Advanced Nursing,* 27, pp. 294–303.

Mental Health Foundation (2002) *Being There in a Crisis: A Report of the Learning From Eight Mental Health Crisis Services.* The Mental Health Foundation & The Sainsbury Centre for Mental Health. London: Mental Health Foundation.

National End of Life Care Intelligence Network (2010) *Variations in Place of Death in England. Inequalities or Appropriate Consequences of Age, Gender and Cause of Death?* Bristol: National End of Life Care Intelligence Network.

Oxford University Press (2017) English Oxford living dictionaries: 'Palliative'. Available at: https://en.oxforddictionaries.com/ (Accessed 2 September 2017)

Pilgrim, D. (2014) *Key Concepts in Mental Health.* 3rd edition. Sage: London.

Reinert, K. G. and Koenig, H. G. (2013) 'Re-examining definitions of spirituality in nursing research', *Journal of Advanced Nursing,* 69, pp. 2622–34.

Scottish Recovery Network (2016) What is recovery? Available at: www.scottishrecovery.net/what-is-recovery/ (Accessed 4 September 2017).

Scull, A. (2016) *Madness in Civilization.* Thames & Hudson: China.

Sidell, M. (1993) 'Death, dying and bereavement', in Bond, J., Coleman, P. and Pearce, S. (eds.), *Ageing in Society,* 2nd edition, London: Sage, pp. 151–79.

Sudnow, D. (1967) *Passing On.* Englewood Cliffs, NJ: Prentice Hall.

Swinton, J. (2001) *Spirituality and Mental Health Care.* London: Jessica Kingsley Publishers.

Swinton, J. (2005) 'Why psychiatry needs spirituality'. *Royal College of Psychiatrists Newsletter 2005.* Available at: www.rcpsych.ac.uk/pdf/ATT89153.ATT.pdf (Accessed 2 September 2017)

Szasz, T. (1961) *The Myth of Mental Illness: Foundations of a New Theory of Personal Conduct,* New York: Harper and Row.

Thornicroft, G., Rose, D., Kassam, A. and Sartorius, N. (2007) 'Stigma: ignorance, prejudice or discrimination?', *British Journal of Psychiatry,* 190, pp. 192–3.

Torn, A. and Greasley, P. (eds) (2016) *Psychology for Nursing.* Cambridge: Polity Press.

Upton, D. (2010) *Introducing Psychology for Nurses and Healthcare Professionals.* 2nd edition. Harlow: Pearson.

Zubin, J. and Spring, B. (1977) 'Vulnerability-a new view of schizophrenia', *Journal of Abnormal Psychology,* 86, pp. 103–26.

To Learn More

National Health Service Scotland. (2009) *Spiritual Care Matters: An Introductory Resource for all NHS Scotland Staff,* Edinburgh: National Health Service Education for Scotland

Swinton, J. (2001) *Spirituality and Mental Health Care.* London: Jessica Kingsley Publishers.

CHAPTER 24

Developing Times

David B. Cooper and Jo Cooper

'Wisdom and compassion should become the dominating influence that guide our thoughts, our words, and our actions'.

(Ricard 2003)

In this book the authors have given their best evidence as to how to practice ethically, day by day. We hope it has stimulated further reading and exploration of how to improve care and practice in your work environment.

> The first dirty little secret of biological psychiatry and of clinical psychology is that they both have given up the notion of cure. Cure takes too long if it can be done at all, and only brief treatment is reimbursed by insurance companies. So, therapy and drugs are now entirely about short-term crisis management and about dispensing cosmetic treatment.
>
> (Seligman 2011, p. 46)

The authors not only appreciate and recognise the immense importance of using the palliative care model to enhance the care of people experiencing mental health problems, but it is significant that they understand the role of this approach and promote the concept of a palliative care approach within mental health as the norm rather than an 'add on' or to be offered only to those approaching their death.

Seligman (2011) provides a very powerful argument in constructing the valid hypothesis of using the palliative care approach in prolonged treatment of mental health problems. Therefore, this approach should be embraced, encouraged and maintained, justifying and typifying compassionate ethical practice.

The caring component of professional practice, the art of caring, is essential and cannot be taught in the classroom. To practice and to care and to do so as one human being to another, we must remain open-minded and reflective of our practice, continually updating and evaluating our knowledge.

As professionals we need to engage our ability to think critically, continually assess each individual, the family unit, the environment, and to plan, implement and deliver care in ethically human and therapeutic surroundings, in order to influence and enhance development of care and practice.

When gathering of information becomes more important than making a connection with the presence of the patient, as nurses, we are diminished in our humanity.

(Long, Long and Smyth 1998, p. 6)

Never presume that what you say is understood. It is essential to check understanding, and what is expected of the individual and or family, with each person. Each person needs to know what he or she can expect from you, and other professionals involved in her or his care, at each meeting. Jargon is a professional language that excludes the individual and family. Never use it in conversation with the individual, unless requested to do so; it is easily misunderstood.

We all, as individuals, deal with life differently. It does not matter how many years we have spent studying human behaviour, listening and treating the individual and family. We may have spent many hours exploring with the individual his or her anxieties, fears, doubts, concerns and dilemmas, and the ill-health experience. Yet, we do not know what that person really feels, how she or he sees life and ill-health. We may have lived similar lives, experienced the same ill-health but the individual will always be unique, each different from us, each independent of our thoughts, feelings, words, deeds and symptoms, each with an individual experience.

We can see within this book how change is taking place. The concept of the book series is to offer a palliative care approach, not necessarily 'palliative care' per se. This approach for people experiencing mental health problems, is no longer conceptual, but is now slowly emerging to become a clinical reality. When we (the editors) committed to the first book, we encountered some difficulty in locating authors who felt justified to write about palliation in mental health, feeling that this approach was outside their remit. Now, a few years on, there is a clearly defined move in attitude amongst practitioners and authors in engaging with this approach and the term 'palliative psychiatry' has been documented by some (Trachsel et al. 2016).

Palliative care approaches offer a mandate for compassionate care; the provision and practice of knowledge, skills and attitudes, ethically to do no harm and to enhance quality of life.

We hope we have argued the case in the series of three textbooks. There is no cost to this change merely a willingness to improve our practice to the benefit of those for whom we care, and for their family.

REFERENCES

Long, A., Long, A. and Smyth, A. (1998) 'Suicide; a statement of suffering'. *Nursing Ethics*, 5, p. 6.

Matthieu, R. As cited in: Föllmi, D. and Föllmi, O. (2003) *Buddhist Offerings 365 Days*. London: Thames and Hudson.

Seligman, M. (2011) *Flourish. A New Understanding of Happiness and Well-Being- and How to Achieve Them*. London: Nicholas Brealey Publishing, p. 46.

Trachsel, M., Irwin, S. A., Biller-Andorno, N., Hoff, P. and Riese, F. (2016) 'Palliative psychiatry for severe and persistent mental illness'. *Lancet*, 3, pp. 1–2.

Index

Please note that page references to Figures are in **bold**, while references to Tables are in *italics*. Footnotes are denoted by the letter 'n' and note number following the page number.